THE WOMEN'S GUIDE TO HORMONAL HARMONY

LACEY DUNN, MS, RD, LD, CPT

DISCLAIMER

This book is not intended for the treatment or prevention of disease, nor as a substitute for medical advice. It contains opinions and ideas of the author and is intended for information purposes only. Any suggestions or guidelines within this book must be followed at the reader's own risk. The author and publisher may not be held liable for any consequences through the addition of or use of, indirectly or directly, the contents of this book.

Please consult with your health care provider before making health care decisions or in the need of medical or health guidance.

The statements and contents of this book have not been evaluated by the FDA. All information and interventions remain for informative and educational purposes only.

CONTENTS

Cover Design by

Graphics by

Interior Design by Homestead Publishing Co. LLC

Hey gorgeous-

I hope you're ready to become the boss of your own body, the master of your metabolism, and the healer of your hormones. In your hands lies every tip and trick you need to reclaim your health and your body. Are you ready to go from "simply surviving" to truly thriving? You better be.

When I sat down to start my book, I knew I wanted to create a resource for women like you. I knew I wanted to pour out every ounce of knowledge, tips, and tricks that I could, slip it into a tangible "bible" for you, and then sprinkle it with magical fairy dust. Why? Because you deserve it. Because I wish I would have had it.

As a Registered Dietitian, I have worked with thousands of women who have lived through the struggles of hormonal chaos, including estrogen dominance, cortisol dysregulation, hypothyroidism, polycystic ovarian syndrome (PCOS), digestive distress, and more. I have spoken with women who are confused, frustrated, and tired of not knowing what to do to feel better, what to eat to reach their goals, and what step to take to finally feel like themselves again.

I have listened to their life stories, their pasts, and their struggles. I have heard them tell me about the countless number of doctors that have dismissed them and their symptoms. I have also had most women tell me that their doctor just threw pills their way. No explanation. No diving into their symptoms. Just shilling pills or saying "eat better" or "sleep more." I am putting my foot down here. Enough is enough!

This book is for you. It's your secret sauce book of knowledge bombs backed by science that can and will produce results. I hope that it empowers you, educates you, and helps you to build the confidence you need to become the true master of your health and body. You will be given the knowledge you need on what your hormones are, how they work, and how they interact. You will learn the truth about what healthy eating really means, what foods will help nourish your body, and how to live a healthy, sustainable lifestyle. I will give you every bit of knowledge that I can. Are you ready to soak it in?

Remember these truths:

-Your diagnosis is not your destiny.

-Your body is not your identity.

-Your worth is defined by you, and you alone- not by others.

Put those reminders on a sticky note and use it as your bookmark as you read this book to remind yourself of them on a daily basis.

My Approach:

You deserve to know not only what is going wrong in your body, but why. This is why I am so passionate about my root cause approach to healing hormonal chaos in the body. Whether it's cortisol dysregulation, a thyroid disorder, digestive distress, or infertility, each scenario and struggle needs an individualized treatment approach that should be fully tailored to fit your needs, symptoms, history, and lifestyle! That's where I swoop in with the fairy dust.

When treating hormonal chaos, conventional medicine sets priority on helping with masking and removing symptoms, instead of solving the root issue. It's common for doctors to "band-aid" situations such as PCOS or irregular menstrual cycles by prescribing hormonal birth control, or providing antidepressants if someone struggles with anxiety or depression. I would be rich if I got a penny for every person with heartburn that was thrown a proton-pump inhibitor (PPI) or statin for elevated cholesterol.

Many times, prescriptions require additional prescriptions, as medication side effects set in. Don't get me wrong, both medica-tions and conventional medicine have their place and can save and change so many lives. However, what if I told you that you can do both? You can fix your hormonal symptoms and find and address the root cause? That is what I am here to do in this book. I am here to help you understand your body, what can go awry and cause chaos, and how you can take steps towards taking your health and hormones back into your own hands! I am here to help you not band-aid the problems, but address them and eliminate them.

This book may give you more details than you asked for. You may find yourself thinking, "But Lacey, just give me what I need to know!". The reason I will not do this is because knowledge is power. You need to understand the what, when, how, and why. If you want to skim the book, feel free to. However, I have made this book as detailed as I can for those that truly want to have as much power over their body and life as possible. We are going to get into nitty gritties. I am not sorry for it.

Here's to you thriving, blossoming, and flourishing. Let's do this thing, girl. It's time to take hold of your power, your health, and your body.

Love,

Lacey

Find me online at:

Website: www.upliftfitnutrition.com

Instagram: @faithandfit

Twitter: @laceyadunn

Podcast: "UpliftFit Nutrition" on most podcast hosting platforms

This book is dedicated to my incredible parents, Mellanie and Brian Dunn, who raised me to become the strong, independent, Jesus loving woman I am today. I can't put into words how thankful I am to have two parents who love me and support me no matter what. I wouldn't be able to write this book if it wasn't for the dedication, passion, and perseverance that you helped me to form. Thank you for being my rocks.

1

YOUR HORMONAL SYMPHONY

"Your hormones are like a symphony. If one is out of balance, it ruins the entire performance."

Your hormones create either a beautiful or disastrous symphony. Have you ever had heavy PMS, cramping, migraines, headaches, painful sex, hair loss, random acne, mid-cycle spotting, or maybe even lost your cycle? Hello- that's the disaster of one component of your orchestra ruining the whole performance of your menstrual cycle!

Hormones are chemical messengers that play crucial roles in regulating your metabolism, appetite, stress response, emotions, mood, immune system, and so much more. The intricate dance of how your hormones interact and influence each other is what makes up your hormonal symphony (or in the case of something being off, hormonal chaos)!

Each hormone has its own job in your body. In fact, most of your hormones have multiple jobs! For example, estrogen is not just in charge of helping regulate your menstrual cycle, it is also in charge of helping regulate your mood, bone health, memory, and cardiovascular function. In order for you to feel your best and achieve optimal health, each hormone needs to be doing its job correctly!

Here is a brief overview of each of your hormones, which we will dive further into throughout this book:

	What it is	What it does
Estrogen:	Manages female reproduction, cardiovascular health, metabolism, memory, maintenance of lean muscle tissues, bone health, and body temperature	Hormone that plays various roles in the body
Progesterone:	Required for a healthy menstrual cycle and pregnancy by regulating the uterine lining, stabilizes mood	The calming or relaxing hormone
Testosterone:	Responsible for the growth and maintenance of muscle tissue, motivation, libido, and energy levels	Produced from DHEA
Pregnenolone:	Responsible for the growth and maintenance of muscle tissue, motivation, libido, and energy levels	Produced from DHEA
DHEA:	A precursor to testosterone that is produced by your adrenal glands & impacted by the stress response	The "anti-aging hormone"
Insulin:	Regulates the use of fuel from your food & directs how your body is to use and store it	Produced by the pancreas in response to glucose levels in the blood to acts as a "key" that allows the glucose to then enter your cells to be used for energy
Ghrelin:	Produced to increase your appetite and hunger levels	The hunger hormone
Leptin:	Affects your metabolic thermostat to manage body fat and body weight and regulates your appetite	Produced by fat cells as a maker of energy availability
Thyroid hormone		The controller of metabolic activity, heart rate, body temperature, digestion, and cognition (really every cell of your body!)
Cortisol:	Regulates as well as your blood sugar, blood pressure, immune function, and anxiety	Controls your flight or flight stress response
Oxytocin:	Helps to facilitate bonding and also stimulates contractions to induce childbirth	The "love" or "feel good" hormone
Vitamin D:	Impacts your immune system, bone health, inflammation, & insulin sensitivity	Serves as a precursor to your hormones from sunlight or dietary cholesterol
Thyroid hormone	Required by almost every cell in order for the body to function optimally	The boss of the metabolism, mood and energy levels in the body

- Estrogen: plays essential roles in female reproduction, cardiovascular health, metabolism, memory, maintenance of lean muscle tissues, bone health, and body temperature
- Progesterone: required for a healthy menstrual cycle and pregnancy by regulating the uterine lining, stabilizes mood, enhances sleep; the calming and relaxing hormone
- Testosterone: responsible for the growth and maintenance of muscle tissue, motivation, libido, and energy levels; Produced from DHEA.
- Pregnenolone: serves as a precursor to your sex hormones as the "mother hormone" and can be converted into progesterone or DHEA; Created mostly by dietary fat and cholesterol.

- DHEA: a precursor to testosterone that is produced by
  your adrenal glands and impacted by the stress response;
  considered the "anti-aging hormone"
- Insulin: regulates the use of fuel from your food and
  directs your body in how to use and store it. Produced by
  the pancreas in response to glucose levels in the blood
  and acts as a "key" that allows glucose to enter your cells
  to be used for energy.
- Ghrelin: the hunger hormone produced to increase your
  appetite and hunger levels
- Leptin: a hormone produced by your fat cells as a marker
  of energy availability; affects your metabolic thermostat
  to manage body fat and body weight, and regulates your
  appetite
- Thyroid: controls your metabolism, heart rate, body
  temperature, digestion, and cognition (really affects every
  cell of your body!)
- Cortisol: largely controls your fight-or-flight stress
  response, as well as your blood sugar, blood pressure,
  immune function, and anxiety
- Oxytocin: provides the "love" or "feel good" hormone;
  helps to facilitate bonding and also stimulates
  contractions to induce childbirth
- Vitamin D: serves as a precursor to your hormones and
  impacts your immune system, bone health, inflammation,
  & insulin sensitivity; is made from sunlight or dietary
  cholesterol

Sadly, you need more than just optimal amounts of these
hormones (darn, there's more? Yes, girl!). You also need optimal
cell receptor function! Your hormones use receptors in the cells of
your body to "dock" on. Think of these hormone receptors as
docks in a harbor. They need to be able to get to where they need
to go in order to do their job. This is where diet quality, genetics,
inflammation, liver detoxification, and mitochondrial health come
into play. You need your hormones to be able to be docked in

order to be used. If hormones can't get into the cell (as in the case of cellular hypothyroidism), are bound too tightly by their carrier proteins (such as estrogen bounded by sex hormone binding globulin), or are unable to be properly used by the cell due to poor cell membrane integrity (as seen in inflammation or low-fat diets), then guess what? They can't do their job!

Each chapter of this book will dive into not only how your hormones work, but how you can optimize them to be the master of your own body. You will be able to understand what hormones do, what influences them, what happens when things go wrong, and how to rebalance them to get back to the vital and energetic woman you deserve to be! You will also obtain a greater understanding for what to eat to balance your hormones, how to optimize your mood and energy levels, and what you can do on a day-to-day basis to be the master of your hormonal symphony, metabolism, and body!

The most common hormonal imbalances that I see in my practice are:

- Low progesterone
- Estrogen dominance
- High (or low) cortisol
- Infertility
- Early perimenopause
- Androgen excess
- PCOS
- Hypothyroidism

Typically, I see multiple imbalances at once, with multiple contributing root causes. This is why I am such a stickler about my "test don't guess" and root cause approach. You want the symphony to be beautiful, right? Well, then you need to assess every factor (what I call root causes) that could be creating the chaos. You need to ensure that every hormonal instrument is playing with the right speed and tune.

Truth is, your hormones don't work by themselves. They are peer pressured to jump off the cliff of harmony together when chaos arrives. Got estrogen dominance? Typically hypothyroidism is there. Have adrenal imbalances? You better bet hormonal imbalances are there too. If you want hormonal harmony, you have to assess and treat each hormonal system, including your adrenal, thyroid, and sex hormones. Not only that, but you need to optimize what influences each system, including your gut, lifestyle habits, and mindset.

I use a holistic and functional medicine-based approach in working with my clients, as well as in this book. What does "holistic" mean? You are probably thinking about gypsy quackery at this point. I am not talking about that. To me, "holistic" means looking at the body as a sum of its parts, accounting for and assessing each system instead of only one. Holistic health and medicine focuses on healing the entire body. Why? Your health is so much more than your adrenal glands, your menstrual cycle, or your digestion. Your health is a combination of your mind, body, and soul. Holistic (and true) health encompasses every system and every part of your being. By addressing your health through a holistic lens, you will be able to achieve better and faster results, and finally secure the secrets to not only surviving, but thriving in life.

So if holistic health refers to the whole body, what does functional health and functional medicine mean? Functional medicine refers to a systems biology-based approach that focuses on treating the whole person, not just the disease. It involves more than just band-aiding symptoms (such as birth control for PMS or an antidepressant for depression), but aims to identify and address the root cause of symptoms in order to promote and achieve health and well being.

Unlike conventional medicine, functional medicine dives deep into a person's past, their story, the physiology and functions attributing to their body's imbalances, and assesses modifiable lifestyle choices such as diet, stress, and relationships. It encompasses patient-centered care, aiming to go beyond simply getting rid of disease, but promoting overall health and vitality. Functional medicine relies on science and research to direct care, which is individualized based on each person's genetics, history, and life story. It's the perfect mix of science and application. Functional medicine is about treating you, not your disease. It's about addressing the cause, not the symptom. Functional medicine is what all medicine should be.

To me, being a holistic and functional medicine dietitian means that I work with my clients in a therapeutic partnership to identify and treat the root cause of their disease and imbalances. I provide them with the knowledge, tools, and confidence that they need to take back control of their own health and body. I am going to be doing that same thing for you in this book. I have created this book as a resource for you. The best resource there is to help you to assess your own potential hormone imbalances, identify the root cause of those imbalances, and make changes to move from what may be your own hormonal chaos, back toward hormonal symphony!

Are you ready to be the master of your own health and body? I hope so. Let's do this!

2

THE QUESTIONNAIRE

This is your magical symptom checklist that can help identify what potential hormonal imbalances you may be suffering from! I have used this questionnaire with hundreds of clients, and now it's in your hands. I even sprinkled magical fairy dust on it. The signs and symptoms listed correlate very well with specific conditions that you may be facing, such as estrogen dominance, hypothyroidism, high cortisol, or androgen dominance. Keep in mind, your hormones work together and influence each other. If one decides to jump off a cliff, others follow (hello body peer pressure)! Also, symptoms can't always be trusted, as a symptom of one condition may also be the symptom of another. This is why some symptoms are listed in multiple places and you may circle them more than once! Keep this in mind, and ensure you are using this questionnaire, along with proper testing, in order to identify your hormonal imbalances, and then dive into them (or it, if you are lucky to have only one!) and why they are there in the first place!

Please read slowly and really question yourself when marking a symptom. As you go through it, count the number of symptoms that you experience in each category. The category with the most symptoms may be an underlying hormonal/adrenal/thyroid imbalance that you face, or may be related to another health condition. Please use this questionnaire for educational purposes and observation use only. It may not be used to diagnose or treat any medical condition. Use your answers, observations, and knowledge acquired in this book to then work with a trusted medical professional (such as an RD like me!). That way, you can ensure that you are doing proper testing (remember my motto "test don't guess"), and that you are receiving an individualized treatment protocol to get you back to healthy, happy, and thriving!

Category A (too much estrogen):

- Heavy PMS or painful periods
- Bloating
- Mood swings and irritability
- Headaches or migraines
- Histamine intolerance
- Anxiety
- Tender breasts
- Irregular menstrual cycle
- Abnormal weight gain (especially around hips and thighs)
- Fibroids
- Acne

Total:

Category B (too little estrogen):

- Hot flashes
- Mood swings
- Fatigue and depression
- Joint pain or muscle aches
- Dry skin
- Frequent UTIs

- Brain fog or memory issues
- Insomnia
- Vaginal dryness
- Low libido
- Bone loss
- Irregular (or loss of) menstrual cycle
- Abnormal weight gain
- Poor skin elasticity or increases in fine lines/wrinkles
- Easy scarring and sun damage to skin
- Muscle loss

Total:

Category C (too little progesterone):

- Hypothyroidism
- Sugar cravings
- Osteoporosis/ Low bone mineral density (BMD)
- Hair loss
- Hot flashes
- Fibroids
- Excess fluid retention
- Heavy PMS or painful periods
- History of miscarriage or difficulty getting pregnant
- Mid-cycle spotting
- Chronic fatigue
- Menstrual headaches or migraines
- Anxiety or depression
- Irregular (or loss of) menstrual cycle
- Irritability or mood swings
- "PCOS" diagnosis
- Depression
- Trouble losing weight

Total:

Category D (too much testosterone):

- Acne or oily skin
- Abnormal facial hair
- Abnormal body hair (such as chest)
- Random weight gain or trouble losing weight
- Darkening of armpits
- Aggression and anger
- Hair loss (especially at front of forehead)
- Deepening of the voice
- Irregular (or loss of) menstrual cycle
- "PCOS" diagnosis

Total:

Category E (too little testosterone):

- Increased belly fat
- Trouble losing weight
- Muscle weakness or loss
- Chronic fatigue
- Low libido or sex drive
- Mood swings
- Anxiety or depression
- Lack of motivation
- Brain fog or poor cognition
- Dry skin
- Hair loss
- Bone loss or low BMD
- Irregular (or loss of) menstrual cycle

Total:

Category F (too little cortisol):

- Chronic fatigue
- Trouble falling and staying asleep
- Salt and/or sugar cravings
- Muscle weakness or loss
- Dizziness when standing up too quickly or orthostatic hypotension
- Low libido
- Exercise intolerance
- Afternoon energy crashes
- Always stressed or anxious
- Getting sick frequently
- Trouble losing weight
- Blood sugar swings
- Lack of motivation

Total:

Category G (too much cortisol):

- Abdominal belly fat
- Brain fog or poor cognition
- Trouble sleeping (tired and wired)
- Hair loss
- Exercise intolerance (or crashes mid workout)
- Sensitivity to caffeine (heart racing & jitteriness)
- High blood pressure
- Body water retention
- Chronic pain or lowered pain threshold
- Always stressed or anxious
- Poor wound healing or recovery from workouts
- High blood sugar
- Second wind at night after mid-day crash
- Waking up in the middle of the night

- Inability to concentrate
- Easily agitated or angered

Total:

Category H (too little thyroid hormone):

- Hair loss
- Brain fog or poor cognition
- Trouble sleeping
- Trouble losing weight or weight gain
- Low heart rate
- Goiter
- Puffy face
- Thinning of eyebrow hair or loss
- Dry skin
- Dry hair that tangles easily
- Constipation
- Poor digestion with gas/bloating
- Cold intolerance (always cold or sensitive to cold)
- Joint or muscle aches
- Chronic fatigue
- High cholesterol
- Hoarse voice
- Lack of motivation
- Anxiety or depression
- Irregular menstrual cycle

Total:

Category I (too much thyroid hormone):

- Shakiness/ trembling hands
- Heart palpitations

- Increased appetite
- Increased heart beat
- Peripheral edema or full body swelling
- Goiter
- Chronic fatigue
- Weight loss or loss of muscle mass
- Insomnia or trouble sleeping
- Excessive sweating
- Heart intolerance
- Irregular menstrual cycle
- Shortness of breath
- Bulging eyes

Total:

Finished? It's time to dive deeper! Now you can flip through the pages of this book to learn more about the root causes of your potential hormonal chaos and take your health and body back into your own hands.

Just so you have further tools for yourself, the following tests are what I use in practice along with this questionnaire to identify and diagnose hormonal conditions. You will learn more about some terms in later chapters.

- DUTCH Complete (hormones only) or DUTCH Plus (if suspected adrenal/cortisol issues)- to order a DUTCH please contact me at laceydunn@upliftfitnutrition.com or work with a functional medicine provider who offers this test, and can read and interpret your report.
- Blood lab markers (you may order through your primary care doctor or self-order through Ulta Labs, MyMedlab, Direct Labs, or Any Lab Test Now). General labs suggested: CMP, TSH, Free T4, Free T3, TPO antibodies, TgAB antibodies, sex hormone binding globulin (SHBG), Estradiol, Progesterone, Free

Testosterone, Ferritin, Serum Iron, % Iron Saturation, TIBC, Vitamin D, Vitamin B12, Iodine, RBC Zinc, RBC Magnesium, Serum Copper

- GI-Map stool test for assessing intestinal permeability, dysbiosis, infections, overgrowths, and parasites
- Hydrogen/Methane breathe test for SIBO
- If thyroid labs are normal but you still have symptoms or suspect cortisol issues, add: Reverse T3, 4 Point Salivary Cortisol, homocysteine, and CRP.

3

MASTERING YOUR SYMPHONY

As a woman, you have 3 main hormones that play distinct roles in regulating your menstrual cycle: estrogen, progesterone, and testosterone. Not only do they work together in the orchestra of your cycle, but they also play critical roles in regulating your metabolism, mood, mental health, and digestion! This chapter will dive into the functions of these hormones and go over what a healthy menstrual cycle looks like. The following chapter will go into why you may be having issues with your menstrual cycle and how to help fix them! **Don't skip this chapter.** This chapter is where the power starts. Knowledge of your cycle is the first step to mastering both it and your body!

Estrogen:

Estrogen is the first queen bee of your hormones. Though men also have estrogen, it's the predominant female hormone responsible for female physical appearance (oh, hi boobs) and reproduction. I like to think of estrogen as the guitar in a rock band. She can either steal the show or ruin it. In either case, she is required for the band to even play!

Estrogen performs hundreds of functions in the body, including:

- Development and maintenance of sex characteristics (breast development, pubic hair, vaginal health)
- The buildup of your uterine lining
- Cholesterol and glucose metabolism (helps to increase insulin sensitivity)
- Maintenance of body temperature
- Bone preservation
- Skin elasticity and youthfulness
- Building and maintenance of lean muscle tissue
- Prevention of estrogen related cancers
- Preserves memory and cognition
- Prevention of vaginal dryness, atrophy, UTIs (urinary tract infections), and cystitis
- Reduction of cardiovascular disease risk

Estrogen gets quite a bad rap these days and is victimized for causing increased water retention, impairment of thyroid function, decreased libido, PMS, increased risk of breast and endometrial cancer, dysregulation of blood sugar, heightened histamine reactions, and mood instability. In reality, yes, estrogen levels in excess can cause a host of hormonal chaos and the symptoms that I just listed. However, it's not estrogen alone that does this. It's an *imbalance* of estrogen. Symptoms and chaos can occur when estrogen is high or low. You need estrogen!

Estrogen chaos occurs when estrogen goes down the wrong metabolic pathways, is too high or too low, or is unable to be detoxified properly in your body. To reiterate, estrogen itself isn't what's bad... having too much estrogen or poor estrogen metabolization is. Please help me spread this truth. Estrogen is not the demon, imbalance is. Your hormones need balance in order to be in harmony. If there is too much or too little of one hormone, that's where the harmony is disrupted.

There are many factors that can influence estrogen's production, metabolism, excretion, and balance. These include: diet quality, lifestyle choices, sleep, medications, gut health, and environmental toxins. Estrogen can also be impacted by genetics, other hormones (such as in hypothyroidism), and by dietary supplements. Don't worry, we are going to dive even deeper. Get your pens ready.

Where does estrogen come from? Estrogen is mainly produced by the follicles in your ovaries after the stimulation of a hormone called FSH (follicle-stimulating hormone). FSH triggers the follicle to release estrogen, which starts day 1 of bleeding in your period. Your estrogen is also produced by your adrenal glands, within fat tissue, and from the aromatization of testosterone (meaning your testosterone also converts into estrogen). Within your fertile years, estrogen largely comes from your ovarian follicles. However, when you reach menopause where your ovarian reserve is diminished or your HPA (hypothalamic pituitary adrenal) axis is malfunctioning, estrogen largely comes from the aromatization of your testosterone. This is because your follicles are no longer releasing estrogen.

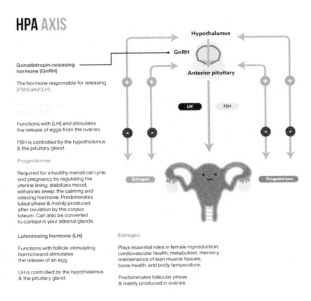

HPA AXIS

Hypothalamus

GnRH

Anterior pituitary

LH   FSH

Gonadotropin-releasing hormone (GnRH)

The hormone responsible for releasing (FSH) and (LH).

Functions with (LH) and stimulates the release of eggs from the ovaries.

FSH is controlled by the hypothalamus & the pituitary gland.

Progesterone

Required for a healthy menstrual cycle and pregnancy by regulating the uterine lining, stabilizes mood, enhances sleep; the calming and relaxing hormone; Predominates luteal phase & mainly produced after ovulation by the corpus luteum. Can also be converted to cortisol in your adrenal glands.

Estrogen

Progesterone

Luteinizing hormone (LH)

Functions with follicle-stimulating hormone and stimulates the release of an egg.

LH is controlled by the hypothalamus & the pituitary gland.

Estrogen

Plays essential roles in female reproduction, cardiovascular health, metabolism, memory, maintenance of lean muscle tissues, bone health, and body temperature;

Predominates follicular phase & mainly produced in ovaries.

The mechanism of aromatization of estrogen is critical to the post-menopausal female, as estrogen is highly beneficial to the body. Remember its job of maintaining bone health, reducing cardiovascular disease risk, and enhancing insulin sensitivity? Without estrogen, you lose insulin sensitivity, develop vaginal dryness, have increased risk of cardiovascular disease and stroke, have increased susceptibility to fractures and osteoporosis, and lose sensitivity to serotonin, leading to increased risk of anxiety and depression. That menopausal weight gain women talk about? That's largely due to low estrogen! I hope this reinstates the benefits of estrogen. Please, no more victimizing our queen bee.

Estrogen predominates during the follicular phase (first 2 weeks) of your menstrual cycle. Though you don't often hear about it, you actually have three types of estrogen in your body: estradiol, estriol, and estrone. Estrone (E1) is a weak estrogen found in small quantities in your reproductive years. It becomes the main estrogen once you hit menopause and is made mostly through the aromatization of androstenedione (one of your testosterone-related hormones). E1 can convert to E2. This is essential for ladies in menopause.

What is E2? Estradiol (E2) is the main estrogen produced in your ovaries from your ovarian follicles. It is the main estrogen that is most commonly mentioned and tested in lab work as well. E2 is the strongest estrogen (aka the super queen bee) and is responsible for the growth of your uterine lining and breast tissue, and contributes to the health of your brain, skin, bone, liver, and your cardiovascular system. E2 estrogen is also one of the main contributors to endometriosis, fibroids, and estrogen-related cancers when in excess.

Estriol (E3) is another weak estrogen which predominates during pregnancy. It is primarily made by the placenta and helps to maintain a healthy uterine lining for the baby. It also functions to assist bone mineral density and to maintain bone health. Unlike E1, E3 cannot be inter-converted. E3 stays as E3, while E1 can become E2.

Estrogen metabolism is a complex and confusing web. Later we will dive into how the different estrogens metabolize in your body. Why? Because not only do type and amounts of your estrogens matter but also how they are metabolized!

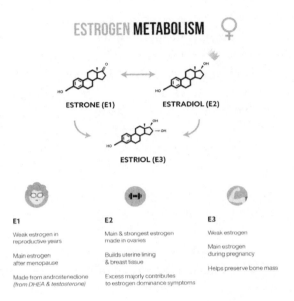

ESTROGEN **METABOLISM**

ESTRONE (E1)   ESTRADIOL (E2)

ESTRIOL (E3)

E1

Weak estrogen in reproductive years

Main estrogen after menopause

Made from androstenedione *(from DHEA & testosterone)*

E2

Main & strongest estrogen made in ovaries

Builds uterine lining & breast tissue

Excess majorly contributes to estrogen dominance symptoms

E3

Weak estrogen

Main estrogen during pregnancy

Helps preserve bone mass

Progesterone:

The second queen bee of your hormones is progesterone. She is the singer in your band, as her presence is imperative for a baby to be made, and she is in charge of the main event of your cycle: ovulation!

Just like estrogen, progesterone also has multiple functions in your body, which include:

- Calming the nervous system and helping the body combat stress
- Thickening your uterine lining
- Helping the body use fat for energy
- Protecting against estrogen-related cancers

- Increasing your metabolism and basal body temperature
- Acting as a natural diuretic
- Promoting a healthy sex drive

Progesterone is the calming hormone in your body, aka the "yin" to your estrogen's "yang". Progesterone interacts with serotonin and GABA, influencing your mood and sleep. This is how low levels of progesterone can increase the risk of anxiety and depression. Low progesterone levels (or high estrogen in relation to normal progesterone, known as relative estrogen dominance), can wreak havoc on your health, hormones, mood, and fertility. Common symptoms of low progesterone include: infertility, mid-cycle spotting, heavy bleeding, crippling PMS, and trouble sleeping.

Progesterone is mainly created by the corpus luteum in your ovaries during the luteal phase (the second half) of your menstrual cycle. However, it can also be produced by your adrenal glands in small quantities. Why is this important? Because it means if you don't ovulate and produce a corpus luteum, you don't produce enough of the progesterone that you need! Ovulation is the release of an egg from your ovaries. After the egg is released, the follicle that once surrounded the egg becomes a temporary endocrine gland called the corpus luteum.. The corpus luteum then produces progesterone while it waits for pregnancy to occur. *If pregnancy doesn't occur,* the corpus luteum breaks down, causing progesterone to fall. This is when estrogen rises again and bleeding occurs (aka the beginning of your period). If pregnancy *does* occur, you don't bleed or have your period, and your levels of progesterone continue to rise until the placenta takes over to produce necessary pregnancy hormones. This rise and continued progesterone production also prevents further ovulation from occurring during pregnancy, preventing the release of another egg from your ovaries.

Now here's the thing– you either ovulate and get pregnant, or you ovulate and have your period. There is no cycle without ovulation or a true period. However, you can have what is called an anovulatory cycle. This is what I mentioned before about a *true* period. An anovulatory cycle is a menstrual cycle where ovulation doesn't occur, meaning progesterone isn't made. This can be seen in women who take hormonal birth control, hormonal imbalances, hypothalamic amenorrhea (due to under-eating or over-exercising), nutrient deficiencies, or in hypothyroidism.

Fun fact- when ovulation occurs, the "explosion" of your egg being released can trigger a mild pain or twinge known as mittelschmerz. This little twinge occurs right near your ovaries on the bottom part of your lower pelvis. Ever felt a tiny twinge in pain during that time of the month there? You could be feeling your ovulation! Mittelschmerz can be used as a tool to assess for ovulation. Not all women can feel it, though. Don't worry- there are other ways you can track and assess for ovulation and we will touch on these soon.

Progesterone can be converted to cortisol in your adrenals. Why is this important? Because in times of chronic stress or in HPA axis dysfunction, your progesterone can over-convert into cortisol, in what is known as the "pregnenolone steal". Though this "steal" really doesn't happen in the tissues, the conversion of progesterone to cortisol is very real, and can leave you having an irregular or lost menstrual cycle, heighten symptoms of PMS and PMDD, alter your mood, cause night sweats, and contribute to anxiety and depression. I will dive more into this, as well as what can cause low or high progesterone, in Chapter 5.

Sadly, many women are not educated about fertility awareness method (FAM) or about their true fertile window. Many think that they can get pregnant any day of the month. If you are just learning about this lie - you aren't the only one. Truth is – you can only get pregnant for about 5-7 days total in your monthly cycle!

Why is this? Pregnancy can only occur when you ovulate. Your egg then has 24 hours to survive and become fertilized. Though your egg has only 24 hours, male sperm have the ability to survive for longer- a period of about 5 days. This means that near your ovulation window, you have the ability to possibly fertilize an egg (and get pregnant) if you choose to have sex near the 5 days before ovulation, or up 2 days after. Mind blowing, right? Unlike what your middle school health teacher told you, you can't get pregnant every day. Here's your permission ladies to have sex when away from these "fertile possible days". This is where something called Fertility Awareness Method (FAM) comes in. You can skip ahead to the "Non-hormonal birth control" section in this chapter for more information. Note- FAM does not have a 100% success rate, but studies have shown that when using FAM correctly, that the failure rate can be as low as 0.6%!

♀ FERTILITY ♂

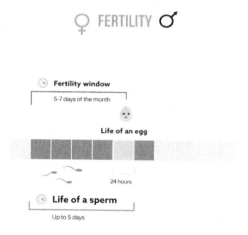

Ovulation is not only a way to track when you can or can't get pregnant, it's also a way to assess for hormonal balance and chaos in your body. If you don't ovulate, you don't produce progesterone. Low progesterone levels lead to symptoms and conditions such as (get ready this is long): chronic fatigue, abnormal or loss of menstrual cycle, mid cycle spotting, irritability, anxiety, depression, mood swings, trouble losing weight, hypothyroidism, sugar cravings, increased risk for osteoporosis and fractures, hot flashes, hair loss, fibroids, heavy PMS, insomnia, and cardiovascular disease. You already know progesterone's beautiful benefits. Now you also know that you only get those if you ovulate.

Don't take ovulation lightly. Don't take not having a period lightly. You want a period (and ovulation) in order to maximize your health and well-being. The next chapter will dive into what can prevent ovulation and wreak havoc on your hormones.

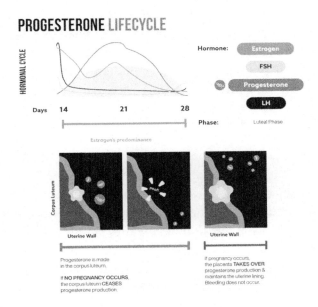

PROGESTERONE LIFECYCLE

Testosterone:

Yes, ladies- you have and need testosterone too! Testosterone is not the "bulky man-enhancing" hormone. Though testosterone plays less of a role in your body than it does in men, it's still an extremely important hormone that you don't want to throw out (like your favorite pair of socks that have holes on them- yes I am talking to my fellow sock hoarders).

Having healthy testosterone levels can help improve your body composition, prevent anxiety and depression, increase your energy, and enhance your libido!

Testosterone plays crucial parts in your body including:

- Aids in mood and cognition
- Helps to maintain and build muscle mass and strength
- Maintains sex drive
- Promotes preservation of bone mineral density
- Helps increase motivation

Testosterone gets a bad rap for causing PCOS (Polycystic Ovarian Syndrome), insulin resistance, and hirsutism (such as excess facial and body hair growth, hair loss, oily skin, and acne). However, it's important to note that these are all conditions that occur when testosterone levels go out of control. Just like any hormone, the imbalance is crucial in order for the chaos to occur.

Testosterone in your body is created by your ovaries and adrenal glands, however half of your testosterone comes from the circulation of two other hormones: DHEA (dehydroepiandrosterone) and androstenedione. This is very important to remember, as DHEA and androstenedione also feed into your estrogen through a process called aromatization. Therefore, not only does testosterone have its own benefits and effects in your body, but it can also heavily impact one of your queen hormones, estrogen! Androstenedione can also form one of two metabolites: etiocholanolone (5-beta preference) or androsterone (5-alpha preference). The preference for which metabolite and "5-beta vs 5-alpha" depends on your 5-Alpha Reductase Activity.

Your 5-Alpha Reductase activity can create symptoms of high testosterone, despite having normal testosterone levels. These symptoms include: scalp hair loss/male pattern baldness, oily skin, acne, facial hair, and increased aggression. Sound familiar?

How does this happen? If you convert and have a higher preference for 5-alpha than for 5-beta, you produce more dihydrotestos-
terone (DHT) in your body, which is three times more potent than
normal testosterone. This means that you can have "normal"
testosterone in labs but experience crippling high testosterone-
related symptoms. 5-Alpha preference can be caused or influenced
by: post birth control syndrome (in which androgens can
rebound), anabolic steroid usage, genetics, PCOS, an inflammatory diet, high insulin levels, chronic stress, adrenal disorders, low
SHBG, endocrine disruptors, gut infections, and nutrient deficiencies. Just like with any hormonal condition, you want to
address *why* you are preferring 5-alpha. Please don't blindly throw
supplements at the problem. Fix the root cause.

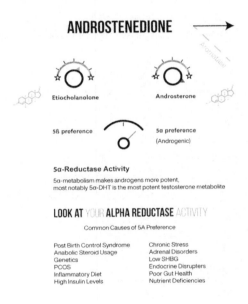

Another important hormone produced that feeds into your testosterone is DHEA. DHEA is produced mainly in your adrenal
glands. It is actually the most potent hormone in your body at all
times! DHEA and pregnenolone are designated as "prohormone"
and are both made by the adrenal glands from cholesterol.

Together, they both serve as precursors to the rest of your hormones.

DHEA, though it doesn't exert power biological effects on its own, feeds into your testosterone and estrogen pathways, and can be a large contributor to hormonal chaos when too high, or too low. As a woman, you don't produce testosterone from testicles, so you have to get it elsewhere. Where do you get it? DHEA! This is where low or high DHEA and adrenal imbalances directly serve into hormonal imbalances. If your DHEA tanks, so will your testosterone (say goodbye to your libido if this happens).

DHEA is commonly referred to as the "fountain of youth hormone" as its levels naturally decline with age. It is my belief that this also contributes to the drops in estrogen and testosterone produced as you grow older, as well as possibly having an influence on the cognitive function loss that occurs with age.

Hormone Transport: The Forgotten Factor

Two of your main hormones, testosterone and estrogen, travel throughout your blood attached to a transport protein made in your liver called sex hormone binding globulin (SHBG). Normally SHBG doesn't cause any issues and is in perfect quantities in your blood. However, if any condition causes SHBG to be too high or too low, this can reduce or increase the amount of free hormones in your body. Cue hormonal chaos! In order for a hormone to do its work, it has to be free (cue me singing *I'm free to do what I want and have a good time*).

Too much SHBG? Free hormones can decrease. Too little SHBG? Free hormones can increase! This is one of the most forgotten lab tests and forgotten factors of hormonal health that I see when working with patients.

What can influence SHBG levels?

What decreases SHBG: insulin resistance, hypothyroidism, low protein intake, obesity, insulin use, PCOS, exogenous androgen use, Cushing's Syndrome, exercise, progestins, prolactin, cortisol

What increases SHBG: pregnancy, hyperthyroidism, liver disease, exogenous estrogen use, birth control, low fat/vegetarian diet

I always suggest if doing full hormone testing, to include an assessment of both your hormones and their transport proteins and forms.

Basic Hormone Assessment Testing:

My suggestions for a comprehensive hormone test assessment (if not completing a DUTCH test) include:

- Thyroid labs: TSH, Free, T4, Free T3, TPO and TgAB antibodies
- Hormone labs: Estradiol, progesterone, free testosterone, SHBG, DHEA-S, prolactin, FSH and LH if trying to get pregnant (test on day 3 for LH and FSH, otherwise 5-7 days before your menstrual cycle)
- Additional markers: CMP (Comprehensive Metabolic Panel), Iron, Ferritin (storage form of iron), Vitamin D, Vitamin B12, Serum Copper, RBC Vitamin A, RBC Zinc, Iodine, and Folate

More in-depth testing should be done if you have any signs or symptoms of menstrual cycle irregularities, or if your health care provider wants to do a more in-depth assessment.

The Symphony of Your Menstrual Cycle- Getting to Know Your Cycle:

Understanding how your menstrual cycle works gives you power and insight in understanding your body and your body's hormonal symphony. Your menstrual cycle is essentially your fifth vital sign. If your body is not functioning optimally, neither is your cycle. Just like how a fire alarm goes off when there is a fire, when havoc occurs in your life or body, your menstrual cycle changes, or even disappears. This is your body attempting to tell you something is wrong! These warning signs show up as symptoms of increased period pain or PMS, heavy bleeding, development of mood swings, spotting, or even the loss of your cycle. Would you ignore a fire alarm going off in your home? I sure hope not! You shouldn't ignore the alarm of an irregular or painful period either.

Whether the disruption in your period stems from too much stress, a nutrient deficiency, or thyroid problems, period problems are not to be ignored. They are your fire alarm telling you to WAKE UP and help your body! Many women think of these symptoms as their bodies hurting them, but in reality, they are really ways that the body asks for help! An irregular or abnormal menstrual cycle is a warning sign of a disrupted hormonal symphony.

The problem with conventional medicine is that women are not taught about this. They are not told what a normal menstrual cycle should look like, what help can regulate it, or what can harm it. Many are just thrown on birth control. You deserve better. Yes, birth control may reduce your symptoms. However, that is ultimately just a band-aid on an open wound. It's simply covering up the symptoms, rather than addressing and fixing the root cause of those symptoms.

Good news is, you have me now. You have this book. You have tools in your toolbox to be the master of your body and hormones. I hope you can learn to read the alarms that your body sends, listen to them, and put out the fires!

Let's dive into what your menstrual cycle should look like, and then we can dive into what can happen to trigger your fire alarms!

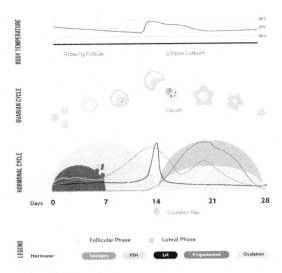

THE MENSTRUAL CYCLE

Stage 1: Follicular Phase

Day one of your period until ovulation marks your follicular phase, which lasts between 1-14 days. The beginning of your follicular phase is triggered by the release of GnRH (gonadotropin-releasing hormone) from your hypothalamus, which stimulates follicle- stimulating hormone (FSH) from your pituitary. FSH then stimulates the follicles in your ovaries to grow, which then releases estrogen, causing your estrogen levels to rise. FSH actually stimulates multiple follicles to grow, anywhere from 3 to 30 total. It becomes a race for the winning, with only a single dominant follicle to fully mature, as only one egg can be released at a time. Throughout the follicular phase, your estrogen stimulates the thickening and growth of your endometrium (the lining of your uterus), which is later shed when your period comes again.

As estrogen levels climb, your brain senses an estrogen peak which triggers your hypothalamus to release gonadotropin-releasing hormone (GnRH). GnRH then signals to the pituitary to release

FSH and LH (luteinizing hormone). This trigger of LH and FSH are what cause ovulation to occur and an egg release from the follicles in your ovaries. Ovulation marks the end of the follicular phase and starts the luteal phase of your menstrual cycle.

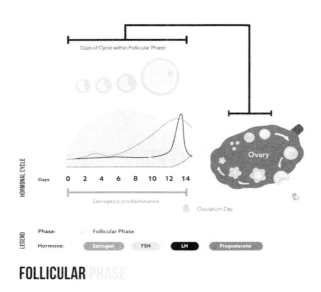

FOLLICULAR PHASE

Stage 2: Luteal phase

Ovulation day marks the start of your luteal phase, which lasts about 14 days or until your period starts. Ovulation is the main event in your menstrual cycle: the true period party to celebrate. Ovulation is required for a true period to happen (versus an anovulatory cycle or withdrawal bleed seen with birth control) and is required for pregnancy to occur. Ovulation is also the only way that you make your progesterone: your soothing, calming hormone and yin to estrogen's yang. Remember the benefits of progesterone? You can only get them if you ovulate!

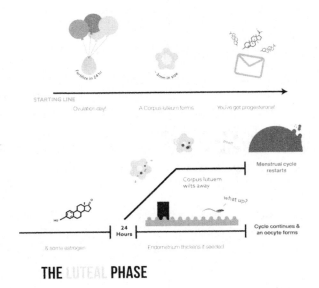

THE LUTEAL PHASE

Ovulation can be described as an "explosion" within the dominant follicle in your ovaries. This "explosion" releases an egg from the follicle and allows it to move from your ovaries, through your fallopian tubes, and into your uterus for possible fertilization and implantation. Your egg has up to 24 hours to be fertilized after being released. This is where ovulation test strips can be used to assess for ovulation timing and aid in fertility planning. They check for your LH surge that triggers ovulation, allowing you to plan for sex within your fertile hours. They can be an incredible part of FAM (fertility awareness method) and in trying for a baby. They also can be extremely helpful to correctly time when you take any at-home hormone test kits that require specific testing days after ovulation.

The leftover follicle becomes the corpus luteum, which secretes your progesterone. This progesterone, as well as some estrogen, acts to maintain the thickening of your uterine lining in hope for egg fertilization. It also causes your cervix to create thicker mucus, preventing sperm from entering the uterus, and increases your basal body temperature. Your rise in basal body temperature serves as another marker used in FAM.

Your endometrium thickening and then stabilization from progesterone is how an egg becomes an embryo and then baby. The egg is nurtured in your uterus after implantation and fertilization. As your luteal phase continues, your progesterone levels maintain your uterine lining for about 10-14 days. However, the length of your luteal phase depends on your "normal" cycle length and is heavily impacted by any disruption in your hypothalamic-pituitary-adrenal axis (HPA axis).

If your egg does not become fertilized and implanted, then your corpus luteum disintegrates like a sad, wilting flower. This decreases progesterone and triggers your endometrium (the lining of your uterus) to shed, starting your period, ending your luteal phase, and restarting a new cycle with day 1 of your next follicular phase. If fertilization of your egg and implantation does occur, your progesterone levels remain elevated to nurture and maintain your uterine lining. Estrogen levels also rise to prevent the maturation of other eggs, allowing for your one fertilized egg to be the "chosen one" to thrive!

*Fun fact- you have the most hormones in your lifetime when you are pregnant.

If your progesterone levels do not rise enough during your luteal phase, this can hinder the thickening of the uterine lining, cease the growth of the corpus luteum, and prevent pregnancy, causing infertility or a missed period. Lack of progesterone can also cause mid-cycle spotting, mood swings, premenstrual headaches or migraines, insomnia, anxiety, and depression. Why? Remember, progesterone is your calming hormone, your singer in the band! Without her, there is decreased GABA and serotonin produced in your brain, which are supposed to help to calm you down, combat stress, and allow you to fall and stay asleep. You also may struggle with fertility, as your uterine lining is not being sufficiently nourished to maintain an optimal environment for your egg.

Side note- testosterone levels also fluctuate during your menstrual cycle, just like estrogen and progesterone. However, the side effects of this fluctuation are largely unnoticeable. Testosterone is lowest in your follicular phase and rises to peak mid cycle, around the time of ovulation. This rise helps with the increase of ovulation energy and enhancement of your libido. It serves as an internal suggestion to "get frisky" when you are most fertile!

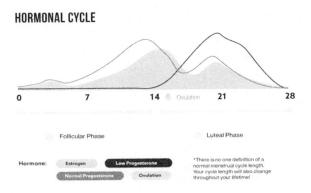

HORMONAL CYCLE

0	7	14 Ovulation	21	28

Follicular Phase   Luteal Phase

Hormone: Estrogen   Low Progesterone

Normal Progesterone   Ovulation

*There is no one definition of a normal menstrual cycle length. Your cycle length will also change throughout your lifetime!

Your Mood and Your Menstrual Cycle

I am sure you have noticed how your mood changes throughout your menstrual cycle. Some days you feel like a complete sloth, other days you feel like an energizer bunny with no care in the world! During "shark week," you may feel like a raging bitch. Excuse my French, no other way to state that fact! Ladies- your menstrual cycle (if not on birth control!), heavily impacts your mood, energy, fuel utilization, and behaviors! It can even influence what kind of men you are attracted to. Interesting, right?!

WEEK 4: CAT PHASE

Decreasing energy & concentration
Sleepiness and fatigue
Increasing craving & mood wings
May have increased anxiety
More reserved & prefer smaller group/isolation

What to do: Self care, rest & sleeping

WEEK 3: PEACOCK PHASE

More energetic and outgoing during ovulation
(1st half of week)
Mellow down. Be more reserved
& more cautious after ovulation
(2nd half of week)

What to do: Socializing & meditation

WEEK 2: DOG PHASE

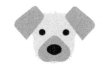

Increased energy & concentration
More social & outgoing
Greater mood stability
More adventuress & creative

What to do: Socializing & activities

WEEK 1: SLOTH PHASE

Decreased energy (but increased strength)
Slower & sleepier
More reserved/inward focused

What to do: More resting & self reflection

Depending on the changes in your progesterone, estrogen, and testosterone levels, when it comes to mood and behavior- estrogen and progesterone are what play the major roles while testosterone greatly impacts your libido, motivation, and energy.

How? Estrogen is highest during your follicular phase (the first day of bleeding on your period until right before ovulation at the end of week 2). It plays a key role in boosting your strength, energy, willingness and desire for adventure and socialization. It makes you feel more confident and motivated! Many women find that during the week of their period, they may feel a bit fatigued, but their strength makes them feel like superwoman. This is the power of your estrogen.

On the other hand, progesterone is highest during your luteal phase (beginning week 3, starting right after ovulation and lasting until the start of your menstrual cycle). It calms or even "sedates" you. This may slow digestion, make you more inward-focused, quieter, and sometimes moody. The rise in your progesterone may help ease anxiety and depression-like symptoms. Too little progesterone? You may not get the anti-anxiety and calming benefits! Too little progesterone is also one of the main causes for your PMS shark week mood swings.

*Fun fact- progesterone puts you at more risk for having blood sugar drops during your luteal phase, as it decreases your insulin sensitivity. This is why it is so important to not skip meals and to have smart snacks ready during this time of your cycle. Some women can also be very sensitive to progesterone, and too much can lead to water retention and breast pain.

The "Animal Faces" of Your Cycle:

I like to think of the fluctuations of your mood and behavior during your cycle as types of animals. Keep in mind, not all women notice these mood and behavior changes, especially since lack of sleep, stress levels, and nutrition can greatly impact them.

Week 1: Sloth Phase

- Decreased energy (but increased strength)
- Slower and sleepier
- More reserved and inward focused

Do More: resting and self reflection

Week 2: Dog Phase

- Increased energy and concentration
- More social and outgoing
- Greater mood stability
- More adventurous and creative

Do More: socializing and activity

Week 3: Peacock Phase

- More energetic and outgoing during ovulation (1st half of week)
- Mellow down and become more reserved and more cautious after ovulation (2nd half of week)

Do More: socializing and meditation

Week 4: Cat Phase

- Decreasing energy and concentration
- Sleepiness and fatigue
- Increasing cravings and mood swings
- May have increasing anxiety
- More reserved and prefer smaller groups or isolation

Do More: self care, rest, sleeping

If you are on any form of hormonal birth control, you won't notice these changes, as your menstrual cycle will not have this natural ebb and flow. Unlike what your doctor told you, the pill won't regulate your cycle. The pill will take it over, including how your mood and behavior naturally change.

Your Menstrual Cycle, Metabolism, and Training:

Your menstrual cycle changes more than just your mood and behavior. It can also change your body's fuel utilization, strength levels, and workout capacity! Dayum being a woman is fascinating, isn't it? Not every female notices these changes in their training. Additionally, research studies are not consistent with their conclusions on how manipulating training for your cycle impacts your progress in the gym or your body composition. Some studies have shown no change in strength or performance between menstrual phases, while others do see a benefit. Sadly, science doesn't focus too much on this connection. We don't yet know the impact on manipulating diet and exercise for enhancing weight loss or muscle gain efforts during the different phases of your cycle, but we do know physiology, so there are some differences that may play a role.

Your Follicular Phase:

- Estrogen increases insulin sensitivity
- Carbohydrates are used more efficiently for energy
- May have increased strength and endurance
- Less reactive to stress

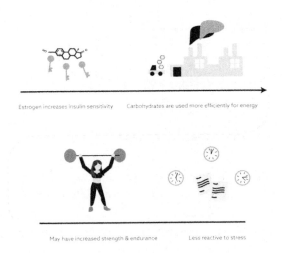

THE FOLLICULAR PHASE

Your Luteal Phase:

- Progesterone increases insulin resistance
- Fats used more efficiently for energy
- Great time for restorative and low impact exercise
- May benefit from increased calorie intake
- Increased basal body temperature due to rise in

progesterone

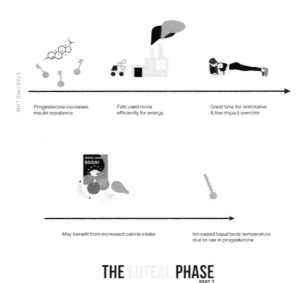

Progesterone increases insulin resistance

Fats used more efficiently for energy

Great time for restorative & low impact exercise

May benefit from increased calorie intake

Increased basal body temperature due to rise in progesterone

THE LUTEAL PHASE
PART 2

So what does this mean for you?

1. If you notice a huge difference in strength throughout your cycle- plan de-loads or low intensity training weeks during your luteal phase. Your luteal phase is when you may feel weakest. Remember- estrogen is highest during your follicular phase, and may increase your strength levels! This may mean that setting PRs and attacking high-intensity activities may be smarter to try to do during the first 2 weeks of your cycle. You may want to hold off on the PRs during your last weeks of your cycle when you may find yourself weaker. Ovulation is another time to be cautious with training as well. The peak rise in estrogen upon ovulation can increase your risk or injury as it decreases muscle tendon elasticity. If you notice tight muscles and lack of mobility around the time of ovulation, I suggest sticking to low intensity movements.

2. Use this knowledge to be kinder to yourself. Lower in energy or not hitting the weights as hard the week before your period? Don't beat yourself up (but also don't be a baby – cue my winky face). Do what you can, listen to your body, and if you need to rest, then rest.

3. Though fuel utilization may be different between phases of your cycle- what matters most is overall diet consistency. If you track macros, I typically have clients remain on the same macros throughout their cycle. I have personally found consistency to work better than baby "menstrual cycle" changes. We don't know the amount of benefit that you may get by switching your fat to carb ratio based on your cycle. However, I do believe that this fuel utilization difference in your luteal phase provides a great opportunity to throw in more refeeds and higher calorie days if you are dieting, especially to help combat cravings that progesterone may create.

What about if you're on birth control? For the most part, your levels of hormones are going to be almost stagnant based on taking hormonal birth control (minus any placebo pills). The effect on your recovery, metabolism, and strength may vary based on the type of birth control that you are on. Some birth control pills show evidence of helping to increase performance and decrease risk of injury. However, that cannot be said for every type.

Your Cycle on the Pill:

There are many, many types of birth control. I swear a new one is being made and sold every day! Not all birth controls are the same, differing in their functions, ratios, dosages, and side effects. I couldn't cover every birth control in this book, even if I wanted to. They come in many forms, from low-dose, extended release, single hormone, and combination hormone... you have a good handful of options. Overall, birth control types work to prevent ovulation (though some allow it) and prevent pregnancy. Each type has its own side effects, risks, and benefits. Birth control can be divided into 2 main categories: hormonal birth control and non-hormonal birth control.

HOW BIRTH CONTROL WORKS:

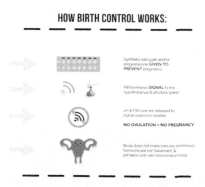

Hormonal Birth Control:

How does the hormonal birth control pill work? The pill works by preventing pregnancy and ovulation. Without ovulation, you can't have pregnancy! Depending on the pill type, it can also thicken your cervical mucus, which blocks sperm movement to the egg, while thinning your uterine lining (preventing the possibility of egg implantation).

The synthetic hormones found within hormonal birth control also work by shutting down the communication between your brain and your ovaries. Your natural hormone production becomes suppressed and the synthetic exogenous hormones take over. This is the reason why birth control is used by many conventional doctors. It takes your cycle and regulates it. However, instead of fixing or balancing your hormones- it shuts them down, takes over, and regulates them itself. You no longer regulate your cycle- your birth control does.

Most birth control pills contain synthetic forms of estrogen and progesterone, in the form of progestin. This is very important to remember, as progestins do not work the same way in the body as progesterone, and in fact, the two have different molecular structures. Some pills are estrogen only, while some are progestin only.

There are also hormonal IUDs (intrauterine devices) that can be implanted in your uterus for pregnancy prevention, such as the Mirena IUD. The Mirena gives off a small amount of progestin, that acts to thin your uterine lining, thicken cervical mucus, and suppress ovulation. This results in preventing pregnancy. Other types of hormonal birth control include implants, injection (such as the depo shot), Nuvaring, and the patch. Either way, hormonal birth control usage will directly impact your hormones and stop your body's own natural hormone regulation.

Let's look back at how your menstrual cycle works naturally, step by step:

Step 1: GnRH in your hypothalamus stimulates FSH to be released from your pituitary.
Step 2- FSH stimulates your follicles to mature, which grow and release estrogen.
Step 3: LH is triggered by a peak in estrogen levels, causing ovulation (though both FSH and LH triggered)
Step 4: Ovulation causes your egg to travel to the uterus. Your corpus luteum forms in the ovary, secreting progesterone.
Step 5: Your corpus luteum continues to secrete progesterone, which helps to maintain your uterine lining and nurture your egg for hopeful pregnancy.
Step 6: If no pregnancy occurs, your progesterone levels drop, and your uterine lining is shed. Your period comes. GnRH triggers FSH again to restart the cycle. If pregnancy does occur, your corpus luteum is maintained in order to nurture a future baby.

In a "cycle" on hormonal birth control, synthetic estrogen and/or progestin (depending on the type) flood your body and tell the brain that it doesn't need to make its own hormones. In turn, your brain does not secrete LH and FSH, so your ovaries do not receive the signal to ovulate. No ovulation means no pregnancy, but also, no progesterone! Which, as you already know, has its own super-powers. Not all hormonal birth controls prevent ovulation (ex. Skyla and Mirena IUDs). However, all hormonal birth control pills do act to prevent pregnancy and shut down your body's own natural hormone production.

Let's clear up some common hormonal birth control myths.

Myth 1: "Birth control regulates your cycle." Slightly False. As I have already discussed, birth control takes over your cycle. Yes, it regulates it. However, this is different from what women think when they are given the pill. They are told it will "regulate their cycle" and assume this means help their body to naturally regulate it. This is false information. The pill can regulate your cycle, but it does this by taking over your hormones.

Myth 2: "Birth control fixes your period problems." False. Birth control cannot truly fix an underlying hormonal issue. It will band-aid it. By taking over your hormones, it will mask estrogen dominance, low progesterone, and even hypothyroid symptoms. Wouldn't you rather know why your period is irregular or painful versus being given a pill to manage symptoms?

Myth 3: "Birth control causes infertility." False. Thousands of women have taken birth control and gotten pregnant. Birth control can disrupt your hormones, and it can take a while to regulate them back to harmony after getting off of it. However, there are no correlations with birth control causing infertility. It will not harm your ovaries, and there has not been evidence to show uterus scarring or damage with IUD insertion.

Myth 4: "Birth control is safe." Slightly false. Yes, safety has been indicated by the FDA, but see the next section for some more truths.

Myth 5: "Birth control causes weight gain." Mostly false. There are no studies to prove this as a correlation for all birth control. Some women do gain weight when going on birth control. There seems to be a larger connection with weight gain and the Depo-Provera shot. However, it is false to claim that all birth control causes weight gain. Birth control can increase appetite and water retention though, leading to weight gain.

Side Effects of Hormonal Birth Control:

As you can imagine, there are some risks to messing with your brain and hormone communication and production. Don't get it twisted. I don't hate birth control pills. I hate the lack of education women are given about it. Most are never told how it works, or even any of its side effects. These side effects can include:

- Increased risk for anxiety or depression
- Digestive problems: including gut dysbiosis, intestinal permeability (also referred to as "leaky gut"), development of IBS (irritable bowel syndrome), and heightened risk of overgrowths and pathogens
- Thyroid disorder: most common being hypothyroidism or the development of Hashimoto's disease
- Decreases in testosterone levels: which for many women coming off birth control, causes a rebound effect leading to post birth control high testosterone levels
- Increases in SHBG (sex hormone binding globulin): this decreases the amount of free hormones in your blood (further impacting testosterone levels)
- Irregular or missed periods depending on the type (which makes it funny that it is prescribed incorrectly to "regulate" a woman's cycle)
- Increased risk of blood clotting
- Nutrient depletions: most common ones include B-vitamins, Zinc, Magnesium, and Folate
- Libido disturbances: this includes a lack of sex drive, vaginal dryness, and pain with sex

- Changes in attraction: It has been found that when cycling naturally, women may find masculine men more attractive, while women on birth control may be attracted to a more feminine partner. This "choice of mate" in my opinion is speculated to be correlated to mood changes as well.
- Shrinkage of vulvar tissue and clitoral tissue (hello- not fun for orgasms!)
- Increased breast and liver cancer risk: in fact, the IARC, International Agency for Research on Cancer, has classified hormonal birth control as a group one carcinogen. Keep in mind research also shows birth control reduces risk of endometrial, ovarian, and colorectal cancers.
- Insomnia and fatigue: this can lead to further hormonal and adrenal imbalances

Don't believe me? Just check the back of the birth control label and warning information. Just like any new medication or drug, you should be informed about it and any side effects. Not all women will have side effects from taking birth control, but all women should be educated on them.

Non-Hormonal Birth Control:

You have many other options methods for preventing pregnancy past hormonal birth control. These include: condoms, spermicides, fertility awareness method (FAM), the Copper IUD, cervical caps, the "pull out" method, and sterilization (called Essure). I hope you are familiar with condoms, as they are the most well-known form of birth control, though the least effective. I am going to skip over the pros and cons of each (I promise I will dive a bit into FAM!), and get straight to the copper IUD here. Please see my resource section if you want more information on the other non-hormonal methods.

Copper IUDs have become a popular option for many women. Just like hormonal birth control, you deserve to know how they work and their side effects. What is a copper IUD? A non-hormonal IUD (intrauterine device) is a flexible piece of plastic shaped like a "T" that contains a copper wire around it. Your doctor surgically places it inside your uterus, where it stays until removal. The inside copper acts to ward away sperm and prevents them from swimming to your eggs. If sperm can't reach your egg, you can't get pregnant. Copper IUDs can be left in your uterus for up to 10 years (depending on the IUD) and have a 99.9% effective rate.

I love non-hormonal IUDs as they still allow for your body to regulate its own menstrual cycle and still allow for ovulation, meaning you get to produce your progesterone! However, just like hormonal birth control, non-hormonal IUDs also have side effects. Common side effects of the Copper IUD include:

- Copper toxicity (which can also contribute to zinc deficiency)
- Nutrient deficiencies (such as B-vitamins, Vitamin C, CoQ10, and Zinc)
- Painful, heavy periods
- Bleeding or spotting between periods
- Potential increased risk for bacterial and yeast infections in the vagina
- Estrogen dominance
- Risk of expulsion and device breakage

I hope that you feel safe and comfortable enough to talk to your doctor about your birth control options, and that he or she is willing to discuss the pros and cons of each with you. If not, I say get a new doctor (yes, I said it). You deserve the best care possible, girlfriend. There is never any shame in what method you choose to prevent pregnancy. It's your body and your life. Just make sure YOU get to make the informed choice based on proper education.

. . .

FAM-Fertility Awareness Method:

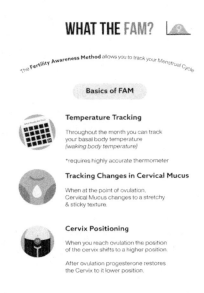

WHAT THE FAM?

The Fertility Awareness Method allows you to track your Menstrual Cycle

Basics of FAM

Temperature Tracking

Throughout the month you can track your basal body temperature (waking body temperature)

*requires highly accurate thermometer

Tracking Changes in Cervical Mucus

When at the point of ovulation, Cervical Mucus changes to a stretchy & sticky texture.

Cervix Positioning

When you reach ovulation the position of the cervix shifts to a higher position.

After ovulation progesterone restores the Cervix to it lower position.

Through fertility awareness method (FAM), you can make use of your body's own biofeedback as a tool to track your menstrual cycle, try for a baby, or prevent pregnancy. FAM incorporates biofeedback including: changes in your cervical mucus, rises in basal body temperature, and cervix position. What is biofeedback? Essentially, it's the signs and symptoms from your body's physiology that allow you to gain a greater awareness of your health and well-being.

FAM can be used for tracking ovulation, aka the main event of your menstrual cycle that is required for pregnancy and the production of your progesterone. Ovulation is stimulated by the rise in LH released from your pituitary after your estrogen levels peak. Remember how your egg can survive only 24 hours, with a sperm life of about 5 days? Tracking your ovulation can be used as a way to assess what days you are fertile or not (aka what days you can, or can't, get pregnant).

A key way to track ovulation is by measuring changes in your basal body temperature (BBT). Your basal body temperature is your waking body temperature and requires a high quality thermometer for accuracy. During ovulation, the rise in your progesterone levels aids to increase your basal body temperature, which stays elevated until you get your period, your luteal phase ends, and a new follicular phase begins. This is where you can track your luteal phase and know when you ovulate! A baby rise in 0.5 degrees F indicates that ovulation occurred. This may take routine practice to assess. I highly suggest investing in a high quality thermometer that tracks temperature to two decimal places for best accuracy.

Though you can use basal body temperature to track this change, it does require measuring your body temperature throughout the month. For best results in using body temperature assessment this with FAM, you would want to track your basal body temperature for at least a few months, along with additional FAM biofeedback markers, prior to using FAM as your sole conception protocol. Why? Your body temperature can also change due to stress, infection, illness, hypothyroidism, alcohol intake, or due to inadequate sleep. Your best friend with tracking your BBT is doing it often, consistently, and tracking it via an app or journal.

Tracking changes in cervical mucus is another tool to track ovulation, fertility, and assess the health of your lady region. Cervical mucus is the liquid discharge you see in your undies throughout your menstrual cycle, or on tissue paper after wiping. Created in your cervix, it's composed of various enzymes and proteins. The mucus-like texture of your cervical mucus helps your man's "swimmers" to swim and fertilize the egg during your ovulation window. If you haven't paid close attention to it, your cervical changes in texture and consistency throughout your cycle! This is how you can use it as another biofeedback marker for ovulation.

What is normal cervical mucus like? Normal cervical mucus will be scentless, and range from a clear and stretchy fluid to a creamy, stretchy white (think egg white texture). During "dry days," your cervical mucus can range from egg white to watery discharge. It may feel lubricative and leave a feeling of wetness in your undies. Some women have completely "dry" days, while others produce small amounts of cervical mucus throughout their cycle. All women are different.

Near ovulation, your cervical mucus changes to a stretchy and sticky texture. This stickiness, along with changes in pH, help the mucus to provide a medium for sperm to easily reach your egg. It helps your man's "swimmers" get to their place of partying. 24 hours after ovulation, your progesterone levels then rise, shifting your cervical mucus back to your "dryer" days. These dry days then last up until your period and end a few days before ovulation in your next cycle.

All women produce different amounts of cervical mucus, and for some, it can be completely normal to have full dry days, while others produce routine mucus throughout the month. However, any changes in color or scent, cottage cheese-like texture, or non-stretchy, watery discharge may indicate abnormalities to your vaginal or cervical health and should be discussed with your doctor. A fishy odor, vaginal irritation or itchiness, or abnormal color may indicate a bacterial or yeast infection. There are various supplements that can increase cervical mucus production, like vitex (chasteberry), or decrease it, such as antihistamines. Keep this in mind when starting or stopping a new supplement and using FAM.

Your cervix position is the last tracking tool to use in FAM. Your cervix is located at the bottom part of your uterus, and is what is responsible for dilating during childbirth, allowing a baby to be born. When you start to reach ovulation and estrogen starts to peak, your cervix shifts to a higher position and softens. After ovulation, progesterone helps your cervix to shift to a lower position and become more firm. Some women don't feel comfortable assessing and tracking cervix position. I get it. If you choose to, you can assess your cervix position by using your middle finger and pressing into your vagina (with clean hands), and touching your cervix to feel for firmness and depth. A great time to do this would be in the shower after washing. I am not the biggest fan of this tracking method, as I find it much less sanitary, but if you choose to use it, just ensure to have clean hands before and after.

Coming off Hormonal Birth Control

When birth control pills or hormonal birth control is stopped, your brain can have a hard time "waking back up" to hormone production, especially if it has been suppressed for a long time. For some women, this can result in what I call "hormonal rebounds" such as in the case for developing estrogen dominance or high testosterone. For others, coming off of birth control can result in blunted and low hormone production.

This is why women coming off birth control can experience "Post-Birth Control Syndrome," or "Post-Pill PCOS," in which they struggle to gain back their cycle and have raging PMS, heavy and painful periods, or gain excess weight. I learned the most about this condition and how to help through Dr. Jolene Brighten (author of Beyond the Pill). She is the queen behind coming off hormonal birth control. Please see the PCOS section for more detailed information about coming off of birth control.

The most important thing to remember here is that what happens when you come off birth control can't be known. There is no single post birth control reaction or protocol to prevent chaos. You must pay close attention to your body and your hormonal symphony, do proper testing, and ensure that you are taking the right steps toward what will be best for you. Please shy away from any claims for "post birth control" protocols. Some may be tearing at your emotions and fear, which in my opinion, is unfair to you and unethical.

Let me put this simply- my issue with birth control lies in the lack of education that women receive from conventional doctors who put them on it to "manage their menstrual cycle." They aren't given the truth on what it does or how it works. They aren't told about the potential side effects. They aren't given a complete list of all their options. I bet some of you reading this haven't even heard of FAM. Birth control hands down is an incredible option to prevent pregnancy and combat hormonal chaos. However it can't cure or fix hormonal imbalances. It doesn't solve the problem behind what causes the hormonal chaos. It simply stops the chaos by taking over. Essentially, birth control becomes the conductor of your symphony instead of you. You should be educated on this. You should be empowered and confident in knowing that your doctor gave you the right information to make your own decision.

No woman should ever feel ashamed for her choice of pregnancy prevention. As a woman, you deserve to be given the details on what the pill or other birth control options do in your body, how they affect your menstrual cycle, and their side effects. You should be given details on how they can affect your health in the short and long term. You deserve to know what you are putting into your body. Remember that fact for any medication you are given.

One more rant from me and then I am done. I constantly see women being prescribed birth control for reasons other than pregnancy prevention. These reasons may include helping with: acne, heavy PMS, period pain or heavy bleeding, PCOS, fibroids, or irregular cycles. Though the pill can be beneficial for many of these conditions such as endometriosis, heavy PMS, PMDD, or inducing a bleed with hypothalamic amenorrhea, it is unethical for doctors to claim that the pill will fix or balance one's hormones in those that suffer with these conditions.

The reality is that the pill can help manage your hormonal symptoms, but simply does so by band-aiding them and blunting your body's natural hormone production. This may be helpful for you at the start, but may wreak havoc in the future! Again, I have no issues with the use of birth control in any situation. You do you, girlfriend. I have issues when you don't receive the education on what you are putting into your body. You deserve to know. You deserve to make your own informed decision.

End rant. Thanks for coming to my TED talk.

Common Types of Birth Control & How They Work:

Name	How It Works	How It's Used	Effectiveness
Hormonal Birth Control Pill	Hormones estrogen and/or progestin are consumed orally & act to prevent ovulation by shutting down signal to your ovaries (LH suppression); Thickens cervical fluid to prevent sperm traveling to egg; Thins endometrium	Oral pill taken daily	91-99%% effective
Hormonal IUD (Mirena, Kyleena, Skyla)	The synthetic hormone progestin prevents ovulation (may or may not prevent ovulation), thins the uterine lining, and thickens cervical fluid to prevent sperm traveling to egg; Changes fallopian tube contractions to make egg travel to uterus more difficult	Inserted by a medical professional into the uterus and lasts 3-12 years	99% effective
Non Hormonal IUD (Para-guard, Copper	Prevents sperm from swimming to fertilize egg through use of copper ions; Prevents egg implantation (allows for normal hormonal creation & ovulation)	Inserted by a medical professional into the uterus and lasts 3-12 years	99% effective
Vaginal Ring (NuvaRing)	Hormones estrogen and progestin released to prevent ovulation.	Inserted personally into the vagina and replaced every 3-5 weeks	91% effective

Birth Control Implant	The synthetic hormone progestin prevents ovulation, thickens cervical mucus to prevent sperm from traveling to egg	Inserted by a medical professional under the skin of the upper arm and lasts up to 3 years	99% effective
Condoms	Prevents sperm from entering the vagina during vaginal intercourse	Placed on the penis before vaginal intercourse	85%-95% effective with typical use
Fertility Awareness Method	Tracking ovulation to identify fertile and non-fertile days	Manually tracking menstrual cycle through cycle length, cervical mucus, and basal body temperature	76-99% effective
Surgery	Follicular tubes are blocked in females or tubes in scrotum are blocked in males to stop motility of eggs/sperm; Ovaries removed	One time, irreversible surgical procedure; May or may not induce early menopause	99% effective
Birth Control Shot (Depo-Provera)	Injected progestin prevents ovulation	Given every 3 months by a medical professional	94% effective
Birth Control Patch	Releases estrogen and progestin to prevent ovulation	Applied to skin and reapplied weekly, with one week taken off each month	91% effective

4

HELPING HORMONAL CHAOS

What does a "normal menstrual cycle" look like?

Facts first. Every woman's cycle may be slightly different. There is no "perfect cycle" or "normal menstrual cycle." Age and body size play a crucial role in the length, duration, and intensity of your cycle, as do your genetics! Just like your body is uniquely your own, your menstrual cycle is too. Your menstrual cycle also changes as you grow older and enter and exit different seasons of your life.

For example, as an adolescent young woman, it's completely normal to have irregular periods with different volumes of period blood loss. As you grow older, your periods typically become heavier and more consistent, until you enter your perimenopause years (ranging from ages 35-45) when they become lighter and infrequent. The heaviness, length, or pain levels of your cycle may mildly change month to month, especially if you go through heavy times of trauma, stress, make changes to your diet, or take any plan B pill.

Slight changes in your menstrual cycle will happen. You may skip a period one month, or have a heavier period another. Don't be overly concerned when this happens. However, if your cycle becomes irregular or changes from your natural "flow" the past two periods in a row, it's time to do some digging. If you notice crippling pains, aches, or heavy bleeding and large clots though, don't wait. Make sure to speak with your medical provider ASAP.

Truths about a "normal menstrual cycle":

1. A pill bleed from hormonal birth control is not a true period. There is no ovulation.
2. Your period should NOT be crippling and cause you severe pain and heavy bleeding. If you need medication to get through your day, something is up.
3. Your period can naturally ebb and flow with different days, and this can and will change throughout your life. Your period will not be the same throughout your life, just like your life won't be the same!
4. Your cycle will change your energy levels, motivation, and mood. This is completely normal.
5. You may miss a cycle, spot one month, or have heavier or lighter bleeding for a month or two. This doesn't mean your hormonal symphony has crashed. It just means something caused an imbalance. Be concerned if this imbalance continues for more than two months in a row.
6. A "normal cycle" can last from 24 to 34 days. What matters, along with length, is consistency in your cycle, blood volume, and pain levels.
7. Ovulation does not always occur on day 14 of your cycle, and will not occur on the same day every month.
8. Your cycle length is primarily determined by your follicular phase. Your follicular phase and when you ovulate are responsible for a short or long menstrual cycle.

9. A typical period will be heaviest at the beginning, and taper off in blood volume as days go by. 25-80 mL of blood is typical to be lost (3-4 tampons a day).
10. Severe PMS, heavy bleeding, heavy clotting, and crippling pain are not normal, though they may seem common.

Type	Definition	Possible Meaning
"Normal" Period	-25 to 80 mL blood loss (3-4 tampons a day or about 2 menstrual cup exchanges- equivalent to 30 mL per cup) -3 to 7 days length -Mild period pain -Bright red to cranberry color	-Your health is probably doing good!
Light Period	-Less than 25 mL blood loss -1-3 days length -Color may be light pink to red	-May not have sufficient estrogen (estrogen builds up uterine lining) -May be only spotting -May be under eating or over-exercising -May have nutrient deficiency -May be stress related -Increased age -Birth control pill bleed
Heavy Period	-80 ML or more blood loss (greater than 4 tampons a day) -3 to 7 days length -May have heavy period pain and crippling cramps -Color may be dark purple -May require changing pads or tampons during the night	-May have too much estrogen (causing excess build up on uterine lining) -May have skipped a period (resulting in excess blood to be shed with your current period) -May be due to endometriosis, fibroids, ovarian cysts, endometrial polyps, thyroid disease, high insulin levels, endometrial hyperplasia, adenomyosis, endometrial cancer, high histamine -May have too little progesterone -IUD side effect -Coagulation disorder -Medication side effects

Putting out the Fire- When Your Cycle is Screaming for Help

Your menstrual cycle is like a fire alarm, alerting your body when it needs help. If your cycle drastically changes in length, flow, or pain, there's an alarm going off in your body saying, "Hey girl, listen to me. Help me!"

Remember, mild PMS is normal. You are going to go through some months with it being worse than others, especially during stressful months. However, crippling and consistent PMS is not normal. If you deal with monthly heavy cramps, heavy bleeding, heightened anxiety or depression, spotting, cycle irregularity, or lose your cycle for more than 3 months, take a pause. It's time to dig deeper.

When your hormones are in harmony and all is well in your body, your hormones are utilized, processed, and then ultimately excreted. In easy terms, you use them, then lose them. Having just the right amount of estrogen, progesterone, and testosterone is needed for your hormonal symphony to be harmonious. Too much or too little of one causes chaos to occur, which can then create a domino effect on your overall health.

Let's go over common scenarios and situations that can wreak havoc on your cycle and health. Then, I will give you my secret strategies to get that period, and your health, back on track.

PMS- The Pre-Period Demon

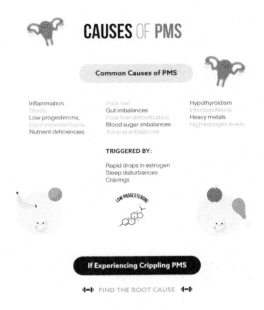

CAUSES OF PMS

Common Causes of PMS

Inflammation	Poor diet	Hypothyroidism
Stress	Gut imbalances	Infection/Illness
Low progesterone,	Poor liver detoxification	Heavy metals
Environmental toxins	Blood sugar imbalances	High estrogen levels
Nutrient deficiencies	Adrenal imbalances	

TRIGGERED BY:

Rapid drops in estrogen
Sleep disturbances
Cravings

LOW PROGESTERONE

If Experiencing Crippling PMS

FIND THE ROOT CAUSE

Just because PMS is common, does not make it normal. We all know the signs and annoyance of PMS- aka Premenstrual Syndrome. (Can we just talk about why women get punished by nature when we aren't pregnant?! Like God, why did you do this?) Common symptoms include: Irritability, headaches, trouble sleeping, anxiety, depression, acne, breast tenderness, water retention, bloating, constipation, cravings, and mood swings.

PMS is defined as any physical or behavioral symptom that significantly impairs your daily life during the 2 weeks before your cycle starts. It commonly includes alterations in pain levels, energy, mood, and motivation. It's estimated that 50-80% of women have mild PMS before their period, and that 2-8% of women suffer from another more severe form called PMDD (premenstrual dysphoric disorder).

When your hormonal symphony is balanced and your hormones are doing their intricate dance together, PMS is mild. However, when your symphony is heading towards disaster, this is where

PMS flares up and crippling symptoms can emerge. Got heavy PMS for multiple months? That's your fire alarm going off, girlfriend!

What causes PMS? The root cause is actually unknown. PMS is greatly associated with hormonal imbalances such as estrogen dominance, low progesterone, nutrient deficiencies, inflammation, as well as serotonin and GABA dysregulation (two of your relaxing brain neurotransmitters). This is why some women are prescribed SSRIs (serotonin reuptake inhibitors) to aid in the management of PMS.

Looking at what can influence your hormones and serotonin levels can give you an idea as to what may influence PMS development. Some potential causes include high estrogen, low progesterone, hypothyroidism, heavy metal toxicity, cortisol dysregulation, endocrine disruptors, inflammation, stress, gut dysbiosis, infection, illness, or nutrient deficiencies.

Though PMS is not desired, it can be normal to go through a few months of bad PMS within a year, as any high stress or trauma can induce it. However, if you experience frequent and recurrent PMS issues, especially ones that cripple you and prevent you from doing day-to-day activities, you need to dig deeper. Your fire alarm is going off. The problem could be as simple as a nutrient deficiency, but it could also be coming from a condition like fibroids or endometriosis.

Luckily, there are some easy changes you can make to help prevent and manage PMS!

My key strategies for being a PMS conqueror include:

1. **Focus on color:** Fill up on all the colors of the rainbow in your fruits and vegetables to increase the amount of antioxidants and polyphenols in your diet. This will not only help you achieve optimal nutrient status, but combat inflammation, which is a heavy contributor to PMS problems.

2. **Power up the cruciferous veggies:** These superpowered veggies can help you to detoxify excess estrogen. They contain indole-3-carbinol, which converts to DIM in your body, which helps to push you estrogen through Phase 1 of estrogen detoxification. Broccoli sprouts are another fantastic addition to your diet, as they contain high amounts of sulforaphane. Sulforaphane helps to combat free radical damage and inflammation in your body, as well as helps to move estrogen through phase 2 detoxification.

3. **Fix your fats:** Focus on consuming healthy fats such as avocado, fatty fish such as salmon, eggs, olive oil, nuts, and seeds. These foods contain rich sources of essential fatty acids (omega-3s and omega-6s) that you can only get from your diet. Lack of essential fatty acids puts you at risk for heavy PMS as well as a whole host of hormonal chaos. These fats are anti inflammatory and work to combat inflammation in your body, which can decrease PMS symptoms. Try to reduce processed vegetable oils that are easily susceptible to oxidative damage and rancidity, which can cause inflammation in your body. These processed vegetable oils include corn, canola, soybean, sunflower, and cottonseed.

4. **Cut the crap:** Avoiding excess added sugars, alcohol, and removing your own food intolerances is crucial to decrease inflammation, which can make PMS a demon. A great goal for sugar is under 10g added sugar per serving for a food, with a total of around 60g per day of sugar total. Reading nutrition labels will allow you to get a better idea for what is in your food and focus on the quality. Note- natural sugars from fruits are always welcome. Eat them to your heart's content! Try to keep your alcohol consumption to 2 drinks per week, though I suggest minimizing this as much as possible. Common food intolerances include gluten, wheat, eggs, nuts, dairy, and soy. Only restrict what you need to and work with a

registered dietitian (like me) to make sure you are on the right path for a sustainable nutrition plan that is best for you.

5. **Focus on fiber:** Fiber helps you to naturally detoxify your estrogen and helps to feed your gut microbiome by feeding your good gut bugs. You need a healthy microbiome for optimal metabolism, mood, and immune function. There really isn't anything your gut *can't* impact. Make sure to utilize different sources and types of fiber based on your needs. Refer to Chapter 7 for more information. A messed up gut can contribute to heavy PMS and pose a threat to your overall health, so make sure to prioritize your fiber.

6. **Drink your water:** Your body is approximately 60% water. (You are pretty much a human cucumber!) Dehydration leads to dizziness, headaches, increased hunger, cravings, and can even be life-threatening. Aim for at least 1 gallon of water per day. Being properly hydrated can positively impact your energy, mood, and metabolism. I suggest setting a timer on your phone to drink water if you struggle with getting it in. You can also try flavoring your water naturally with fruit or even using natural water flavoring agents. My favorites are made with stevia and also include electrolytes.

7. **Balance your blood sugar level:** An imbalance of blood sugar in your body can leave you hit with hanger. Ever noticed periods of shakiness, sweaty palms, anger, irritability, and brain fog? That's a sign of low blood sugar. Going up and down in a blood sugar rollercoaster can heighten your PMS. Especially if you are progesterone-sensitive. Be mindful of your carbohydrate sources and choose whole grains if possible. Always pair your carbs with a fat or protein to help stabilize your blood sugar (I call these smart snacks), & avoid skipping meals or going more than 4 hours without eating (unless doing planned intermittent fasting).

8. **Remove endocrine disruptors:** these chemicals will disrupt your hormonal symphony and wreak havoc on your health. Hands down, they can cause and worsen PMS. See Chapter 6 for more information.

9. **Supplement Smartly:** Supplements can be highly beneficial to help reduce your risk of PMS and decrease inflammation. Any nutrient deficiency will wreak havoc on your health, so ensuring to supplement smartly is critical. My favorite supplements for PMS include:

Favorite Supplements for PMS	
Supplement Name	Dosage per day
Magnesium Glycinate	300-400mg
N-acetyl-cysteine (NAC)	600-1200mg
Curcumin	1000mg
Vitex/Chasteberry	200-800mg/day
Myoinositol	2-6g/day
Ashwagandha	600-1200mg/day
Vitamin B6	50-100mg/day
Omega-3 fatty acids	1000-2000mg/day
Vitamin D	1000-5000 IU/day (depending on Vitamin D levels)

There are many other herbs, vitamins, and minerals that may help to decrease symptoms of PMS. Make sure to always speak with your dietitian or medical professional before starting or stopping a supplement.

10. **Manage Stress:** High stress levels and lack of self-care will lead you to PMS problems. Focus on ensuring you have proper stress reduction practices in place, practice healthy sleep hygiene, and make sure to allow yourself periods of rest and relaxation. Stress is one of the most common culprits leading to PMS prob-

lems. See Chapter 9 for more tips on stress and why I call it the demon of health.

Estrogen Dominance:

Though estrogen is the queen bee of your hormones, you don't want her in a full dictatorship! If estrogen becomes a dictator, this results in estrogen dominance, which can be due to high estrogen levels alone, or due to low progesterone in relation to estrogen (aka relative estrogen dominance).

Do these symptoms and conditions sound familiar? If so- you may have estrogen dominance:

- Painful periods
- Heavy periods
- Bad PMS or PMDD
- Tender breasts
- Mood swings
- Migraines and headaches (especially the week before your period)
- Abnormal weight gain
- Bloating or water retention
- Acne
- Fibroids

There are many reasons you can become estrogen dominant. These include:

- Endocrine disruptors
- Nutrient deficiencies
- Poor diet (high in added sugars, refined carbs, and alcohol being the most common diet culprits)
- Heavy metal toxicity (especially copper toxicity)
- High histamine levels

- Excess aromatase activity (your conversion from testosterone to estrogen in fat cells)
- Poor liver health
- Defects in estrogen detoxification (can be Phase 1, 2, or 3)
- High insulin levels
- Hypothyroidism
- Infections (such as Epstein Barr Virus, Lupus, Lyme disease, or even mold)
- Gut dysbiosis
- Inflammation
- Low progesterone
- Hormonal birth control or post birth control rebound
- Obesity or high body fat levels

How can you improve estrogen dominance? First things first. You need to figure out why estrogen is high in the first place. Doing a comprehensive assessment on your diet quality, the potential endocrine disruptors in your day-to-day life, and assessing your gut function is step 1.

The Estrogen Dominance Solutions:

1. **Fix your diet:** Reduce the amount of added sugars and refined grains in your diet that don't provide you with enough vitamins and minerals and may cause blood sugar imbalance. Focus on whole grains, a variety of fruits and vegetables, and healthy sources of dietary fat. If you can, choose organic over conventional meats, as they have been shown to be higher in essential fatty acids.
2. **Reduce alcohol:** Alcohol can disrupt both your hormones and liver function. If you are going to drink and have estrogen dominance, stick to 1-2 glasses of wine per week. I suggest eliminating alcohol if possible.

3. **Reduce environmental toxins:** See Chapter 6 for more information. Reducing endocrine disruptors will reduce inflammation, help to balance your hormones, and support your liver (helping to reduce its toxic burden).

4. **Focus on Fiber:** Aim to consume at least 25 g fiber per day- with 35-45 g being an even better range. Adequate fiber intake helps you to detoxify and eliminate excess estrogen. It also helps to reduce the levels of intestinal beta-glucuronidase activity that can cause havoc with your phase 2 estrogen detoxification (preventing it from being excreted).

5. **Promote a healthy gut microbiome:** This is where fiber plays a major role to help your good gut bugs produce short-chain fatty acids, B vitamins, and vitamin K. Why is this important? They help modulate your immune system, protect your gut lining, reduce inflammation, combat pathogens, promote healthy cholesterol levels, and enhance your mood and cognitive function. Other adjustments to help promote a healthy gut include diversity in the plants in your diet, reducing intake of artificial sweeteners, and removing food intolerances.

6. **Prioritize sleep:** Lack of sleep will disrupt both your hormones and adrenals. Focus on getting at least 7-8 hours of sleep per night. Make sure to have a healthy sleep routine, which includes blocking blue light at least 2 hours before bedtime, stopping electronics 30 minutes before sleep, sleeping in a cool, comfortable environment, and avoiding high strenuous exercise before bed.

7. **Focus on self care:** I can't say this enough. You need to fill up your cup to be able to pour out into others. Lack of self care will wreak havoc on your mental, physical, and emotional health. Go to Chapter 9 for the science on why.

8. **Supplement smartly:** Just like with PMS, supplements can help you in rebalancing your hormones and fixing nutrient deficiencies. With estrogen dominance, I do like to see my clients do a DUTCH test to look at their Phase 1-3 estrogen detoxification. Why? There are certain supplements that can downregulate or upregulate specific pathways. For example, DIM and Indole-3-carbinol help to push you *down* Phase 1. If you have trouble with phase 2 and phase 3, then you can't get rid of your estrogen, and taking these supplements can make your estrogen dominance worse.

Favorite Supplements for Estrogen Dominance	
Supplement Name	Dosage per day
DIM	100-300mg/day
N-acetyl-cysteine (NAC)	600-1200mg
Calcium D-Glucurate	200-2000mg/day
Vitex/Chasteberry	200-800mg/day
Myoinositol	2-6g/day
Broccoli seed extract or sulphoraphane	100-200mg/day
Hops	50-100mg/day
Milk thistle	100-300mg/day
Resveratrol	100-300mg/day
Vitamin D	1000-5000 IU/day (depending on Vitamin D levels)

Again, please make sure to speak with your dietitian or medical provider before starting or stopping any supplement. I also find quercetin and micronized, oral, or transdermal progesterone highly beneficial for symptom management in estrogen dominance.

9. **Reduce Inflammation:** Inflammation will upregulate cytokines and prostaglandins in your body, causing increased period pain, body aches, and increase the risk of heavy menstrual bleeding. Inflammation also further increases aromatase activity in

your body, which converts your testosterone to estrogen. This can further drive estrogen levels higher. You can reduce inflammation by following all the previous tips suggested, plus making sure to incorporate omega-3 fatty acids, reduce caffeine intake, and add anti-inflammatories such as curcumin (the active component of turmeric), Boswellia, or cat's claw in your life. If you carry excess body fat, losing weight will also help to decrease aromatase activity and decrease inflammation.

10. **Exercise for energy:** Yes, you read that right. Your exercise and workouts should not drain, but instead energize you. Focus on finding a fitness routine that you enjoy and that you can stick to. Moderate intensity weight training is a great option, as it will help to increase insulin sensitivity and preserve lean muscle mass. I also suggest yoga, power walking, and small amounts of running or high intensity cardio. Be cautious on the runs and cardio because if you have adrenal imbalances, this can cause even worse hormonal chaos.

Estrogen Detoxification:

In order to best balance your hormones and prevent estrogen related chaos, you need to understand how your estrogens are detoxified in your body. No, I am not talking about the bull crap detox teas that are basically laxatives. I am talking about detoxification that happens naturally in your body through your liver, skin, lungs, and digestive system! There are three main phases of estrogen metabolism in your body. These phases follow your body's natural detoxification process. Let's dive into each phase and discuss their importance in relation to not only estrogen, but to all toxins that your body handles.

Your estrogens are conjugated through a series of reactions that make them go from being fat soluble to water soluble. In fun science terms, conjugation helps your estrogen go from being hydrophobic to hydrophilic. This is what allows them to be eliminated out of your body. What is conjugation? Conjugation is a fancy term for "the transfer of hydrophilic compounds," allowing for enhanced excretion by the body.

Remember, estrogen isn't bad. It's when you have too much, too little, hang ups in estrogen detoxification, or if increased levels of estrogen are pushed down the wrong metabolic pathways, that havoc happens in your body. This havoc then ruins your hormonal symphony and can put you at risk for a multitude of health hazards.

"Detoxification" can be defined as the removal of toxic, unneeded, or unnecessary substances found within your body. There is a lot of fear mongering, lies, and misleading marketing surrounding the world of "detoxing." From companies using misinformation to sell "liver cleanses" and "detoxes" to skinny teas and supplement sales, the world seems to think that detoxing is something you need to buy something in order to do! Newsflash- your body can and does do this for you! Most people have no issues with detoxification, however, with poor diet (including too many processed foods or nutrient deficiencies), poor liver health (due to genetics, diet, or medication or supplement-induced), or too much of a toxic burden (let's be real- there are a lot of toxins in this world!), your body can need some help. The truth here lies in understanding how detoxification works, and ensuring that you get the necessary nutrients to help your liver, limit toxin exposure, and get a good sweat and poop in daily!

Detoxing of drugs, environmental toxins, hormones, chemicals, water, air, and even the food you eat is mostly performed in your liver, but detoxing also occurs through your digestive tract, kidneys, skin, and lungs! Each phase requires specific vitamins and minerals to power various enzymes that transform toxins (and estrogens) in your body from their fat soluble forms to water-soluble forms, allowing them to be excreted through your bile, urine, and feces.

Your liver is critical to maintaining a healthy immune system, metabolism, and digestion. It plays the superhero role of detoxification! Without your liver, you cannot convert food into energy, make immune system molecules, or process and eliminate medications or environmental toxins. The liver is found in the upper right-hand side of your abdomen. It's snuggled up underneath the ribs, and is actually quite large, around 3 pounds. In some cases, it can actually be the size of a large football!

Doctors will typically physically examine your abdomen in the area of your liver to see if it's enlarged. This may be a first clue to whether or not there are any true issues going on! Most enlarged liver cases stem from alcohol use, fatty liver (fat deposition in the liver- better known as nonalcoholic fatty liver disease or NAFLD), viral infection, liver cancer, or congestive heart failure. Most healthy individuals have a normal sized liver though, and just because it isn't enlarged doesn't mean it doesn't need some love and care!

How exactly does your liver work? Well, it has a long laundry list of tasks to complete daily. It stores glucose (and releases it!), metabolizes protein, carbs, and fats, detoxifies toxins, produces bile (which helps to digest fats and carry waste products out of your body) and cholesterol, synthesizes plasma proteins and blood clotting factors, processes hemoglobin to use its iron content, activates enzymes, and even fights infections by making immune factors! With all of these jobs, your liver is a legit superhero organ. It's an extremely vascular organ as well and receives 25% of the heart's blood output each time that it beats from what is called your hepatic artery and hepatic portal vein. This allows the liver to gather particles, nutrients, and toxins from the blood.

Liver detoxification (or "detoxing" as you hear it) is divided up into two phases, resulting in end products that are sent to other organs and parts of your body for excretion. Once your liver has gone through all three phases, the byproducts are excreted into bile or blood for their removal out of your body. This removal can occur through bowel movements or your urine. All while this is happening, you are also detoxifying through your breath, kidneys, spleen, and skin!

Let's dive into the three phases of liver detoxification. Phase 1 detoxification involves a process called "bioactivation" and is largely performed by hepatocytes, aka the cells of your liver. During this phase, a series of reactions occur including oxidation, reduction, hydrolysis, hydration, and dehalogenation. During these reactions, Cytochrome P450 enzymes (CPY450) convert fat soluble toxins and various "materials" mentioned, including estrogen, medications, environmental pollutants, and waste materials into more water-soluble metabolites.

In doing this, however, reactive oxygen species called reactive intermediates are produced, making the intermediate potentially more harmful than its precursor! This is where ensuring to include antioxidants in your diet comes in, as they can combat these reactive oxygen species from causing damage, as well as ensuring that you can get through phase 2 of detoxification. You have to be able to transform the reactive intermediates in Phase 1 into even more water-soluble compounds through phase 2 in order to properly excrete them. How can these intermediates damage your body? They can generate oxidative stress, inflammation, and DNA adducts, which can cause DNA and tissue damage! Most people have no issues with Phase 1 detoxification, however poor liver health, certain genetic mutations in the CYP family, and nutrient deficiencies can hinder Phase 1 from happening.

DEPURINATING ADDUCTS

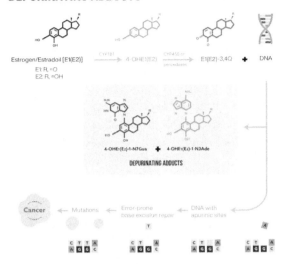

Your diet can ensure that this phase is performed properly. Antioxidants in your diet are the true superheroes that come in to prevent damage from the reactive intermediate This includes something called glutathione, which can be considered your master antioxidant! These super hero antioxidants include: Riboflavin (Vitamin B2), Niacin (Vitamin B3), Pyridoxine (Vitamin B6), Folic acid, Vitamin B12, flavonoids, Vitamin A, ascorbic acid (vitamin C), and tocopherols (vitamin E). Nutrients such as selenium, copper, zinc, manganese, Coenzyme Q10, thiols (found in cruciferous vegetables), and silymarin (better known as milk thistle) also play a role. An easy way to help ensure Phase 1 detox is achieved is to get a wide variety of nutrients in your diet with lots of colorful fruits and leafy greens and to help your liver by lowering your overall toxic burden, including limiting exposure to environmental toxins, not overloading your body with supplements or medications, and eating a balanced healthy diet.

Note- there are also many substances, nutrients, and drugs that can influence the function of the CYP enzymes that are in charge of Phase 1. This can be from the inhibition or induction of their activity, and can greatly influence how you detoxify, which is very important if you're on any medications because speeding up or slowing down drug metabolism can either heighten or diminish their ability to work! Therefore, you should be very cautious if you are on a medication and using any food, food components, or supplements that alter CPY enzyme activity. Beyond the ones addressed above, additional substances include: DIM and indole-3-carbinol (found naturally in cruciferous vegetables), resveratrol, quercetin, green tea, red wine, carrots, celery, grapefruit, and herbs such as dill, parsley, and thyme.

CYP Inducers:

- Soy
- Curcumin
- Garlic
- Fish oil
- Rosemary
- Resveratrol
- Chicory
- Astaxanthin

CYP Inhibitors:

- Raspberries
- Blueberries
- Black currants
- Pomegranate
- Peppermint
- Quercetin
- Daidzein
- Grapefruit
- Dandelion

Special note for estrogen! In Phase 1 detoxification, estrogen can go down 3 pathways: the 2-OH (favorable pathway), 16-OH (less favorable), or 4-OH pathway (least favorable). Ideally, you want about 60-80% of your estrogen flowing down the 2-OH pathway. The 4-OH pathway is what is deemed the "problematic pathway." It's there that estrogen metabolites can create reactive quinones, that can increase oxidative damage, inflammation, and create DNA damage.

What can make you favor the wrong estrogen pathway? Inflammation, nutrient deficiencies, endocrine disruptors, genetic mutations, and gut infections or overgrowths. Addressing the cause can help address the pathways! This is where a test such as the DUTCH (dried urine hormone test) can be highly beneficial, as it allows for the evaluation of your hormone metabolism to be seen, including the pathways of estrogen metabolism.

After Phase 1 detoxification, Phase 1's bioactivation production of reactive metabolites are then neutralized in Phase 2, where they are made more slightly water soluble, to more water soluble. It is here where they are conjugated (which basically means another substance is added to them), and undergo a complex series of reactions including: sulfation, glucuronidation, glutathione conjugation, acetylation, amino acid conjugation, and methylation. This conjugation makes the reactive intermediate less harmful and ready to be excreted through Phase 3 detoxification. Phase 2 detox is quite detailed and confusing (just like your ex boyfriend).

Just like Phase 1, Phase 2 requires specific nutrients in order for the enzymes within each reaction to perform optimally. You need to get through Phase 2 in order to get to Phase 3, where the toxins and estrogen in your body can be fully excreted. These nutrients include glycine, taurine, glutamine, N-acetylcysteine (NAC), cysteine, and methionine. They also require choline, inositol, and sulfur-containing compounds such as MSM and Sam-E. Just as in Phase 1, ensuring a healthy, balanced diet can most of the time ensure a healthy functioning Phase 2. Adequate protein intake is required (as many require Phase 2 nutrients come from protein!), as well as dietary fat, which is needed to mobilize the required fat-soluble vitamins used. Though diet plays a key role for ensuring adequate nutrients to perform Phase 2, just like in Phase 1's enzymes, problems can arise if there are "roadblocks" affecting any of the methylation steps.

Methylation is one of the conjugation reactions within Phase 2 detox. As previously described, your estrogen can flow down 3 different Phase 1 pathways, and once down Phase 1, the fate of Phase 2 is largely affected by your ability to methylate your estrogen. This methylation is performed by your COMT enzyme (catechol-o-methyltransferase).

The COMT enzyme is responsible for the degradation and elimination of not only your estrogen but also the norepinephrine and epinephrine in your body (aka your flight-or-flight response). Homozygous ++ mutations in the COMT gene can slow elimination, especially in the presence of nutrient deficiencies, causing higher risk of elevated levels of estrogen, norepinephrine, and epinephrine due to decreased clearance. Homozygous - - mutations can enhance metabolism and elimination, however causing increased metabolism and elimination of these hormones. What does this mean? It means that someone with a slow COMT has a higher risk of estrogen dominance or slowed estrogen clearance and more trouble eliminating and combating stress, while someone with a fast COMT may have increased risk for lower estrogen levels but better stress management. The COMT enzyme requires nutrients such as vitamins B12, B6, magnesium, betaine, folate, and methyl donors like SamE and MSM. Trouble with methylation can play a critical final role in reducing proper detoxification of estrogen.

If COMT is slow due to poor methylation, estrogen can recirculate back into the body to elevate estrogen levels, possibly sending estrogen down the cancerous 4-OH-E1 pathway, especially in the presence of reactive oxygen species and low glutathione levels. Glutathione is your master antioxidant and works to combat free radical damage, protect your tissues, and enhance your immunity!

Liposomal glutathione is a great option but you can also take N-acetylcysteine (NAC), which serves as its precursor. See my supplement reference guide at the end of the book for recommendations.

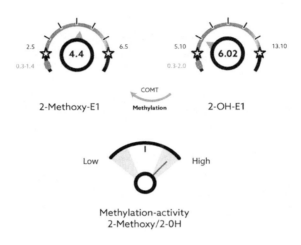

In addition to a slow or troubled COMT, estrogen can also be prevented from excretion through trouble with further conjugation reactions. Once methylated, your estrogens are able to undergo sulfation and glucuronidation, which is the final step to make them water soluble so they can be cleared and eliminated from the blood and sent into the urine and feces for excretion. High levels of beta-glucuronidase in the gut can deconjugate your estrogen, unbinding them and allowing them to recirculate back into your blood. Think of this process like a present and a bow. Upon methylation, your estrogen is neatly packed into your present with a cute little box on top to hold it all together for giving. However, high levels of beta-glucuronidase can come in and unravel and steal your bow, causing the estrogen to not get to go where it needs to go, to your friend/family or in this case, out of your body!

High levels of beta-glucuronidase can be caused by symbiosis, bacterial overgrowths, slowed gut motility, and chronic constipation, and can be heavily influenced by genetics, lifetime exposure (known as the exposome), the diet, medication and antibiotic usage, and environmental factors such as toxins, pollutants, and xenobiotics. To prevent this, it's imperative to address your gut function, treat your body like the temple it is, avoid endocrine disruptors, and ensure gut microbiome diversity!

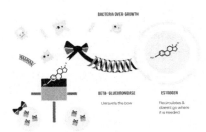

Your Detox Bathtub

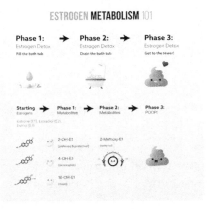

Phase 1 and 2 detoxification are like a bathtub. Phase 1 involves the filling of your bathtub, while Phase 2 involves draining. You have to get Phase 2 to occur in order for the "water" in Phase 1 to get out. If both Phase 1 and Phase 2 occur, then Phase 3 can happen.

The final step in Phase 3 estrogen detoxification involves the neutralization of metabolites and excretion through your bile, feces, or urine. This is where constipation can cause issues or lack of bile production from the liver! Lack of bile can reduce the ability of estrogen to bind within bile acids, which reduces the amount that gets excreted, while constipation can cause estrogen to remain in the large intestine for an extended period of time, causing its reabsorption into the body. Both constipation and lack of bile flow are additional contributing factors to estrogen dominance! Therefore, it's essential that you focus on getting adequate fiber intake (in general 25-45g per day), prioritize your gut health, and be kind to your liver!

	Nutrients involved	Foods to support
Phase 1	B vitamins, folic acid, glutathione, amino acids, flavonoids, phospholipids	Broccoli sprouts, flaxseeds, raw carrots, green tea, curcumin, garlic, berries, cruciferous vegetables, rosemary, green tea
Phase 2	Glycine, taurine, cysteine, methionine (amino acids), glutathione, magnesium, B12, sulfur, choline, calcium-d-glucarate, MSM	Eggs, collagen or bone broth, leafy greens, organ meats
Phase 3	Fiber	Digestive bitters, flaxseeds, fiber, pre and probiotics

In summary of estrogen metabolism:

- Phase 1: estrogen becomes more water soluble and becomes 2-OH (most beneficial), 4-OH (least beneficial), or 16-OH (less beneficial)
- Phase 2: estrogen is methylated and conjugated to become more water soluble. The COMT enzyme and MTHFR play a critical role in this phase.

- Phase 3: Estrogen is eliminated out of the body through bile, urine, or your poop.

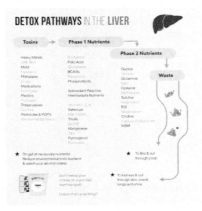

I am always a fan of getting fiber from food sources, if at all possible. However, some people may need an extra supplemental boost of prebiotics or fiber in certain cases. Partially hydrolyzed guar gum (PHGG) is a soluble fermentable fiber that is clinically shown to help speed up digestive transit time (helping with constipation), support beneficial gut flora, reduce bloating in IBS, and help improve lipid and glucose metabolism. Lignans, found in foods such as whole grains, seeds, fruit, vegetables, and legumes are also a great source of fiber which can be taken supplementally. Lignans can act as weak phytoestrogens that can help lower aromatase expression and shift estrogen towards Phase 2-OH and 16-OH pathways, helping reduce estrogen dominance and supporting healthy estrogen levels. Flaxseed powders are fantastic as well to help with enhancing Phase 1 estrogen detox and Phase 3, however keep in mind that the safety of flaxseed is determined by rancidity. Make sure to use freshly ground flaxseed or utilize whole flax seeds. You can freshly grind and freeze your flaxseed to prevent rancidity.

Diet Modulators of Estrogen Metabolism: from Metagenics

Estrogen Metabolism	Nutrient Modulators
Production- goal to reduce body toxic burden, support the microbiome and estrobolome, ensure proper Phase 3 detox	Flaxseeds, flavonoids (chrysin, resveratrol), zinc, isoflavones (soy), calcium-d-glucarate, dietary fiber, prebiotics (guar gum), probiotics
Systemic Estrogen Pool- circulating estrogen	Fiber, lignans (flax seed), isoflavones (soy, red clover)
Receptor Sensitivity and Binding- related to quinone production	Isoflavones, lignans, indole-3-carbinol, DIM, hops, curcumin, B6, rosemary, resveratrol
Detoxification- promoting Phases 1-3	Cruciferous vegetables, I3C, rosemary, isoflavones, curcumin, vitamins A, E, and C, NAC, green tea, alpha lipoic acid, flavonoids, superoxide dismutase, folate, B vitamins, glycine, magnesium, adequate dietary fat and protein

Common Causes of Estrogen Dominance:

- Low progesterone: Low progesterone levels in relation to estrogen levels can cause women to have estrogen-dominance symptoms, despite having normal estrogen levels- this is where the ratio of estrogen to progesterone causes issues
- Chronic stress: High cortisol levels can reduce the body's ability to produce progesterone, which in turn can lead to an imbalanced estrogen to progesterone ratio
- Endocrine Disruptors: Environmental toxins, pesticides, herbicides, and heavy metals can bind to estrogen receptors and also mimic the effects of your body's hormones, causing increased levels and estrogen dominance. Examples of endocrine disruptors include plastics, BPA, mercury, copper (found in the copper IUD or copper pipes!), phthalates and parabens found in skin care, fragrances, sulfites, sulfates, dioxins, and more!
- Poor Diet: Nutrient deficiencies can cause inflammation and prevent the body from creating progesterone, causing estrogen dominance, or can inhibit the body's conversion of food for energy, worsening symptoms & stopping the metabolism and detoxification of your hormones. Also-

poor diet can lead to inflammation and weight gain, which can increase fat cells that can produce estrogen, further heightening levels, or decrease SHBG, leading to excess free estrogen in the blood.

- Excess Alcohol intake: this can lead to increased estrogen levels, oxidative stress, and liver damage
- Thyroid Disease: too little thyroid hormone can create increasing amounts of SHBG. Too much SHBG can increase the amount of free estrogen in your blood, leading to estrogen dominance

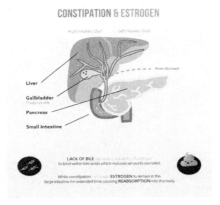

CONSTIPATION & ESTROGEN

PCOS:

PCOS, aka Polycystic Ovarian Syndrome, is a common hormonal disorder diagnosis (and misdiagnosis!) given to women with an abnormal menstrual cycle. Sadly, it has become what I call an "umbrella diagnosis." Why? The criteria for PCOS are very broad and based on the Rotterdam criteria, which involves having 2 of the 3 following symptoms:

1. Abnormal menstrual cycle- defined as oligomenorrhea (can be defined as long cycles or fewer than 9 cycles in a year)
2. Hyperandrogenism (aka excess testosterone), which

includes symptoms such as oily skin, acne, increased facial and body hair, hair loss, and deepening of the voice (these can also be referred to as androgenic alopecia and hirsutism)

3. Presence of polycystic ovaries confirmed on ultrasound

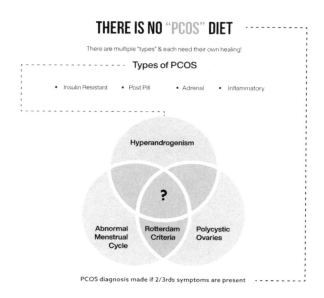

THERE IS NO "PCOS" DIET

There are multiple "types" & each need their own healing!

Types of PCOS

• Insulin Resistant   • Post Pill   • Adrenal   • Inflammatory

Hyperandrogenism

?

Abnormal Menstrual Cycle   Rotterdam Criteria   Polycystic Ovaries

PCOS diagnosis made if 2/3rds symptoms are present

If you have 2 of the 3 criteria, you can be diagnosed with PCOS. The problem with this? First, women naturally have polycystic ovaries. Follicles in your ovaries grow monthly, forming cysts. Secondly, abnormal menstrual cycles have become quite common, especially in our high-stress, workaholic US environment (though just because they are common does not make them normal!). A woman may lose her cycle for a reason not related to high testosterone levels and yet becomes diagnosed and thrown into the "PCOS box."

This is why the PCOS diagnosis can be very troublesome. It potentially puts women into a box that they may not fit in! Many clinicians, and even registered dietitians, shill out specific "PCOS diets" or "PCOS protocols" for women diagnosed with PCOS to follow. These diets are mainly tailored towards the androgen-based symptoms of PCOS, which is commonly caused by insulin resistance and inflammation. The people pushing these diets like to suggest the elimination of carbs, fruit, or avoidance of specific types of foods such as dairy and gluten.

This is an issue not only because restrictive diets should not be followed or pushed unless medically necessary, but also because there are a wide range of root causes that can cause PCOS! Really, anything that can cause an abnormal menstrual cycle can potentially lead to a diagnosis of PCOS if polycystic ovaries are caught on ultrasound. Hypothalamic Amenorrhea (HA) is even misdiagnosed as PCOS in many cases.

Hypothalamic Amenorrhea – NOT PCOS

What is hypothalamic amenorrhea (HA)? HA is a condition caused by suppression of the HPG (hypothalamic-pituitary-gonadal) axis, and many times is a result of stress, under-eating, over exercising, or nutrient deficiencies.

Main causes of HA:

- **Anorexia:** an eating disorder that stems from a desire to be thin or have control, causing food restriction, food fears, and body dysmorphia. This can result in seeing yourself as overweight when you are at a healthy body weight and can be a life-threatening disease.
- **Bulimia:** an eating disorder also characterized by a desire for thinness and control, but also tied to feelings of shame, inadequacy, and restriction. Bouts of purging through excessive laxative use, over-exercising, vomiting, or excessive fasting are used.
- **Orthorexia:** a disorder classified by obsessive control and concern over one's health, fear of "unhealthy"

ingredients, and inability to eat anything not "clean or pure." Though not classified as an eating disorder, it very much is one and shares common symptoms of anorexia.

- **Over-exercising:** whether intentional or not, over-exercising in any form, even with adequate food intake, can lead to HA. This is a common cause of HA seen in college athletes, runners, and bodybuilders.
- **Low body fat or body weight:** inadequate body fat or low body weight causes too little thyroid or sex hormones to be produced. Those with this type of HA may eat sufficiently and balance healthy exercise, but are unable to maintain a normal menstrual cycle due to insufficient body fat levels.

With HA, there are alterations in the release of your hormones within your HPA axis that lead to low sex and thyroid hormones. This causes you to have an irregular menstrual cycle, lose your cycle, or have an anovulatory cycle (in which you don't ovulate but still bleed). Sadly, it's common in women with HA for a cycle to be lost for six months or more. This can create trouble with fertility, as well as produce undesired side effects due to low hormones, including bone loss and increased risk of anxiety and depression.

The reason I want to distinguish the difference between HA and PCOS is because PCOS, though it can be stress induced, is a completely different animal. It does not follow the complete loss of ovulation and is not simply caused by low energy availability (i.e., over-exercising and/or under eating) like HA is. PCOS and HA are separate diagnoses with different root causes, so they require different treatment approaches. To treat HA, you need to address the low energy availability, bring sex and thyroid hormones back to normal, and eliminate stress.

The Types of PCOS

In her book, *The Period Repair Manual,* Dr. Lara Briden coined four types of PCOS that are commonly seen in women. Remember, PCOS is an umbrella diagnosis. These four types are the most common reasons why women may be diagnosed with PCOS. Each type requires its own healing approach. There is no single "PCOS protocol" because PCOS is not a disease, but rather a cluster of specific symptoms.

If you are a fellow cyster, you may have already had testing for PCOS and know what your PCOS type may be. If you have not, and suspect PCOS, I warn you to make sure that you do proper testing prior to starting any suggestions in this book. I also encourage you to work with a healthcare professional to help guide you on the right road for your body!

What are common symptoms of PCOS?

Weight gain or trouble losing weight, irregular menstrual cycle or fertility issues, blood sugar imbalances, ovarian cysts, oily skin and acne, increased facial or body hair (hirsutism), hair loss from the head, mid-cycle spotting, heavy menstrual bleeding, heavy menstrual cramps, low sex drive, and chronic fatigue. Note- not all women have the same symptoms, as symptoms depend on the root cause of the condition!

The 4 main types of PCOS:

1. Insulin Resistant PCOS (includes Androgen dominance):

With insulin resistance PCOS, the body becomes resistant to the hormone insulin. This means that the body is unable to utilize carbohydrates for energy sufficiently, which can result in weight gain, hormonal imbalances, blood sugar dysregulation, and inflammation.

What is inulin? In a healthy metabolism, insulin acts like a key, "unlocking" your cells to allow the glucose in your bloodstream to enter, so it can be used for energy. However, when your cells become insulin resistant, the key is unable to unlock the cell to allow glucose to enter! This means insulin can't do its job. The key lock is faulty. Instead of the glucose getting inside your cells to be used for energy, glucose then remains in your blood. This blood sugar elevation can cause your blood to become "sticky" like honey, which slows down your blood flow through your body and further causes inflammation. If your blood glucose remains elevated chronically, this can ultimately lead to the progression of Type 2 Diabetes.

When you have elevated blood sugar, this causes your pancreas to secrete more and more insulin. This is an attempt for your body to get your blood sugar levels back down to normal. However, if insulin can't do its job, blood glucose remains elevated, and the pancreas continues to output insulin. The extra insulin plus the high levels of blood sugar lead to hormonal and metabolic chaos in your body. This causes inflammation along with abnormal fat and glucose metabolism, which contributes to weight gain, fertility issues, the development of Type 2 diabetes, as well as cardiovascular disease.

I commonly see insulin resistance PCOS be caused mostly by poor diet or lifestyle choices. A high intake of refined grains, added sugars, excessive alcohol consumption, or a sedentary life-style can pull the trigger on developing insulin resistance. However, insulin resistance can also be developed through a genetic predisposition to abnormal glucose metabolism, inflammation (as in the case for a gut or viral infection, heavy metal toxicity, or mold exposure), nutrient deficiencies, and can also be induced by medications such as corticosteroids or antidepressants.

To help diagnose insulin resistance PCOS, you can test your fasting blood glucose, Hb1c (a marker of the the average level of glucose within your red blood cells for a period of 2- 3 months), as well as fasting insulin levels. I also find that those who are insulin resistant are unable to go three hours without eating and have frequent bouts of blood sugar crashes. Abdominal concentrated weight gain is another marker that you can use, as well as symptoms that include: skin tags, frequent urination, poor wound healing, tingling in the hands or feet, extreme thirst or hunger, sleepiness after meals, increased blood pressure, sugar cravings, weight gain, or trouble losing weight.

Remember the discussion on androgens with a PCOS diagnosis? This is where insulin resistance, androgen dominance, and inflammation all come together to create the "PCOS picture." Together, they contribute to the overproduction of your androgens. This leaves you with high testosterone levels or can potentially cause abnormal androgen metabolism. Excess insulin decreases your sex hormone binding globulin (SHBG), which can further result in higher free testosterone levels. Too much insulin can also lead to the impairment of ovulation, as it can cause disruptions in LH secretions from your pituitary.

Have you had your bloodwork done and your doctor claimed your testosterone levels were normal, yet you still struggled with androgen dominant symptoms of hair loss, oily skin, acne, aggression, or facial hair? This is because you have issues with androgen metabolization. Specifically, problems with 5-Alpha Reductase.

Ladies, your total testosterone level isn't the only thing that matters- it also matters how you metabolize it. We are about to get geeky. Your 5-Alpha Reductase enzyme converts your testosterone into two metabolites, which can be influenced by a 5-alpha (5A) or 5-beta (5B) pathway preference. These metabolites include etiocholanolone (5B preference) or androsterone (5A preference). If you convert and have a higher preference for 5-alpha, you actually produce DHT, which is three times more potent than normal testosterone! This means that you can have "normal" testosterone in labs but experience crippling high testosterone-like symptoms!

A 5-Alpha preference can be caused or influenced by: post birth control syndrome (in which androgens can rebound), anabolic steroid usage, genetics, altered GnRH pulses from your hypothalamus, an inflammatory diet, high insulin levels, chronic stress, adrenal imbalances, low SHBG, endocrine disruptors, gut infections, or nutrient deficiencies. Any of these factors can also lead to high testosterone levels.

Do you suspect issues with DHT? This is where a DUTCH test is highly suggested to assess your hormonal pathways and gain insight into how your hormones are metabolizing. Bloodwork is fabulous as well, however it will not assess your 5-Alpha Reductase activity.

What can help to decrease your 5-Alpha Reductase activity and promote your 5-beta pathway? Reducing inflammation, insulin levels, endocrine disruptors, and excess body fat are the first steps, along with a nutrient-dense diet! Supplements that may also help include: Sam palmetto, stinging nettles, zinc, EGCG (green tea extract), reishi mushroom, inositol, spearmint tea, Vitamin C, plant sterols, black cohosh, pygeum extract, PUFAs (polyunsaturated fats), ketoconazole (anti-fungal used for male pattern hair loss), and vitex. Common drugs that are used include Finasteride, Dutasteride, and Spironolactone.

Please, don't ever start or stop a new supplement or medication without medical supervision. Many supplements can increase or decrease other hormonal or metabolic pathways in your body, and if you are not careful, taking one thing for one pathway can wreak havoc on another! (Yeah, I know... not what you wanted to hear.)

Remember, testosterone is also a precursor to your estrogen. Having high testosterone also puts you at risk for high estrogen levels, especially if your aromatase enzyme is upregulated. What can help block the aromatization of testosterone to estrogen? The same lifestyle factors of blocking 5-Alpha Reductase can help, along with the monitored use of supplements such as zinc, flaxseed, isoflavones, EGCG (from green tea), chrysin, damiana, and stinging nettle. Reducing alcohol intake, improving blood sugar balance, liver support, weight loss, lowering inflammation, avoiding endocrine disruptors, and adequate stress management also are essential in helping prevent over-aromatization. I would be very cautious and only manipulate aromatase under medical supervision.

Here's my issue again with PCOS. Many conventional doctors will say to "just lose the weight." They claim this is the easiest way to help increase insulin sensitivity. Though yes, that will help, the problem is that those with insulin resistance struggle to lose weight. Many times there are additional hormonal imbalances that need some work along with the insulin resistance. Plus- there is typically a reason why insulin resistance is there to begin with and sometimes losing weight won't fix the issue! My suggestions to help increase insulin sensitivity are focused less on weight loss, and more on changing lifestyle habits. The goal is to address and target the root cause.

My suggestions for helping to increase insulin sensitivity are simple! Make sure to follow the overall PCOS suggestions as well.

1. Stay Active: Incorporate weight training and moderate intensity cardio into your life at least three times a week. This will enhance insulin sensitivity in your body, specifically by increasing the amount of GLUT4 receptors (what helps glucose enter your cells) in your cells and number of mitochondria. What does this mean for you? Help with insulin sensitivity, fuel utilization, and a happy metabolism!

2. Fix your diet: Avoiding refined carbohydrates, added sugars, processed vegetable oils, and trans fats. Pay attention to what foods you are eating and focus on filling up your plate with 1/2 fruits and vegetables at each meal, the other 1/4 complex carbohydrates, and then 1/4 lean sources of protein. Strive to follow a whole foods, anti-inflammatory diet outlined in my nutrition chapter.

3. Balance your blood sugar: This is essential to help regulate your blood sugar and insulin levels. To do this, make sure to always pair a carbohydrate with a good source of protein (about 15 g) and/or a fat (about 10 g). A great smart snack idea would be half of a banana with 1.5 tbsp almond butter, or 3 oz berries with ½ cup low fat Greek yogurt. Find foods that you enjoy and that make you feel good. Try to eat every 4 hours unless you practice a specific type of intermittent fasting.

4. Contemplate trying intermittent fasting (IF). There are many ways to do this, including an 8 hour feeding with 16 hour fasting window, alternate-day fasting, or 2/5 fasting. Check out my nutrition chapter for more information. If your blood glucose levels are extremely elevated, I suggest combining IF with a lower carb diet under medical supervision to help with increasing insulin sensitivity. Fasting can be powerful to quickly aid in blood sugar levels, however it can also cause hypoglycemia (low blood sugar) if not done correctly or extended for too long. Make sure to work with a dietitian, medical professional, or trusted health coach if you want to dive into IF.

5. Supplement smartly: My favorite supplements for blood sugar include Myoinositol (6 g/day), Berberine (500-1000 mg/day), Magnesium (300-400 mg/day), Chromium (200-400 mg/day), Zinc (20 mg/day), Alpha lipoic acid (100-200 mg/day), Vitamin D (2000-5000 IU/day) and Gymnema Sylvestre (500-1000 mg/day). Many companies make "glucose disposal agents" that incorporate insulin sensitizing herbs and dietary ingredients that may help the body to use glucose. These can be helpful and some are clinically effective. However, I suggest focusing on diet, inflammation, and lifestyle changes before attempting any supplementation. Supplements, especially those that enhance insulin

sensitivity, can have undesired side effects, including gastrointestinal upset, headaches, fatigue, and may cause low blood sugar. Make sure to speak with a healthcare professional before starting any new supplement!

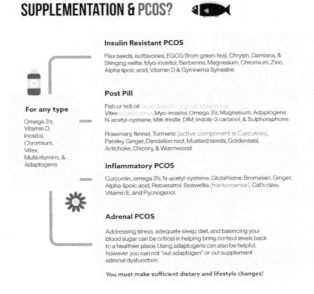

SUPPLEMENTATION & PCOS?

For any type

Omega 3's,
Vitamin D,
Inositol,
Chromium,
Vitex,
Multivitamins, &
Adaptogens.

Insulin Resistant PCOS

Flax seeds, isoflavones, EGCG (from green tea), Chrysin, Damiana, & Stinging nettle. Myo-inositol, Berberine, Magnesium, Chromium, Zinc, Alpha lipoic acid, Vitamin D & Gymnema Sylvestre.

Post Pill

Fish or krill oil *(a plant based is a great alternative)*
Vitex *(chasteberry)*, Myo-inositol, Omega 3's, Magnesium, Adaptogens N-acetyl-cysteine, Milk thistle, DIM, Indole-3 carbinol, & Sulphoraphone.

Rosemary, fennel, Turmeric (active component is Curcumin), Parsley, Ginger, Dandelion root, Mustard seeds, Goldenseal, Artichoke, Chicory, & Wormwood.

Inflammatory PCOS

Curcumin, omega 3's, N-acetyl-cysteine, Glutathione, Bromelain, Ginger, Alpha-lipoic acid, Resveratrol, Boswellia (frankincense), Cat's claw, Vitamin E, and Pycnogenol.

Adrenal PCOS

Addressing stress, adequate sleep, diet, and balancing your blood sugar can be critical in helping bring cortisol levels back to a healthier place. Using adaptogens can also be helpful, however you can not "out adaptogen" or out supplement adrenal dysfunction.

You must make sufficient dietary and lifestyle changes!

Insulin Resistance PCOS Labs:

- **HgA1c (Glycated hemoglobin):** this test measures your average blood sugar over the past 2-3 months and is commonly used to diagnose Type 1 or Type 2 diabetes. Anything below 5.7% is considered normal. 5.7-6.4% indicates prediabetes, while 6.5% or higher indicates diabetes.
- **Fasting Glucose:** this test measures the glucose in your bloodstream after an overnight fast. A normal fasting glucose should be 100mg/dL or less. A fasting glucose from 100-125mg/dl may indicate prediabetes and insulin resistance. If a fasting glucose on two occasions is great

than 126mg/dL, diabetes may be present. Anything under 70mg/dL is considered hypoglycemia or low blood sugar.

- **Fasting insulin:** this measures the amount of insulin in your blood to assess for how your pancreas is producing insulin. Normal ranges should be between 5-10 mIU/L. Insulin levels are typically low in Type 1 Diabetes, and may be low, normal, or elevated in Type 2 Diabetes or insulin resistance.
- **2 Hour postprandial (after meal) glucose:** this measures your blood sugar response to a sugar drink consumption and helps assess your ability to produce insulin and respond to glucose. After 2 hours, if your blood sugar is less than 140mg/dL, your blood sugar is normal. If more than 200mg/dL, diabetes is often diagnosed.

Androgen Dominant PCOS Labs:

- **Free Testosterone:** measures unbound testosterone levels and what is free and able to be used by the tissues.
- **SHBG:** measures the amount of sex hormone binding globulin in the blood which carries testosterone and estrogen to the tissues.
- **Total testosterone:** measures total testosterone levels, both free and bound in the blood.
- **DUTCH Test:** measures a combination of all sex hormones including all 3 estrogens (estrone, estriol, estradiol), testosterone, DHEA, testosterone metabolites, progesterone, cortisol (both free and metabolized), cortisone, and markers of nutrient organic acids (B12, B6, VMA, HVA, melatonin, and glutathione).

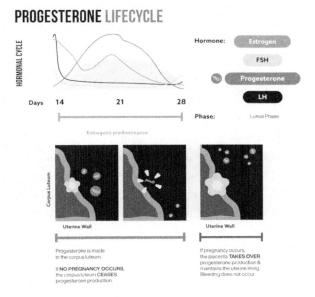

PROGESTERONE LIFECYCLE

2. Post- Pill:

Many women can have abnormal cycles or no cycle for months after getting off of hormonal birth control (or even after the use of IUDs like the copper IUD). This does not always happen, and some women can get their cycle back right away. However, I find that the longer someone is on BC, the longer it can take to normalize their cycle when coming off. Additional factors that play a major role into returning to a normal menstrual cycle include: the reason for getting on birth control to begin with (as any hormonal issue pre-BC can resurface or exacerbate post-BC), genetics, alterations in thyroid or gut health, nutrient deficiencies, diet, and stress. See the Chapter 3 for more information on birth control, how it works, and its effects on your body.

Treatment for post-pill PCOS (which can also be referred to as post-pill amenorrhea) involves 3 key steps: Replenishment, Removal, and Reinoculation. I also suggest assessment of thyroid and liver function which can be affected by BC.

Step 1- Replenishment: This includes replenishing the micronutrients that are commonly depleted by hormonal birth control. This includes: Zinc, Magnesium, B6, Vitamin C, and Folate. An anti-inflammatory diet with sufficient energy intake is imperative, as under eating (i.e., dieting) for many can hinder your cycle from returning. However, this is not always the case! If someone is overweight with insulin resistance, weight loss may be beneficial. This is where replenishment and food intake is person-by-person dependent. A great way to replenish is to take a prenatal supplement (with methylated folate which is more readily absorbed) and to optimize your diet with plentiful (and a variety of) fruits and vegetables! Focus on at least 2 cups a day of vegetables and ½ cup of fruit. The more the merrier! Just make sure to not overload your gut with lots of roughage and fiber or you may have gastrointestinal upset like gas, bloating, or even constipation or diarrhea. You should also increase your omega-3 consumption by choosing high omega-3 fatty foods such as salmon, sardines, walnuts, olive oil, flaxseed, chia seeds, grass fed beef, and soybeans. If you do not consume fatty fish at least twice a week, I suggest supplementing with a high quality fish or krill oil. If vegan or vegetarian, ALA to EPA and DHA conversion is quite low, so you will need to stay on top of your omega-3 intake and ensure that you are taking a high quality vegan omega source (I am a fan of algae based).

Step 2- Removal: This is where you want to focus on removing the synthetic estrogens and/or progestins within your BC. You can do this through natural liver support! No, I don't mean a detox (many are just glorified laxatives!). Natural, healthy, liver support can help in the elimination of synthetic hormones, toxins such as endocrine disruptors, and improve drug metabolism as well as the elimination of heavy metals. Liver support may include N-acetyl-cysteine, milk thistle, DIM, indole-3 carbinol, and sulforaphane. The key to optimizing your liver lies in optimizing the micronutrients and co-factors that it needs to do its job! Natural foods that help enhance liver detoxification include: cruciferous vegetables, garlic, onions, raw carrots, berries, citrus fruits, leafy greens, flaxseed, walnuts, beets, green tea, and apples. Herbs can be powerful aids as well, including milk thistle, rosemary, fennel, turmeric (active component is curcumin), parsley, ginger, dandelion root, mustard seeds, goldenseal, artichoke, chicory, and wormwood. Again, please speak with a healthcare professional before starting any new supplement.

You also want to focus on removing your specific food intolerances as well as endocrine disruptors from your environment. These can greatly impact your hormones and inflammation in your body. Everyone has potential different food sensitivities, and any gut infections or dysbiosis can create "pseudo-intolerances." See Chapter 10 for more information. I suggest becoming aware of endocrine disruptors and what toxic ingredients are in your household, beauty, and skin products. See my lifestyle chapter for more information! Common endocrine disruptors include: BHA, BHT, BPA, parabens, phthalates, fragrances, sulfates, sulfites, plastics, and dioxins. Other things to reduce, but not necessarily completely remove, include processed vegetable oils, added sugars, and of course, negative people in your life. Let's focus on surrounding ourselves with people (and things) that improve our lives rather than tear us and our overall health down!

Step 3- Reinoculation: This step can be a hit-or-miss for some. I am strictly talking about reinoculating your gut in this step. Birth control can cause alterations in your gut microbiota as well as potentially impact your gut motility. With any dysbiosis, gut infection, overgrowth, or gut damage, you want to make sure that you are working with a healthcare professional so that you are taking smart steps to get your gut health and function back on track! If you have any potential dysbiosis, overgrowth, or infection, the wrong reinoculation approach may be like throwing gas on a fire! Please, make sure if you have any signs or symptoms of gut distress or question any gut-related issues, that you work with a professional. Common reinoculation involves high dose probiotics (greater than 30 billion CFUs), specific strain probiotics, and the use of fermented foods like kefir, sauerkraut, and pickled vegetables.

Additional supplements that are helpful for post-pill PCOS include: vitex (chasteberry), myoinositol, omega-3s, additional magnesium, and adaptogens.

3. Adrenal PCOS:

This type of PCOS can be caused by any alteration or dysfunction in your HPA axis, and includes conditions such as hypothalamic amenorrhea (though it is not PCOS- it is commonly misdiagnosed as so), and cortisol dysregulation. Adrenal dysfunction can result from either high cortisol, low cortisol, or a combination of the two, called adaptive cortisol. See Chapter 9 for details and specifics on what can cause adrenal dysfunction and what you can do for help! Symptoms of adrenal dysregulation include: trouble falling or staying asleep, feeling "tired but wired" at night, chronic and constant fatigue, blood sugar crashes, mood swings, body fat concentrated around your abdomen, and constant salt or sugar cravings. In general, addressing stress, ensuring adequate sleep, prioritizing your diet, and balancing your blood sugar can be critical in helping bring cortisol levels back to a healthier place. Using adaptogens can also be extremely helpful, however you can not "out-adaptogen" or out-supplement adrenal dysfunction. You have to make sufficient dietary and lifestyle changes! I cover adaptogens and adjustments for adrenal dysfunction in Chapter 9.

4. Inflammatory PCOS:

In this case, inflammation is the root cause of your menstrual cycle irregularities. Inflammation can come from the diet via:

poor micronutrient intake, inflammatory foods (such as processed vegetable oils, fried foods, excess added sugars, processed meats, too much saturated fat), intake of individual food intolerances (or supplement intolerances- yes they exist!), or excessive food intake. Inflammation can also come from your gut dysbiosis or infection, as well as your environment, endocrine disruptors, heavy metals, mold, pollution/exhaust, and excess minerals such as fluoride, calcium, or iron. Infections or viruses, especially stealth infection like Epstein Barr or Lyme disease, can cause underlying low-grade systemic inflammation. Commonly, inflammation does not have one sole root cause. Inflammation is like a little cup that will continue to fill up, then produce havoc and symptoms when the cup overflows. The key is to reduce what you can from adding into your cup! The treatment for inflammation depends on the source. However, it's also important to follow an anti-inflammatory diet, focus on stress management, ensure adequate sleep, balance your blood sugar, and use exercise to help instead of harm your body (as inflammation can be from over-training or under-recovering). Helpful supplements for lowering inflammation include: curcumin, omega-3s, N-acetyl-cysteine, glutathione, bromelain, ginger, alpha-lipoic acid, resveratrol, Boswellia (frankincense), cat's claw, vitamin E, and pycnogenol. Having low levels of vitamin D and magnesium may also contribute to inflammation. By decreasing inflammation, you can potentially decrease the aromatization to estrogen (which may be causing estrogen dominance in your body), dropping down insulin levels (which could be causing insulin resistance), as well as decreasing systemic inflammation (that could be preventing proper nutrient absorption and thyroid absorption), which all affect your fertility and health!

Though I outlined four main "types" of PCOS, please know that you do not ever fit into a box and please - do not try to "cure" your PCOS yourself. Always work with a healthcare professional to ensure you are getting the right treatment for you based on your own symptoms, labs, history, and genetics! Keep in mind, hormonal issues and thyroid trouble go hand-in-hand, and any thyroid trouble can also go hand-in-hand with digestive trouble, so make sure to invest in yourself and do testing as needed.

Overall, the best PCOS supplements for any type include: omega-3s, vitamin D, inositol, chromium, vitex, multivitamin, and adaptogens.

Favorite Supplements for PCOS	
Supplement Name	Dosage per day
N-acetyl-cysteine (NAC)	600-1200mg
Curcumin	1000mg
Vitex/Chasteberry	200-800mg/day
Myoinositol	2-6g/day
Ashwagandha	600-1200mg/day
Omega-3 fatty acids	1000-2000mg/day
Vitamin D	1000-5000 IU/day (depending on Vitamin D levels)

5

WHEN YOUR CYCLE CHANGES

As previously discussed, there are many reasons why your menstrual cycle can change month to month! Stress, trauma, changes in your diet or exercise, or changes in medications can greatly affect the length, duration, and intensity of your menstrual cycle. It's completely normal for your cycle to be missed on a random month, as stress can prevent ovulation from occurring, or for one month to be heavier or lighter than another. However, if you notice any abnormal findings such as extreme heavy bleeding, blood clots, or severe pain and cramps, I highly recommend you see your healthcare professional to rule out fibroids, cysts, or ectopic pregnancy. My rule of thumb- if it's pain free and doesn't result in many symptom changes, wait for at least 2 months of a change before you fret. However, if you have crippling symptoms, heavy bleeding, or pain, don't wait!

Let's discuss specific reasons why your menstrual cycle can change. Common conditions include: high estrogen, low estrogen, low progesterone, high testosterone, low testosterone, high cortisol, low cortisol, high thyroid, low thyroid. Remember, any imbalance or stressor on your body can result in an altered or missed cycle.

Your body's inner fire alarm is going off asking for help! Common fire alarm signals and what could be occurring include:

Skipped or missed period:

Amenorrhea (a missed period) can be used as just one marker of assessing your overall health! There are 2 main types of amenorrhea: primary, in which one has never had a period, or secondary, in which a period goes missing after the onset of menses for more than 3 months at a time.

Many times, a random missed or skipped period is simply due to increased stress, which prevents ovulation from occurring, and is not something to cause concern or alarm. This is your body's safety response to the stressor, which can be emotional, physical, or mental! Your body can not distinguish between types of stress and sees them all as a threat to the body. This threat can result in lack of ovulation from occurring, as the body strives to put energy into preservation instead of reproduction. A healthy pregnancy wouldn't be advantageous for you or a baby if there was danger, therefore, a missed or skipped period serves as a response to aid in your, and a future baby's, safety. Ovulation doesn't occur without a period (unless pregnancy occurs). No ovulation, no progesterone, no period! (see Chapter 9 for more on this progesterone and cortisol/stress connection)

Common stressors that can cause a missed period include nutrient deficiencies, lack of sleep, over-exercising or too high intensity workouts (the amount each women can handle is quite individualized), under eating or chronic dieting, low body fat, emotional stress (such as a break up or job deadline), trauma (such as the loss of a loved one or pet), or change in medication. Estrogen dominance, low progesterone, cortisol dysregulation, thyroid disorders, pituitary dysfunction, stealth infections (such as Epstein Barr Virus (EBV) or Lyme Disease), gut infections (such as SIBO- small intestinal bacterial overgrowth, Candida, or H. Pylori), insulin resistance, and environment toxins can also play a role and be a root cause of a missed or skipped period. Ultimately, any acute or chronic stressor may impact your menstrual cycle.

A missed period may also be due to inadequate FSH and LH secretion. FSH and LH are both brain hormones secreted by your hypothalamus that aid to signal ovulation. High FSH with low estrogen may be caused by lack of ovarian function, as seen in primary ovarian failure. High prolactin levels may also prevent ovulation and cause a missed cycle. Prolactin does this by blocking FSH secretion, and in turn, blocking ovulation. This may be due to hypothyroidism or a pituitary or brain tumor as well as PCOS. Amenorrhea may also be caused by low GnRH (gonadotropin-releasing hormone), which signals the brain to produce FSH and LH. As you can see, there are many reasons why you can miss a period! That is why it is very important to be in tune with your body, do proper testing and assessment, and not blindly follow a "Period Repair" or "Get Your Period Back" program. Your root cause of amenorrhea needs its own treatment approach. One woman may need to eat more to get her period back due to previous chronic dieting or over-exercising, while another woman may need to eat less and exercise more to reduce high insulin levels in order to get her period back. I always suggest having a second eye to help whenever you struggle with any hormonal, adrenal, or thyroid imbalance to ensure you are taking steps to help yourself, not wreck yourself more!

Post-pill amenorrhea is another form of amenorrhea that occurs. Because birth control naturally shuts down your own hormone production, it can take a few months for some women to get their cycle back after stopping birth control. Some women also experience a hormonal rebound after stopping, which further causes chaos for their hormones, especially if they struggled with period problems before starting it. It may take weeks, or even up to months, to regulate your menstrual cycle after coming off of birth control. See the "Post-Pill PCOS" information previously discussed to help aid in post-pill amenorrhea.

. . .

Longer or Late Period:

There is no one definition of a normal menstrual cycle length. Your cycle length will also change throughout your lifetime! Teenagers may have longer cycles, while older women entering their 40s may have shorter cycles. When looking at your cycle length, it's important to always compare your length with your cycle's history and not to someone else's. In general, a healthy menstrual cycle may range from 24 to 35 days. The length of your follicular phase is what will dictate an earlier or later period, as it is what is in charge of building up your endometrial lining. Your luteal phase then transforms your uterine lining and is controlled by the growth of your corpus luteum and increased progesterone levels, which stimulates the maintenance of your endometrial lining.

A longer cycle or late period can be caused due to a chronic or acute stressor. Just like in a missed period, this is your body's safety response! This lengthened cycle or late period occurs through delaying ovulation. When ovulation is delayed, this can extend your follicular phase, which extends the time estrogen is at its highest as well. This can result in both a longer and heavier cycle, as estrogen helps to thicken your uterine lining. Just like a missed period due to stress, any stressor can potentially cause this to happen. Whether it's a big move, traveling, or even planning your own wedding, stress is stress.

Another reason for a late period, if you are late and have not tested for pregnancy, it could, of course, actually be pregnancy!

Shorter or Lighter Period:

The definition of a "light period" differs woman to woman, but overall, a light period can be described as less than 3 days of bleeding or only light spotting. Having a short or light period may be due to stress, post-birth control, a nutrient deficiency, dieting, under eating, low body fat, over-exercising, or a hormonal imbalance such as hypothyroidism or low estrogen.

Remember, estrogen is what helps to build up your uterine lining. Lack of estrogen means your build up is not created or sustained, which can lead to low blood volume and a shorter, lighter cycle. Many women get thrilled when this happens. However, your cycle is your fifth vital sign. If something changes your cycle drastically, it's a huge sign something is wrong. A short or lighter cycle is a sign that your body is not ready to conceive, and this should be a red flag to you and you should question why.

A shorter period may also be caused by: lack of ovulation, hypothyroidism, peri menopause, uterine fibroids, ovarian cysts, high prolactin levels, illness, or infections. Stress is stress in your body (see Chapter 9 for more details), and this will manifest in changes in your menstrual cycle. Cue a potentially shorter period, or even skipping a period.

HORMONAL CYCLE

| 0 | 7 | 14 | Late Ovulation | 21 | 28 |

Follicular Phase   Luteal Phase

Hormone:	Estrogen	Low Progesterone
	Normal Progesterone	Ovulation

*There is no one definition of a normal menstrual cycle length. Your cycle length will also change throughout your lifetime!

Another cause of shorter cycles is a luteal phase defect, which is a common cause of infertility and miscarriages. In a luteal phase defect, adequate progesterone levels are not created.

Some conventional doctors will just smother on some progesterone cream, give you a progesterone pill, or put you on birth
control for a light period. I say this is a disservice to you and your
health. You deserve to know why your period is light and be told
the alternatives to naturally balance your hormones versus just
being given a band-aid.

How can you naturally avoid a shorter or lighter period from occurring and ensure to help improve your fertility?

- Avoid under eating or over-exercising. If you are dieting,
  ensure that you are taking diet breaks and refeeds, as well
  as not dieting for long periods of time. Losing your cycle
  or getting a lighter period more than 3 months in a row
  would be a great sign that dieting is not suggested at this
  time for your body.
- Ensure you are consuming adequate micronutrients and
  dietary fat. Dietary fat and cholesterol are the makers of
  your hormones. Without them, you will not have
  adequate hormone production. You need a foundation to
  build a house - that is, fat and cholesterol for your
  hormones. Aim for healthy fats such as omega-3s from
  fatty fish, nuts, seeds, unprocessed oils like olive, avocado,
  and coconut, as well as healthy animal fat sources such as
  eggs, organic meats, and full-fat dairy.
- Prioritize sleep and stress management. Your body needs
  to be in a safe zone in order to have a "normal" menstrual
  cycle. Stress and lack of sleep are a perceived threat to the
  body. Your body responds by shifting its energy away from
  baby production and into body preservation! (This is the
  same reaction with any stressor such as under eating- see
  Chapter 9 for more on stress and cortisol's effects on your
  hormones.) Self care and proper nutrition are the
  fundamentals of a healthy menstrual cycle. Make sure to
  prioritize them, and yourself.

- For herbal therapies, you may add in vitex agnus-castus (also known as chasteberry) and myoinositol to help balance estrogen and progesterone. These herbs may also encourage ovulation and aid in the brain to ovary communication. Please make sure to discuss with your doctor or registered dietitian before starting any supplement. Remember, supplements are not magic and always have to be taken with caution (and patience). I highly suggested avoiding vitex if you have or suspect low prolactin levels, as vitex may block prolactin secretion. Recommended doses: 400-800 mg vitex and 4-6 g of myoinositol.

Mid-Cycle Spotting or 2 Periods in 1 Month:

If you experience bleeding when you aren't expecting a period, you may have gotten your period early, or you may be experiencing mid-cycle spotting. This occasionally may happen and is not something to be concerned about, however if you notice this occurs for two to three consecutive months at a time, you need to speak with your doctor. The difference between a period and mid-cycle spotting may be confusing to you. What distinguishes the two is the amount of blood and color! If you are able to fill a couple tampons or soak through a pad with bright red or dark red blood, it's most likely a period. If your bleeding does not soak a tampon or pad and is brown or light pink, it is more likely to be spotting.

What can cause two periods in one month? Endometriosis (in which uterine tissue grows outside your uterine lining), uterine fibroids (noncancerous growths outside of your uterus), hypo- or hyperthyroidism, nutrient deficiencies such as iron deficiency, peri menopause, and acute or chronic stress.

Symptoms of iron deficiency include: fatigue, weakness, hair loss, shortness or breath, irregular heartbeat, dizziness (especially upon standing quickly), and headache.

What can cause mid-cycle spotting? For some women, spotting can occur during ovulation as estrogen dramatically declines, causing shedding of the endometrium (the lining of your uterus). This is coined a "ovulation bleeding," and may or may not happen in all women or be a case for concern. Typically ovulation bleeding coincides with changes in BBT (basal body temperature) and cervical mucus, marking ovulation.

However, if outside of ovulation or purely random spotting occurs, there may be an underlying issue causing it. Mid-cycle spotting may be caused by acute or chronic stress (including under eating, over-exercising, dieting, trauma, emotional distress), nutrient deficiencies such as iron deficiency anemia, sexually transmitted diseases (usually accompanied by additional pain and abnormal discharge), PCOS, cervicitis (inflammation of the cervix), and even pregnancy.

If you suspect pregnancy or had missed a previous menstrual cycle, it's very important to test and assess whether the mid-cycle spotting could be due to a miscarriage or ectopic pregnancy (in which a fertilized egg is implanted into the fallopian tube or outside your uterus). Spotting may also be due to implantation bleeding, which could be confirmed using a pregnancy test. A pregnancy test will test for positive levels of hCG (human chorionic gonadotropin) in your urine, marking a state of pregnancy. This is a hormone produced by the placenta after egg implantation, and if pregnant or due to implantation, its presence can rule out other potential causes of spotting.

If you notice irregular spotting a few weeks apart, this may indicate lack of ovulation, which could be due to any stressor or condition that prevents progesterone from being created. It can also occur when starting birth control or there are changes in birth control usage, in which the mid-cycle spotting is called "breakthrough bleeding." If your spotting lasts more than a few days, causes severe cramps or pain, or is accompanied by abnormal discharge or smell, make sure to speak with your medical care provider.

Heavy or Painful Periods:

Do you constantly go through super tampons, refill your menstrual cup several times a day, or reach towards anti-inflammatories like ibuprofen or Midol for relief from pain during your period? You may have a heavy period, known as "menorrhagia," or severe menstrual cramping, known as "dysmenorrhea," which can both be quite crippling and annoying! Dysmenorrhea may be followed by additional symptoms such as back pain, nausea, diarrhea, headaches, muscle weakness, and fatigue. Not all women experience the same symptoms, and the level of blood flow and pain that you exhibit may be different compared to other women. It's always important to compare your pain and blood flow with yourself and your history, not another woman's. One woman's normal may be your heavy period!

Many times having a heavy cycle out of the blue can be related to stress or inflammation. Whether you had a crazy work week or lost a loved one, this can manifest in increased PMS symptoms such as pain, cramping, and fatigue, as well as increase your menstrual blood flow volume. If you had more inflammatory foods than normal, such as dairy, processed foods, added sugars, alcohol, or if you ate foods you are intolerant to, this can increase inflammation in your body, which worsens your PMS and menstrual flow. This may be "normal" as a stress response if it happens randomly, however if you consistently struggle with heavy periods (with blood flow greater than 80 mL per day or need to frequently change super tampons every few hours), you may have estrogen dominance! Just a quick note, if you notice large blood clots and heavy bleeding, unfortunately it is possible that you had a miscarriage. Please speak to your doctor if you have any painful, heavy bleeding with clotting and suspect a potential miscarriage.

Estrogen is your hormone in charge of building up your uterine lining. Too much estrogen can cause excess build up of your lining, which then increases blood volume during your cycle, and can also create increased clotting and prostaglandin production, contributing to more inflammation and pain. Prostaglandins, which are created to help shed the uterine lining when no pregnancy is present, cause the uterus to perform contractions that are meant to speed along shedding of your uterine lining. When you have too many prostaglandins, this increases cramping and pain!

Other causes for having a heavy menstrual cycle include: endometriosis, fibroids, ovarian cysts, endometrial polyps, thyroid disease, high insulin levels, endometrial hyperplasia, adenomyosis (in which the uterine lining attaches to the muscle tissue of your uterus), endometrial cancer, infections, high histamine levels, low progesterone, medication side effects, or a nutrition deficiency such as iron, omega-3 fatty acids, magnesium, B12, or B6. Heavy periods can also be an undesired side effect from birth control and IUDs, especially if IUD placement is affected. The copper IUD is commonly known for causing heavier periods. If you have an IUD, make sure to speak with your doctor if your periods are or become painful or heavier, and ensure that you rule out any other causes or contributing factors, as well as ensure your IUD is in place!

What may help to alleviate a heavy or painful cycle (minus finding the root cause!):

- Natural anti-inflammatories: Curcumin, Omega-3 fatty acids, Boswellia (also known as frankincense), Ginger, Bromelain
- PMS alleviating nutrients: Magnesium, B6, Zinc
- Alternative therapies: yoga, meditation, and massage

- Lifestyle management: stress reduction, sleep hygiene, exercising, avoiding alcohol and smoking

Your Period & Digestion:

Have you ever noticed yourself being more constipated or having trouble pooping the week before your menstrual cycle? Have you noticed an increase in bowel movements or a "clear out" when you period comes? Welcome to the land of period poops!

Period poops are a result of shifts in both progesterone and prostaglandins. Progesterone, made after ovulation (the release of an egg and the start of your luteal phase), is what helps build up the uterine lining in hopes of a pregnancy. It rises mid-cycle and is lowest during your period (the start of the follicular phase). This progesterone SLOWS down your digestion by decreasing levels of motility in your gut, contributing to slower fecal movement, trouble pooping, and constipation. You may also notice more gas and bloating, as food takes longer to digest and has more time to ferment in your gut, producing gas along the way (oh, what a joy to be a woman!).

When progesterone drops at the start of your period (day one of your follicular phase), this causes increases in motility and reductions in fecal transit time. Hello poop finally moving! This is further influenced by prostaglandins, which help the uterus to contract and shed blood. These contractions can aid in digestive contractions as well, leading to more frequent bowel movements.

If you struggle with constipation or trouble pooping during your luteal phase, the following tips may be helpful for moving things along and preventing discomfort:

1. Get enough fiber! 25-40 g in women per day is suggested, with at least 14 g for every 1000 calories consumed. Find your fiber "sweet spot." Both quantity and type of fiber

can play a role in your digestion, so play around with what amount you feel best with. Make sure to also focus on insoluble fiber if you struggle with constipation, as this is the type of fiber that will help bulk up your stool and help alleviate constipation. Refer to the appendix to see a fiber chart! Keep in mind, too much fiber can constipate you too. Be willing to see what amount you feel best with.

2. Get enough sleep and water! Lack of sleep will further slowdown gut motility, as well as a lack of water. When you are dehydrated, your colon responds by further increasing the uptake of water from your intestines, causing harder poops that may be difficult to pass. If you have low electrolyte intake, that can worsen constipation, as electrolytes are what help in the movement of materials in and out of your cells.

3. If fiber, sleep, water, and electrolytes are already optimized and don't aid in constipation, magnesium citrate (last resort) may help at 400 mg. I suggest trying a hot coffee or tea first, as coffee and caffeine can help stimulate the bowels to move things along. Magnesium citrate should not be used routinely. If you continue to have constipation issues, there may be a deeper cause to your poop issues, such as hypothyroidism, nerve damage to your gut, low neurotransmitters, a gut infection or overgrowth, or intestinal blockage. Make sure to speak with your doctor if you struggle with constipation on a weekly basis.

Peri Menopause

Peri menopause is referred to by many women as "the years of hell." From mood swings, hot flashes, and difficulty sleeping, to chronic fatigue, the symptoms can be quite crippling! Now don't let me scare you! Peri menopause is not well understood and is heavily demonized by women that don't have this book in their hands. But you do! The years of peri menopause don't have to be a disaster. Whether you are about to be, or are already in, those years, I am going to give you the tools and knowledge you need to be in control.

What is peri menopause? Peri menopause is a natural transition in your life. I like to call it "entering the age of wisdom." The eggs of your ovaries have their last chance to be released as you go from your fertile to non-fertile years. As you enter peri menopause, your hormones go through this transition period, which can roller-coaster your hormones on a day-by-day, week-by-week, and month-by-month basis. Peri menopause is not due to one single hormone, but is caused by the symphony of your hormones changing tune permanently.

It's quite common for women to have major hormonal fluctuations like a rollercoaster ride during this time. Cue symptoms such as an irregular menstrual cycle, hot flashes, difficulty sleeping, vaginal dryness, mood swings, irritability, breast tenderness, fatigue, migraines, and low libido. You may notice increased cravings (as lower estrogen also drops your natural serotonin levels), increased feelings of anxiety or depression (as less happy neuro-transmitters are produced), and trouble losing weight or main-taining your body composition (as your metabolic rate naturally decreases). Add in the fact that you are at increased risk for cortisol dysregulation with lower progesterone and serotonin, and a hormonal storm can erupt!

Why does this occur? Remember that progesterone is only produced when you ovulate, and that estrogen is largely created within your ovaries. As your ovarian reserve (aka egg reserve) diminishes, your progesterone and estrogen levels slowly dimin-ish as well. In fact, your testosterone also takes a dive. Bad news is you can't stop peri menopause from happening. Good news is that you can manage it and reduce symptoms!

HORMONE LEVELS

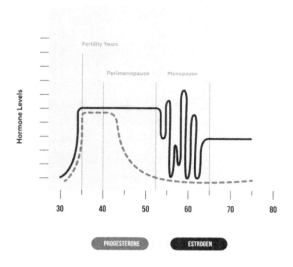

Peri menopause can last several years and typically occurs between the ages of 35-50. During this time of your life, your periods can become heavier, irregular, or even skipped. You will notice months where you feel energized and "normal," and then months where you are moody, exhausted, and dealing with the spikes and dips of your fluctuating hormones (hello hot and cold flashes!). This is what I call the "peri menopause rollercoaster." This is important to remember, because many "peri menopause" or "menopause" support supplements have specific modes of actions, which can help in certain situations, however they are not tailored to your individual needs and where your hormonal peri menopause roller coaster is currently at. For example, some work to help increase estrogen, while some help to decrease it. Some help in Phase 1 detoxification, while some help with aromatization of testosterone to estrogen. This is where it is extremely important for you to be aware of your symptoms, test, don't guess your hormones, and ensure you speak with a healthcare professional prior to stopping or starting a new supplement.

Lifestyle changes such as focusing on self-care, stress reduction, getting adequate sleep and ensuring proper sleep hygiene practices, reducing environmental toxins and endocrine disruptors, staying active, and maintaining a healthy body weight can be critical components in helping to reduce the chaos of peri menopause. Diet also plays a huge role, and ensuring to eat an anti-inflammatory diet with a focus on reducing added sugars and processed vegetable oils can help to reduce inflammation, which can exacerbate symptoms. Focusing on nutrients such as omega-3s, B-vitamins, zinc, magnesium, and vitamin E is also important! I have found in practice that some women also benefit from a moderate to low-carb diet as estrogen levels drop because low estrogen decreases your body's ability to utilize glucose.

My favorite supplements to help peri menopause include:

- **Black Cohosh:** can decrease hot flashes and improve mood
- **Vitex:** can improve mood and fatigue by balancing estrogen and progesterone
- **Flaxseed and soy:** can help increase progesterone and estrogen, reducing symptoms (no, soy does not have the same effects as estrogen because it binds to different receptors) -Phytosterols: can help balance estrogen and reduce symptoms
- **Vitamin D:** low levels greatly contribute to fatigue, insulin resistance, and bone loss. Adequate Vitamin D, K2, and calcium intake are essential to prevent bone loss (low levels of estrogen increase risk for bone loss and osteoporosis)
- **Ashwagandha:** helps to combat fatigue and nourish the adrenals. Also helps to improve T4 to T3 (inactive to active) thyroid conversion.
- **Special note-** St. John's Wort is a commonly suggested supplement but I am NOT a fan because it has so many drugs, nutrient, and supplement interactions!

- **Digestive enzymes:** as estrogen lowers, this can decrease the release of digestive enzymes, creating more gas and bloating and trouble digesting food.

Some women do well using bio identical therapy or DHEA, however that is a case-by-case basis and please speak with a clinician about those, because that is beyond the scope of this book. I do want to note that you should be extremely careful with supplementing purely with progesterone. Progesterone should be in a delicate balance with estrogen! If you have low estrogen, and are supplementing with progesterone, you can create a state of high progesterone, which is actually a hormonal state of pregnancy. Side effects may include bloating, reflux (as progesterone relaxes your esophageal sphincter), and constipation! Think of your hormones like a cupcake here. Frosting yourself with progesterone is not the answer. You need the cake (estrogen) to create the full cupcake! THEN you can slather on the icing.

After peri menopause occurs, you enter into the wise age of menopause! The indication of a transition from peri menopause to menopause can be confirmed by the loss of your menstrual cycle after one full year. This transition marks the end of your reproductive and fertile years! This also marks the end of the peri menopause rollercoaster, and it's during this time that estrogen and progesterone levels stay low and do not come back up again. Remember the roles of both estrogen and progesterone in your body beyond their functions for reproduction? Estrogen is powerful in preserving bone mineral density and reducing the risk of cardiovascular disease. Progesterone increases your metabolism, helps your body use fat for energy, and enhances your sex drive.

Losing the power of these two hormones naturally results in an increased risk of cardiovascular disease and osteoporosis, which estrogen levels protect during reproductive years, as well as an increased risk of endometrial cancers and reduced metabolic rate, which result from the reductions in your progesterone levels. Additional changes common during menopause include increased levels of abdominal body fat, loss of lean muscle mass, increased levels of cholesterol, higher blood pressure, increased occurrence of UTIs (urinary tract infections), and urinary incontinence. Your vaginal microbiome also changes, and you may notice an increased risk of bacterial or yeast infections, pain or loss of lubrication during sex, along with low libido. This can also occur in premenopausal women with low estrogen! I am a firm believer that no woman should have to go without good orgasms just because of their age. Take the steps you need and speak with your health care provider if you experience these symptoms.

6

ENDOCRINE DISRUPTORS
FROM HELL

What you choose to cook and clean with your skin and beauty products, your water quality, and the air you breathe can all play crucial roles in impacting your overall health. How? They can expose you to environmental toxins. Environmental toxins come in the form of hundreds of different chemicals that can impact your hormones, metabolism, and mental health. Your health is more than what you eat. It's also what surrounds you.

The most common environmental toxins that you may face are endocrine disruptors. Endocrine disruptors have been defined by the US Environmental Protection Agency (EPA) as "exogenous agents that interfere with the synthesis, secretion, transport, metabolism, binding action, or elimination of natural blood-borne hormones that are present in the body and are responsible for homeostasis, reproduction, and development process." In simpler terms- they disrupt your hormones. Endocrine disrupters can go in mimicking your own hormones, block hormone receptors, or alter hormone pathways, leading down to hormonal chaos is your "toxic bucket" overflows.

Conditions associated with disruptions in hormones due to endocrine disruptors include PMS, PMDD, fibrocystic or painful breasts, estrogen dominance, dysmenorrhea (painful periods), uterine or ovarian cancer, endometriosis, infertility, cervical dysplasia, and systemic lupus erythematosus.

We come into contact with endocrine disruptors on a daily basis and actually can't fully avoid them! Don't freak. There are simple swaps you can make to help reduce your environmental toxin and endocrine disruptor load. Just like your stress bucket, making small changes to reduce your exposure and overflow of your "toxin bucket" allows you to reduce your risk of their consequences. The more droplets in your bucket, the more risk you have of these chemicals impacting your health. Therefore, if you can reduce the exposure and drops added to your toxin bucket, you can reduce their harmful effects on your health!

Endocrine Disrupters include:

1. BPA and BHT
2. Dioxin
3. Atrazine
4. Phthalates
5. Perchlorate
6. Fire Retardants
7. Lead
8. Arsenic
9. Mercury
10. Perfluorinated chemicals
11. Organophosphate
12. Glycol ethers
13. Plastics
14. Parabens
15. Fragrances

Some endocrine disruptors cause specific hormone disruptions. Xenoestrogens are one of these. They mimic estrogen within your body and swoop in as uninvited guests, adding to your body's estrogen pool party. Cue estrogen dominance and hormonal chaos!

A common devilish form of a xenoestrogens is Bisphenol-A (BPA). BPA can be found in canned food linings, plastics, store receipts, and some dental sealants. You can even be exposed to it through inhalation or transdermally (through your skin). Because of its ability to be easily absorbed by the body and disrupt hormone function, BPA has been banned in infant feeding materials and formulas.

BPA can build up in the body, specifically in fat, liver, and reproduction tissues. It can also build up within a mother's breast milk. Not good for mom or baby. BPA exposure has been correlated with increased obesity, diabetes, late puberty onset, and behavioral issues in children. It is also linked to a child's development of mood and hyperactivity disorders. In adults, BPA has been linked to both male and female infertility, reproductive cancers (such as breast and prostate cancer), hormone imbalances, insulin resistance, and high blood pressure.

How can you reduce exposure? Choosing BPA free products is a great step. Common BPA containing products include plastics and cans. Luckily, many plastic and canned products are now BPA-free. By switching your plastic containers, bowls, glasses, and cups to glass, porcelain, or stainless steel, you are making a simple swap to reduce your exposures.

Another way to reduce your BPA exposure is to choose to receive email vs paper receipts. This way, you're saving yourself from the BPA exposure, while also saving the environment. I mentioned the shift from plastics to glass, porcelain, and stainless steel- not just BPA free plastics. Why? There has yet to be safety established for BPA substitutes (including BPS and BPF). These other plastic products should be used with caution and are not guaranteed to be safe for use (just like the term "natural"). To me, it's better to make swaps that could benefit you the most. Regardless of being

BPA-free or not, please never microwave plastic. Ever. This can cause the chemicals in the plastics to leach into your food. Do you want to eat those chemicals? I don't think so.

When it comes down to lowering your exposure to other endocrine disruptors, it's the dose that makes the poison. Since you can't fully eliminate exposure, think about simply reducing it. You don't need to start with doing a complete overhaul - that can be very overwhelming. Take small steps, such as assessing your cookware or skincare products. Read the labels of what you currently have and use. Then, start by purchasing safer, non-toxic options as you run out of your previous ones. A great first step is to start swapping your favorite laundry detergent or face wash.

I know the process of reducing endocrine disruptors and environmental toxins can seem daunting and annoying. Remember the reasoning behind the changes. Think about the benefits to your health and what you may gain from the change. After switching to cleaner products, reducing fragrances, and eliminating excess use of plastics, I have had hundreds of clients transform their health from the inside out. From increased mental clarity, eradication of migraines and headaches, clearer and smoother skin, to significant hormone improvements and body composition changes, the work put in to reduce environmental toxin load can make a huge impact. I want you to be able to feel those changes too.

I used to love being doused in scents. I grew up with my daily sprays of flowery perfume and lavender lotions. When I finally took the initiative to get rid of these fragrances, it helped to lift away my brain fog, clear up my skin, and aided in reducing my hypothyroid symptoms! Now when I walk down the laundry detergent or candle aisle, or get stuck in a man's whiff of excessive cologne, my throat closes up. I instantly get a headache. The truth is- you don't know how these chemicals can actually impact you unless you try eliminating them. Do yourself an experimental test. See how you feel after reducing their exposure. You won't regret it.

· · ·

Special Note on Skincare:

Did you know that your skin is your largest organ? It can soak in both the good and bad into your body! Think about that when you choose to slather on skincare products. Not only may those products sit on and affect the integrity of your skin, but they also may be soaked into the pores and into the bloodstream. Don't believe me? Think about how women are given estrogen or progesterone creams to help balance their hormones. Yes- the skin can absorb these and more!

Skincare products are largely unregulated, and therefore it is up to you as a consumer to utilize trusted companies and thoroughly read ingredient lists prior to trying a new product. Skincare products are never guaranteed as safe, and even dermatologist prescribed products may cause reactions, especially if you have sensitive skin. I always suggest spot testing on your skin prior to using a new product, as well as assessing for the common endocrine disruptors that may be within their ingredient profile. Websites such as Skin Carisma, EWG (the Environmental Working Group), GoodGuide, and Think Dirty can be extremely helpful!

I am a firm believer in assessing your exposure, experimenting with reduction, and eliminating what you find causes or heightens your health or hormonal symptoms. Reducing environmental toxins has become a hyped and taboo topic, and though it excites me to see them discussed since education is power, I also see issues regarding fear mongering and greenwashing. What do I mean by this? Companies have started to come out with new "clean," "natural," or "safe" product lines, increasing pricing to profit off of this demand or using scare tactics in marketing to try to make the consumer purchase their product vs another based on fear. We cannot claim that a natural product is safer, and we also cannot claim that products are "clean." I would be very cautious when purchasing products and ensure to assess their ingredient profiles, not their marketing claims. Choose to be a precautionary, but smart, consumer.

Heavy Metals

Heavy metals are a sub-component of endocrine disruptors that, in low amounts, are safely excreted through your kidneys. However, increased exposure and lack of elimination can lead to soft tissue deposit in the body, which can cause poisoning, adverse health reactions, and be a hidden cause of chronic inflammatory conditions. Heavy metals can also be an underlying cause of digestive distress and tough cases of dysbiosis. If the heavy metals aren't removed, the dysbiosis and gut infection can't be either. The most common heavy metals that can accumulate in the body include mercury, lead, arsenic, aluminum, chromium, cadmium, and copper.

Exposure to heavy metals can come from unfiltered water, dental fillings, water pipes, occupational exposure such as in glass or car manufacturing, industrial plant working, artistry such as pottery or painting, or even high consumption of fish! In the case of mercury, this is why pregnant women are recommended to avoid high-dose mercury fish such as king mackerel, shark, swordfish, tuna, and tilefish. The mercury in these fish build up within their bodies over time, and can be consumed and then built up in a mother's body, causing complications to pregnancy or adverse health outcomes to the baby, such as the development of neuro-logical problems or failure to thrive.

Chronic Heavy Metal Poisoning symptoms include brain fog, headaches, chronic fatigue, visual disturbances, muscle or joint pains, hypothyroidism, burning or tingling sensations, chronic infections, chronic digestive issues, poor immunity, and trouble sleeping.

To reduce your heavy metal exposure, I suggest making sure to use a high quality drinking water filter, such as a Berkey or reverse osmosis system. If you suspect heavy metal toxicity, there are 3 ways to test: blood, urine, and hair. The verdict is still out on which method is best and most reliable. Blood and urine testing will give you one-day snapshots in time of your exposure, while hair will give you more of a three month marker (depending on how fast your hair grows). Both have their pros and cons.

Cons to Urine and Blood: requires a provocation agent such as DMSA (a short-term radioactive isotope) to pull metals from tissues; only reveals a snapshot in time of recent and acute exposure

Cons to Hair: not clinically validated for use; easily affected by chemical treatment of hair, shampoo/conditioner usage, and testing protocols

If you suspect heavy metal issues, I suggest working one-on-one with a clinician instead of toying around with a heavy metal hair test. No need to cut your hair off alone. A general safe and gentle way to detox heavy metals would be, of course, pooping, however you could also (under guidance) utilize binders such as activated charcoal, modified citrus pectin, bentonite clay, humic acid, zeolite, and chlorella.

Mold Toxicity

This topic opens up a large can of worms. Mold toxicity can be a true demon to your entire body.

Symptoms of both acute and chronic mold toxicity include:

1. Fatigue and weakness
2. Headaches, light sensitivity
3. Poor memory, difficulty finding words or concentrating
4. Mood swings
5. Sharp pains, morning stiffness, joint pain
6. Unusual skin sensations, tingling, and numbness
7. Shortness of breath, sinus congestion, or a chronic cough
8. Appetite swings

9. Issues with body temperature regulation- includes night or cold sweats
10. Increased urinary frequency or increased thirst
11. Red eyes or blurred vision
12. Abdominal pain, diarrhea, bloating
13. Metallic taste in your mouth
14. Static shocks
15. Vertigo, feeling lightheaded

The most important thing to do if you suspect mold is to check your environment and then get out of the exposure! Do you feel better or worse at home or at work? Do you notice your symptoms go away when you go out of town? Do you notice you feel worse when going into older buildings? Ask yourself these questions to see if your health may be affected by mold!

I highly suggest hiring a professional mold inspector and/or doing a ERMI mold test if you suspect mold. A VCS (Visual Contrast Sensitivity) test may be a great start with symptom analysis before you bite that bullet. Some practitioners may recommend a urine mold test, such as Great Plains MycoTox, however I find that the results may tell you that mold is present, but not reveal where it's coming from. If you can't find and eliminate it, you can't get healed from it!

My top tips for mold healing include:

- Get out of the environment- you can't heal staying in the same environment that you got sick in.
- Test, don't guess- you need to know where it's coming from.
- Clean up your air- using a high quality HEPA air filter such as an Air Doctor or Austin Air may help to reduce 99% of endotoxins, mold particles, airborne viruses, volatile organic compounds (VOCs), dust, allergens, and airborne pollutants. If you suffer from asthma or

environmental allergies, you should have one regardless of mold being an issue or not.

- Use a dehumidifier- this will reduce the moisture that mold needs to grow. It can't get rid of the mold, but can help prevent it.
- Reduce your intake of moldy foods- these may include coffees, boxed/canned/packaged foods, packaged grains, yeast containing foods such as cheese, alcohol, condiments, mushroom products, cured meats, and dried fruits. I also suggest reducing your sugar intake, which mold would love to feast on.
- Use gentle natural detox methods. Stay active and sweat daily, get in an infrared sauna, and optimize your digestion. Remember detoxing comes from exhalation, sweating, and pooping. Power up the fiber in your diet and make sure to optimize your poop health. Dry brushing or lymphatic massage may enhance lymphatic flow, however I find active exercise is the most beneficial to get your body's blood flow circulating. You can also use liver support such as NAC (n-acetyl-cysteine) or liposomal glutathione with gentle binders, however I suggest working one-on-one with a professional for this and therefore will not give direct recommendations.
- Remediate and clean up your life- you have to get rid of more than just the visible mold, but the invisible mold spores as well. Just because you can kill visible mold with diluted bleach, borax, vinegar, and biocides does not mean that you will get rid of all the mold spores. I suggest getting rid of items that have large pores, such as rugs, furnishings, mattresses, bedding, and pillows. Make sure to clean up your entire environment, including air vents, counters, and floors. Make sure to have your vehicle cleaned as well as you can take mold spores from one place to another.

Menstrual Health Products:

Ladies, your skin is your largest organ system. The thin, absorbent tissues around your vagina, vulva, and in your vaginal canal are an open door for soaking in any chemical you put on or in it. I want you to really think before using pads, tampons, douches, creams, or lubricants. Think about any self pleasure tools you may be using as well. Chemicals and fragrances in these products can easily enter your bloodstream and negatively impact not only your vaginal flora but also your hormonal health!

This doesn't mean you have to go choose all organic tampons or menstrual cups, as we do not yet know the safety or benefit to these switches. Truth is, your vagina doesn't care what type or tampon or cup you use- it only cares about the ingredients in them. I suggest ensuring that your menstrual cups, tampon applicators, and self pleasure toys are BPA free, switching to hypoallergenic lubricants, and avoiding any fragrances, flavors, or aromas.

Have you struggled with yeast infections, smelly discharge, or vaginal burning? Take a look at the feminine hygiene products that you are using! (As well as your gut- hello Candida and SIBO!) You don't need to use douches or vaginal wipes. Your vagina is designed to clean itself. If there are smells or abnormal discharge, you should be seeing a gynecologist, not masking with fragrances! Please, please use plain, fragrance-free soaps on your lady parts. Using douches and wipes can disrupt your vaginal bacterial flora and set you up for endocrine disruptors, heading right into your bloodstream.

The Toxin Reduction Plan

Though I cover nutrition in greater detail in the next chapter, the foods that you eat can increase or decrease your toxin load. Why? Some foods are more heavily sprayed with pesticides, herbicides, and have a higher risk of being contaminated with heavy metals!

Have you heard of the "Dirty Dozen" and "Clean Fifteen?" The EWG (Environmental Working Group) produces an annual list of the top foods sprayed with pesticides from the USDA and FDA's Pesticide Testing Program. This includes a thorough analysis of common produce options that have higher or lower pesticide content. Though I don't 100% trust them and the lists (I won't dive into details here, but to keep it short: 1. They don't test all agricultural products; 2. They don't assess organic foods (yes- they have pesticides too!); and 3. They seem to be very selective with what and where they test from).

I have come up with my own list of higher or lower "toxin load" foods and products that I hope you find helpful. Don't treat this like a bible. Remember, in the end, it's your toxic bucket over-flowing that creates havoc. By making small changes and reducing the "drops" going into your bucket, you can reduce your toxic load!

If you struggle with symptoms of thyroid disease, hormonal imbalances, gut distress, or have cognitive-related disturbances, you may want to think of following my toxic load reduction plan. You don't have to be strict- focus on only removing what you need to. The goal is to be as liberated as possible!

Toxic Load Reduction Plan - Foods		
	Foods to Eat	**Foods to Limit**
Protein	Organic meats, wild-caught fish, liver, sardines, pastured poultry, organic eggs, organic soy	Shellfish & fish heavy in toxins (see seafoodwatch.org); processed meats (cold cuts & hot dogs); non organic soy products (tofu, tempeh, etc.)
Grains	Organic grains- including rice, quinoa, wheat, organic corn; gluten-free oats	Conventional grains and corn; gluten if intolerant
Sweeteners & Sugar	Stevia, maple syrup, blackstrap, molasses, monk fruit (all in moderation i.e., 1 tsp)	Brown, white, & cane sugar; evaporated cane juice; agave nectar; corn syrup; artificial sweeteners (saccharin, aspartame, & sucralose)
Legumes, Nuts, & Seeds	All legumes, pumpkin, flaxseed, sesame, sunflower seeds, almonds, walnuts, brazil nuts, pine nuts	Pre-ground flaxseed (easily oxidizes); If you experience GI symptoms after eating beans, consider eliminating them.
Fats & Oils	Olive oil, coconut oil, coconut butter, avocado oil, lard, tallow, duck fat, grass-fed butter, ghee, extra-virgin olive oil, flaxseed oil, sesame oil, walnut oil, MCT oil	Processed vegetable oils- Canola oil, soybean oil, corn oil, sunflower, safflower, cottonseed oil; trans fats or partially hydrogenated fats (avoid completely)
Dairy	Coconut, almond, & hemp milk; coconut or cashew yogurt; grass-fed butter, organic dairy	Cow, goat, & sheep milks; soymilk, yogurt, & cheese; oat milk, dairy-based cheese, yogurt, kefir
Fruit & Vegetables	All fruits & vegetables	N/A- may choose to limit conventional if you fear pesticides (which can be washed off)
Beverages & Additives	Filtered water, sparkling water, herbal teas; natural flavors and colors	Coffee, caffeinated teas, alcohol, juice, & soda; food dyes, preservatives, and artificial colors/flavors

Toxic Load Reduction Plan—Household, Personal Care, & Lifestyle		
Good	***Better***	***Best***
Household		
Remove all synthetic air fresheners from your home & open windows often	Vacuum frequently with a HEPA filter & change A/C & heater filters regularly	Use a high-quality air purifier equipped with a HEPA filter
Remove bleach-containing cleaning & laundry products	Swap home-cleaning products for ones that don't contain bleach, synthetic fragrances, or harsh chemicals	Make your own cleaning products using water, vinegar, essential oils, baking soda, & other natural ingredients
Throw out your plastic bottles and switch to glass or stainless steel; Bring your own reusable shopping bags; throw out Aluminum and Teflon based cooked ware; stop accepting receipts unless paper (contains BPA)	Use safe cookware; replace plastic wrap with reusable wraps & silicone lids; replace plastic containers with glass; replace plastic sandwich bags with reusable silicone	Avoid takeout foods that come in plastic containers; avoid BPA lined canned foods
Personal Care & Lifestyle		
Swap your conventional lipstick or lip glass, face lotion, & liquid/powder foundation for fragrance and paraben free products	Swap your shampoo, conditioner, & hair styling products for fragrance and paraben free products	Look deeper at ingredients of your products for harsh ingredients and utilize EWG
Choose local and fresh produce options; switch to organic dairy	Choose organic produce options, keeping to the Clean 15 in conventional products; switch to organic meats	Choose organic produce, dairy, and meats
Exercise in a way that makes you sweat for 30 minutes 1-2 times per week	Exercise in a way that makes you sweat for 30 minutes 3-4 times per week	Use an infrared or regular sauna or steam room a few times a week.

7

CONQUERING YOUR NUTRITION

Science Over Opinions

I am sure you have had everyone and their mother try to tell you what diet is best for health, weight loss, longevity, or digestion. Everyone always has an opinion and wants to share it with the world! Karen from work may have backed you into a corner to discuss her new ketogenic protocol, or Susan, your mom's friend, may have Facebook messaged you about a new weight loss shake that "really works".. I will never reprimand someone for their opinion, and we all have freedom of speech. However, science doesn't care about opinions, and pushing opinions can confuse people. The reality is that there is no "best diet" or "one size fits all" approach to nutrition. You have your own metabolism, genes, gut microbiota, and dietary preferences that must be taken into account in order to find the best diet for you!

How does what you eat make you feel? What foods do you enjoy and what pre-existing medical conditions may you have or be at risk for? What about your genes? Have you dieted in the past, especially with yo-yo dieting? There are so many factors that can play into what your nutritional needs are, and these needs will change and evolve over your lifetime - just like you do! For example, an adolescent girl may have a sky rocket high metabolism, with no issues consuming calories or digesting her favorite pizza. Being super active in sports, she may be burning through calories. As she grows older, her metabolic rate naturally decreases, hormones change, and her environment and lifestyle changes as well. So do her nutritional needs and her diet! We lose the ability to fully digest lactose with older age, the output of digestive enzymes decreases, as well as our basal metabolic rate. Therefore, this teen could potentially not be able to eat that same pizza later down the road, and may actually develop an intolerance to dairy. She may develop PCOS from endocrine disruptors in her environment in combination with stress from an intense workload in her career. This may further decrease her metabolism, cause her to gain weight, and change her nutritional needs. Your nutrition and diet will need to be transformed as you grow, and change throughout your lifetime. Nutrition is never static, and neither are you.

Food is Code

Food communicates directly with all the cells in your body. What you eat and drink isn't just fuel, it's a chemical messenger within you. Your messengers can tell your cells to store or burn fat, preserve or lose muscle, communicate with your nervous system to increase "feel good" hormones, tell inflammation to rage or be calm, and encourage your immune system to be over- or under-active!

The foods that you eat can tell your body: "Hey, we've got enough fuel" or "Hey we need more fuel!" If you eat too much, too little, make poor food choices, or are unable to digest and absorb your food efficiently, this then impacts your energy, motivation, stress, sleep, libido, hormones, digestion, and overall health.

Food also talks to your epigenome (a group of chemical compounds that tell your genes what to do), helping your body turn on or off genes! You heard that right- Food is code! Just like a computer writing code, your body is always writing. Your DNA is being transcribed, translated, and expressed. Every moment and every meal allows you to become a programmer, writing HTML for all your body's functions. If you want a glitching body, write bad code. If you want good health and vitality, write good code. The foods that you eat, your lifestyle, your digestive health, and the inflammation levels in your body all influence your code-writing ability.

The Facts

In the United States, many people are overfed, yet undernourished. Overall food availability isn't scarce, and access to highly palatable, highly processed foods makes it easy for someone to grab hold of high-fat and sugary foods. Think frozen pizzas, Doritos, and McDonald's hamburgers. Cheap, highly processed, and high-calorie foods that not only have low overall nutritive value in regards to vitamin/mineral content, but also ignite the brain's inner reward systems, causing the consumer to go back for more and more. This is where nutrition fails us. This is where the food industry fails us. The truth is- all food is fuel. However, how our body responds to this fuel can either harm or help our health!

Let's go into the basics of what we eat and why quality (not just quantity) matters. Knowing the what's, why's, and how's of nutrition will allow you to not only better decipher through the "jungle of diets," but will also allow you to better understand your body and how it works! Knowledge is power. The more you know about what you eat, the more you can ensure you are fueling your body with what it needs to not just survive, but thrive!

.   .   .

Calories are King

All food is made up of calories. What exactly is a calorie? A calorie is a measurement of energy! The calories in your food, when digested and absorbed into your bloodstream, are used by the cells of your body to create what's called adenosine triphosphate (ATP). This ATP is utilized to perform thousands of functions in your body, and therefore, calories are what give us energy to live, breathe, rebuild tissues, and thrive as humans!

When counting calories and assessing energy needs, nutritional labels use kcals (also known as kilocalories) that in the world of physics just means "the amount of energy required to raise 1 kilogram of water by 1 degree Celsius." For you specifically, it just means fuel for your body and serves as a numerical form of your energy needs! Everyone needs calories to survive, however, calorie needs change based on a variety of factors including activity level, age, sex, height, weight, overall health, as well as hormone levels.

Your ability to maintain, lose, or gain weight is essentially controlled by your basal metabolic rate and total energy expenditure. In general, too many calories over your total energy expenditure produce weight gain, while too little produces weight loss. A net balance of calories in versus calories out is what produces weight maintenance. This control of "calories in vs calories out" is much more complex than just calories themselves, and your metabolism is much more complex than calories in vs calories out! Why?

- Your body is an ever-changing organism, not a car with one set fuel-need and way to run. You have hormones that can increase or decrease your metabolism, specifically thyroid hormone!
- Just because you eat a calorie, does not mean that you properly digest and absorb it.
- Calories are not created equal. Yes- all calories are technically equal, as all measures of energy are equal,

however the nutrients that come from the calories you eat differ in quality, digestibility, and can have different impacts on your immune response.

The Pieces Factored Into Calculating Calorie Needs:

The amount of calories you need depends on several factors including age, gender, activity level, height, and weight. Your needs are also impacted by diet history, hormones, and overall health status. I am going to walk you through how to estimate your calorie needs for maintenance step-by-step, but I want you to keep in mind that this will be just an estimation. No calorie calculators will be perfect, even in a clinical setting. I am sure you have seen hundreds of calculators on the internet, and I promise, they won't ever be spot on. They don't know your history of yo-yo dieting, under-eating, the medications you take, or your health concerns that may greatly impact your needs. Use this as a guide, and then you can adjust based on how your body responds!

Let's start with the *what*. In order to calculate your calories, you need to understand the components of the equation that yield your total daily energy expenditure (aka TDEE). These include your BMR, NEAT, and TEF.

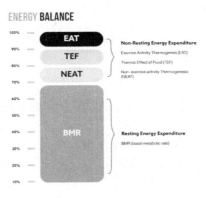

ENERGY BALANCE

EAT
TEF
NEAT

Non-Resting Energy Expenditure
Exercise Activity Thermogenesis (EAT)
Thermic Effect of Food (TEF)
Non-exercise activity Thermogenesis (NEAT)

BMR

Resting Energy Expenditure
BMR (basal metabolic rate)

Your BMR

We each need a certain amount of calories per day to survive. This amount is known as your basal metabolic rate, or BMR. Your BMR is the amount of energy that you need to survive lying down all day in bed. Basically, it's how many calories you need to just survive as a human while doing absolutely nothing. Your BMR makes up about 60-75% of your TDEE and in general, it depends on your body weight, height, age, and lean body mass (aka muscle mass).

Your BMR can change based on any disease state (such as hypothyroidism, HIV, cancer), illness (such as strep throat or the flu), infection, injury (such as a broken leg or burn), and even medications. It also can be affected by caloric restriction, as the body will downregulate to preserve energy. This is what is referred to as metabolic adaptation. In simple terms, metabolic adaptation is your body's survival response to dieting. It does not want to diet! Your body will decrease hormones (such as your sex hormones and thyroid hormones) in an attempt to maintain body weight and survive. These changes can lower your metabolic rate and BMR, which is why, as you diet, you have to continue to drop food or add cardio in order to lose weight. Not only do you lose body fat that burns calories, lowering your BMR, but your body's metabolic thermostat is downregulated.

Good news is you can help negate metabolic adaptation. In the coming chapters, I will dive into this!

Your NEAT

NEAT, or non-exercise activity thermogenesis, includes activities that you do that are not workout or exercise activity. These include activities such as walking throughout the day, playing with your kids, cleaning, making dinner, using the stairs to get to work, or random fidgeting. Your NEAT can significantly impact your

TDEE and is one of my favorite tools for manipulating caloric burn without adding intense exercise. NEAT can range from 300 up to 1000 calories, depending on the person.

I am sure you have seen fitness step trackers used as a way to help increase activity during the day. Daily steps add up and increasing your step count is a great way to increase your NEAT! Though step trackers are far from accurate, they are a useful tool to help motivate an increased step count and NEAT activity. The more steps done, the higher your potential NEAT. Don't get it twisted and go out with a bang on your step count, but aiming for at least 10,000 steps a day may be a way to help keep your NEAT higher.

NEAT is the most common neglected component of energy balance, and many times is not taken into account with online calculators. NEAT is also heavily impacted by dieting and influenced by metabolic adaptation, as the body naturally tries to reduce NEAT levels to preserve energy. Your body will try to "cheat" and conserve its energy. Commonly in dieting, this results in taking fewer walks, not taking the stairs, doing less cleaning, or lessening general subconscious movements. On the other hand, as someone adds food into their life, they may notice enhanced NEAT and want to walk more, dance to music, or explore. This is the body adapting again, but this time in a positive manner!

Therefore, maintaining NEAT levels and knowing where your NEAT levels are is a powerful way to stay on top of your daily TDEE, and can be helpful to further manage your daily total calorie burn, fat loss, or muscle gain goals.

Your TEF

TEF (thermic effect of eating) is the amazing component of your TDEE that includes the calories that you burn from eating. Yes, that's right. You burn calories eating. It takes energy to digest your food and extract the calories from it. About 10% of your TDEE comes from your TEF. Though you can't adjust this much, some foods do require more energy to break down, increasing the caloric burn when eating. For example, it takes more energy to digest an ounce of almonds than it does to digest two tablespoons of almond butter. Why? Your stomach has to break down the almonds more, while the almond butter is already partially broken down and more readily absorbable. The breakdown of your food requires energy! In general, foods higher in fiber and protein have a higher TEF. Whole foods also typically have a higher TEF than those that are ultra-processed.

Your Physical Activity

Your physical activity (PA) includes planned workouts, which may be your weight training, cardio, dance sessions, or yoga. Though fitness trackers can estimate the calories you burn during exercise, they are again far from accurate. How many calories you burn during exercise depends on duration and intensity. It can also depend on the environment, as you will potentially burn more calories in the heat sweating than in a cool and comfortable environment. As you diet, metabolic adaptation will lower the amount of calories burned from physical activity. This is where I like to use NEAT as a strategic way to increase total calories burned without adding significantly more cardio or workouts.

Overall- your calories needs are based on: TDEE = BMR + NEAT + TEF + PA

ENERGY BALANCE

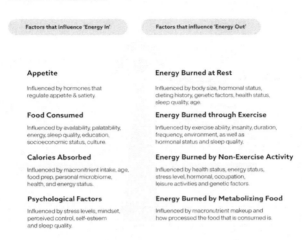

Factors that influence 'Energy In'	Factors that influence 'Energy Out'
Appetite	**Energy Burned at Rest**
Influenced by hormones that regulate appetite & satiety.	Influenced by body size, hormonal status, dieting history, genetic factors, health status, sleep quality, age.
Food Consumed	**Energy Burned through Exercise**
Influenced by availability, palatability, energy, sleep quality, education, socioeconomic status, culture.	Influenced by exercise ability, insanity, duration, frequency, environment, as well as hormonal status and sleep quality.
Calories Absorbed	**Energy Burned by Non-Exercise Activity**
Influenced by macronutrient intake, age, food prep, personal microbiome, health, and energy status.	Influenced by health status, energy status, stress level, hormonal, occupation, leisure activities and genetic factors.
Psychological Factors	**Energy Burned by Metabolizing Food**
Influenced by stress levels, mindset, perceived control, self-esteem and sleep quality.	Influenced by macronutrient makeup and how processed the food that is consumed is.

Your TDEE and overall energy balance can vary day to day based on daily activity, workout intensity, and the foods you eat. As you can see, energy balance is influenced by things out of your control, including changes from metabolic stress, disease, hormones, and trauma. Additional factors that can change your energy expenditure include cold-induced thermogenesis (CIT), which is your body's response to make heat in the cold, growth (such as in childhood or pregnancy), as well as any impact from medications.

Your TDEE will also change as you age and as you go through dieting phases, reverse dieting, or have changes to your health, such as stress, infection, or hormonal imbalances. More on this later and how to adjust!

How to Calculate Your Calories Needs:

My favorite calculator is the Mifflin-St Jeor equation. No equations will be perfect, though I find this is one of the easiest and more accurate calculators to use. You can do this yourself, or use a general handy dandy calculator at: https://www.calculator.net/bmr-calculator.html

Step 1- Calculate your BMR

Sex	Calculation
Men	BMR = (10 × weight in kg) + (6.25 × height in cm) − (5 × age in years) + 5
Women	BMR = (10 × weight in kg) + (6.25 × height in cm) − (5 × age in years) − 161

Step 2- Calculate your Activity Level and Multiply your BMR by it

Activity Level=

- **1.2:** If you are sedentary (little or no exercise) = BMR x 1.2
- **1.375:** If you are lightly active (light exercise/sports 1-3 days/week) = BMR x 1.375
- **1.55:** If you are moderately active (moderate exercise/sports 3-5 days/week) = BMR x 1.55
- **1.725:** If you are very active (hard exercise/sports 6-7 days/week) = BMR x 1.725
- **1.9:** If you are extra active (very hard exercise/sports & physical job or 2x training) = BMR x 1.9

Step 3- Try it out!

Follow your calculated calories for at least 2 weeks. Be consistent. Remember, this is an estimation of your needs. I highly recommend estimating your needs and sticking to these calories for at least two weeks prior to changing. You need to estimate your maintenance calories first before diving into muscle gain or fat loss! How to know if you're in maintenance? Weigh yourself and use measurement tape! If after two weeks you lose weight or inches, you are in what's called a caloric deficit and have found your weight loss calories. If you gained weight or inches, you found what is called a calorie surplus - the calories needed to gain muscle or bodyweight.

You Calculated Maintenance Calories and Found Them- Now What?

This is where you can decide to stay at maintenance, focus on fat loss, reverse diet, or choose to gain muscle or weight. What you choose to do is up to you! Before you set your needs for macronutrients, you need to set your caloric needs first.

Your Caloric Budget

I want you to think about your calorie needs like a budget. If you make $2,000 and spend $2,000, your net balance is zero. This is like your overall metabolism! Calories are like money. You can over- or underspend them.

For example- if you make $2,000 (your TDEE is 2,000 calories), then you can "spend" $2,000 and maintain a zero balance in your bank, or have zero net gain or loss in weight. If you decide to "coupon clip" and save $500 (or 500 calories), then your net balance is now $500 left in your bank of 500 calories unspent. What happens with the unspent calories? That becomes your caloric deficit!

On the other hand, if you go overboard online shopping on Amazon and spend $500 more than you should, your net balance becomes -$500. What does this mean for your weight? This is what puts you into a caloric surplus and can contribute to fat or muscle gain. This is very overgeneralized, but I hope it gives a little perspective to your calorie needs. Just like you have to set a budget for your expenses with inputs and outputs, you have to set a budget for your calorie inputs and outputs as well! This is the beauty of tracking calories (and macros!); you can keep yourself from over- or underspending on your "budget."

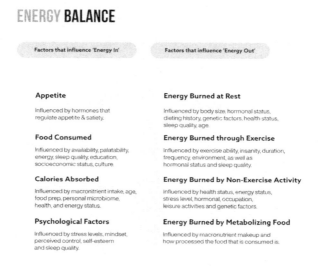

ENERGY BALANCE

Factors that influence 'Energy In'	Factors that influence 'Energy Out'
Appetite Influenced by hormones that regulate appetite & satiety.	**Energy Burned at Rest** Influenced by body size, hormonal status, dieting history, genetic factors, health status, sleep quality, age.
Food Consumed Influenced by availability, palatability, energy, sleep quality, education, socioeconomic status, culture.	**Energy Burned through Exercise** Influenced by exercise ability, insanity, duration, frequency, environment, as well as hormonal status and sleep quality.
Calories Absorbed Influenced by macronutrient intake, age, food prep, personal microbiome, health, and energy status.	**Energy Burned by Non-Exercise Activity** Influenced by health status, energy status, stress level, hormonal, occupation, leisure activities and genetic factors.
Psychological Factors Influenced by stress levels, mindset, perceived control, self-esteem and sleep quality.	**Energy Burned by Metabolizing Food** Influenced by macronutrient makeup and how processed the food that is consumed is.

Changing Calorie Needs Based on Goals

For Fat Loss

First, you need to decide your *rate* of weight loss. I recommend a rate of loss of 0.5 to 1.0% of body weight per week to minimize muscle loss, strength loss, and prevent hormonal disturbances. In general, I like to see a maximum of 2 lbs lost per week. The more you weigh, the more you can lose per week without potential repercussions. Slow and steady wins the race! Remember- a quick weight loss typically results in a quick rebound and increases your chances of losing muscle.

The scale is not all that matters. To measure progress, use a combination of the scale, body measurements, and how your clothes are fitting. The scale will bounce up and down based on markers such as stress, lack of sleep, hormonal changes like during your menstrual cycle, digestion, and changes in your salt and water intake. You want fat loss- not just weight loss, right? Then focus on what matters: changes in your total body composition! Use the scale as one indicator of progress, not the only one. Stay clear from home fitness scales that claim to measure body fat levels because they are largely inaccurate. Instead, if you want to truly measure changes in your body composition, think of doing a DEXA scan every 3-6 months to assess your progress!

If you can afford a dietitian or coach to help you in your journey, I highly suggest hiring one. If not, you can use these general guidelines to help you!

You may have read about the 3500 calorie rule. "3500 calories roughly equals 1 lb of fat. Therefore, if you drop 500 calories per day (500 calories x 7 days a week = 3500 calories), then you'll drop roughly 1 lb per week."

This is an oversimplification of your metabolism and does not account for the changes in your BMR, NEAT, PA, dieting history, individual metabolism, or metabolic adaptation. Though it can be used in general to guide how to create a deficit, it again does not take into account your beautiful and unique self. My suggestion? Start slow. Then adjust as you go.

Want to lose weight faster? Start with a 250 calorie deficit. Not dropping? Drop another 100-250 calories or add in a cardio session.

Want to lose weight more slowly? Start with a 100 calorie deficit. Not dropping? Drop another 100 calories or add in a cardio session.

If you calculated your maintenance at 1750 calories, this may mean consuming 1550-1650 calories as your starting point for weight loss, with maybe 1-2 moderate intensity cardio sessions per week. Didn't lose weight? It may mean you should add another cardio session like 15 minutes of HIIT (high intensity interval training), a moderate intensity session, or LISS (low intensity steady state) to help increase daily caloric burn, or you could drop to 1550 or 1450 calories. Again- go slow. Make baby adjustments. The snail wins the fat loss race.

In the hundreds of clients that I have worked with and helped achieve successful fat loss, I have even seen great rates of consistent weight loss with 100 calorie drops alone. Some people have what I call "adaptive metabolisms" and need larger deficits in order to lose weight (up to 500 calories), but this is where a second eye to help in adjustments and individuality come into play. What macronutrients you drop can also play a potential role. However, metabolic ward studies show that the macronutrient breakdown for the best fat loss does not make a difference as long as calories and protein are equated. In my experience with clients, however, this is not the case, and each person responds differently.

You can adjust your calories to create a calorie or energy deficit by either reducing caloric intake, adding workouts or cardio, increasing NEAT, or a combination of all the above. My suggestion is to make one single adjustment if you can, and to try to keep cardio as low as possible with food intake as high as possible when trying to diet. Why? It will not only help prevent metabolic adaptation and preserve lean muscle mass, but it will also help keep you sane and help in managing hunger and stress levels. Nobody wants a hangry dieter near them. You also don't want to create hormone imbalances for yourself or lose healthy and potentially hard-earned muscle tissue!

Weight Training vs Cardio vs Diet Alone

You need a caloric deficit to lose weight, which you can achieve through diet, workouts, cardio, or a combination of all the above!

So which is best? What matters most? They all do! Your best friend for fat loss and preserving lean muscle is going to be weight training and maximizing the quality of your diet. Not only does weight training help to preserve lean muscle tissue, enhance insulin sensitivity, and increase mitochondrial efficiency, but it will also help to preserve your bones and may also help enhance your cognition! Weight training and cardio may burn the same amount of calories, but the differences in the metabolic benefits to cardio vs weights are fundamental truths you should always remember.

Your truths:

- A consistent calorie deficit is key to losing body fat, but adding regular resistance training into the mix can have a greater impact than diet alone
- Resistance training alone is not sufficient to shed body fat without a calorie deficit, but it can help to increase lean body mass
- When it comes to body recomposition (more information soon on this), resistance training should be incorporated
- Resistance training alone may be an effective tool to lose fat if the body is in a caloric deficit
- Resistance training can help to preserve lean muscle tissue that may be at risk for loss during a caloric deficit
- Diet alone may be sufficient to lose weight, but at the risk of losing muscle mass as well
- Diet plus cardio plus resistance training combined together can be more beneficial for fat loss than one modality alone

What Type of Cardio Is Best?

Cardio type and duration for fat loss should depend on personal preference, cardiovascular endurance, need for recovery, and total health status. You wouldn't want to program in a HIIT sprint session if someone can barely walk for 30 minutes. You also wouldn't plan a long endurance cardio session for someone struggling with an autoimmune disease (in which their body is more susceptible to flares from too much stress). Find what you enjoy doing, what helps you recover the best and feel your best, and what keeps your body happy- including your joints, digestion, and mental health!

LISS (low intensity steady state) or MICT (moderate intensity continuous training) can help increase your daily caloric burn, act as a recovery agent, and limit interference with weight training recovery. However, both can be time consuming. Typical LISS or MICT sessions can vary from 10 to 60 minutes. Examples of LISS include incline walks, swimming, the elliptical, steady rowing, yoga (yes, for some this can count as cardio!), and leisure bike riding. Examples of MICT include: the stairmaster, hiking up hills, steady state runs, or moderate intensity or hilly bike rides.

HIIT (high intensity interval training) is another type of cardio that can be used for fat loss, however special attention must be made to its potential detrimental effects on recovery. HIIT is very taxing on the adrenals, as well as the body as a whole, as it requires more power output and muscle activation. Though HIIT saves time and can alleviate "cardio boredom," HIIT may reduce strength, impair workout recovery, and it relies on the oxidation of carbohydrates for fuel (whereas LISS relies more on fat oxidation). True HIIT is typically performed in 15-20 seconds of all-out intensity activity, with 45 seconds to 1 minute of rest for a total of 10 to 15 min. If done correctly, you should not be able to sustain HIIT for longer than 15 minutes. A small but potentially significant benefit to HIIT comes from the slight increase in metabolic rate that occurs afterwards. This metabolic rate increase does not happen with LISS or MICT. Does this mean you should do HIIT? Not necessarily. HIIT will hinder your recovery and add more stress to your system than a lower intensity session.

Your cardio choice should be made mostly by personal preference and the time you have available. LISS, MICT, and HIIT provide similar benefits on body fat reduction when the caloric burn is equated, and the choice of either type of cardio also does not appear to affect energy intake throughout the day (though some people find that one type may make them hungrier later on in the day than others). What may play a potential role, however, is how exercise intensity and duration change the selection of the fuel source used by the body. This may or may not make a big difference in the scheme of fat loss, however I still would like you to have the background information.

What do I mean by fuel source use? Higher intensity, short duration activities use an ATP (aka energy) system that relies on anaerobic metabolism. Essentially, your body in these short spouts of activity such as HIIT, cardio, or CrossFit will rely mostly on your body's carbohydrate "bank" that includes the glucose in your blood or glucose from your muscle and liver glycogen stores. During these activities, your body's preferred method of fuel is carbohydrates.

During lower intensity or longer duration activity, such as walking, distance running, swimming, general weight training, or biking, your body relies more on fat for energy. Why is this? The time goes on, your body switches from using up liver glycogen stores and blood glucose for energy, and switches to use plasma free fatty acids and muscle triglycerides. Basically, you rely more on fat oxidation for energy than carbohydrate oxidation. However, more fat oxidation does not necessarily mean more fat loss.

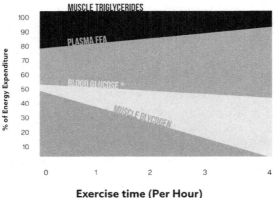

Exercise time (Per Hour)

What about fasted cardio? Fasted cardio does not have any benefits over fed cardio and can be detrimental if you are trying to preserve muscle mass or if you have adrenal imbalances. Why is this? Fasted cardio forces your body to rely on muscle and liver glycogen. If these sources become depleted, you are at risk for muscle loss.

What about cardio timing? My suggestion is performing all cardio AFTER resistance training to ensure all energy and strength is utilized in the weight training prior. Some people like to break up their workouts into a lifting or yoga session and cardio session. Do what works with your schedule and helps you perform your best. Be sure to choose cardio that is easy on your joints, allows you to recover in between sessions, and is something you can somehow enjoy!

Final note on fat loss: keep in mind again, your BMR, NEAT, and PA will downregulate as you diet and lose weight. You will need to adjust your fat loss calories, and/or your workouts, cardio, and NEAT. As you lose weight, your body will need fewer and fewer calories, and will burn fewer and fewer calories. This is why it can continue to be harder to lose weight the longer you diet, and why it can be hard to maintain weight loss post-diet, as your maintenance calories are now lowered. (A great reason to reverse diet post-diet!)

Why You Aren't Losing Weight

Let me step on my soapbox real fast. Weight loss is hard. There are genuine reasons why you can not be losing weight that may truly be out of your control, such as a hormonal imbalance, hypothyroidism, cortisol dysregulation, or even a metabolic abnormality.

However- and I know I'm not going to be everyone's favorite person with this statement, but here it goes- for MOST PEOPLE, the reason you aren't losing weight is not because of your hormones, thyroid, or cortisol. It's because you aren't really in a caloric deficit and you're not being consistent.

Whether that's because you are:

- Not tracking accurately (or not tracking your intake at all)
- Being consistent over the week but blowing it on the weekends
- Not sleeping enough
- Stressed to the max and burning your candle at both ends
- Eating highly processed foods and not enough micronutrients
- Not pushing enough in the gym to grow the muscle you want to see
- Subconsciously reducing your NEAT levels, dropping your daily TDEE and pulling you out of a deficit

THESE are the top reasons you're not losing weight.

Y'all know I am team functional nutrition and am ALL about balancing hormones, cortisol, gut health, thyroid, etc. Half of my book is on these topics. I work with clients on a day-to-day basis fixing these things that are REAL STRUGGLES for them, their health, and their physique goals. I post about how these struggles can impact your goals. BUT- I want to emphasize that for MANY people, the issue is actually quite simple. Most people need accountability, consistency, and patience- they don't need any "hormone balancing" protocol. If you have conquered the above, you're consistent, and you're truly taking every step to take care of your health through the foods you eat, fixing your sleep and stress, putting the effort in, and THEN still not losing weight... that's when you can start blaming hormonal and cortisol influences. I hope you still love me.

How to Lose the Fat and Keep It Off?

That's the magical question I know you want answered. The hard truth is that you will have to sustain your workouts and NEAT or the pounds will pack back on. You will need to continue to monitor your food intake or the pounds will pack back on. Especially since post-diet, your fat cells are primed to gain the weight back.

When you lose weight or body fat, you actually lose the lipid content within your fat cells. You can't get rid of those cells! They only shrink. Post-diet, those cells are ready to fill back up again with fat.

Your body was not made to diet. It was made to survive. If you were dieting before and then all of a sudden there was food available, the first thing your body would try to do is attempt to try to store it for future use. In a way, your body goes into full "let's hibernate!" mode. This is a survival response. The more you activate this survival response (especially with chronic yo-yo dieting), the more the body will activate its survival response as well. There is evidence that shows that the more you weight cycle or yo-yo diet, the more difficult it can become to lose weight, and the more weight you end up gaining over time.

This is where many people end up: grinding and grinding (and grinding into the ground) with little food and lots of exercise, yet producing no results! Your body says "NOPE!" Hormones deplete, your metabolic rate goes down, hunger hormones climb, and you end up spinning your wheel with no return on your "investment."

Weight loss being hard to maintain sucks, but in reality, it's your body trying to help you, not harm you. Remember that! I highly recommend after a dieting phase to reverse diet by slowly weaning down your workout and/or cardio training and slowly increasing your food intake. See the section on reverse dieting for more information. Working with a dietitian or coach can be extremely helpful to sustain fat loss and continue any habit changes you made in the process.

True diet success and keeping the weight off comes from sustaining habit changes and preventing post-diet regain. This requires manipulating the hormonal adaptations that occur with dieting as best as you can.

Remember these principles of metabolic adaptation:

- Dieting decreases your BMR as thyroid and sex hormones drop
- The calories you burn from PA go down as you lose weight (less mass to require energy)
- Your NEAT drops down with dieting and less body weight, further lowering your TDEE
- Hunger hormones go up as a safety mechanism, making it harder to eat less

REALITY: WEIGHT LOSS PROGRAMS

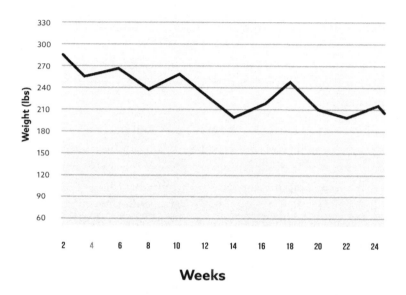

But- "Diets Don't Work"

Yes, they do - when done in a healthy, sustainable manner and when the body is not stressed and hormones are optimized. Most "diets" do *not* work because they are unrealistic. They set you up for failure from the get-go. They don't tell you how to continue your weight loss or what to do after the diet. Take the South Beach Diet, for example. Cool- they give you food that puts you into a caloric deficit. But what happens as your BMR goes down and your body needs less food? What happens after the diet? Do you know what to do? Are you told how to change your diet to maintain your new weight loss? No. There is no game plan, accountability, or nutrition education. You are left lost and alone and *hangry*.

I don't believe everyone needs to diet. I also believe that our bodies truly do have a "set point" that they like to stay at. However, to simply say "diets don't work" is false. Millions of people have been able to successfully lose weight in this world and have also been able to keep it off.

For Reverse Dieting

I know you are asking "what is reverse dieting". You got questions, I got answers! You may have heard "reversing" as being a way to "eat more without gaining weight", or "eat more to lose weight". I hate to burst your bubble, but though it can do both, it's not meant to. Reverse dieting is a methodical way of slowly increasing calories and lowering cardio to help bring the body's metabolism and hormones back to a healthier homeostasis.

Here's the truth about reversing- it's not meant for everyone, and it doesn't promise any specific outcome.

Benefits to reverse dieting may include:

- More food intake
- Higher energy levels
- Improvements to your metabolism
- Improvements to sleep & stress levels
- Ability to lose weight at higher calories in the future
- Improvements to your menstrual cycle, thyroid, and adrenal health
- Less restriction and food focus
- Less cardio and more time to do what you love
- Increased strength and gym performance
- Better mood and libido
- Increased TEF (thermic effect of food), and increased NEAT (non exercise thermogenesis), therefore increasing

the amount of food you can eat while maintaining your body weight

Is this you? If so, you may be a candidate for reverse dieting:

- You have been in a dieting phase for more than 3 months and stalling, despite refeeds and diet breaks
- You are starting to see signs and symptoms of a hormonal imbalance despite being in a mild deficit or maintenance calories
- You're always hunger, energy is low, sleep and recovery are suboptimal, and your motivation is trash
- You have reached your goal physique or goal weight and you're ready to focus on maintaining or adding back in more food
- You have been yo-yo dieting for months to years and can't seem to see progress

Remember- dieting causes down regulation of your thyroid, sex, and leptin hormone through metabolic adaptation, which leads to drops in TEF, NEAT, and your BMR. By doing a reverse dieting phase post diet, you can help to mitigate the metabolic adaptation and negative hormonal consequences of dieting. In fact, you can use metabolic adaptation now to your advantage (whether you were dieting or just choose to jump into a reverse) How? As you increase calories and food, your TEF and NEAT will increase, allowing you to expend more calories on daily basis, increase your workout intensity and capacity, and raise your BMR. Metabolic adaptation goes both way- it can help and harm you. Use it to your advantage with reverse dieting!

Why reverse diet post dieting? What you do NOT want to do post diet is just go back to eating what you were eating before your diet. Cue unwanted, and uncontrolled fat gain. Remember, dieting decreases your metabolism, dysregulates your hunger hormones, and sets you up for the creation of new fat cells. You need to work your way back up to your previous food intake if you want to maintain your weight loss efforts or maintain your current body composition. Post diet you can not trust your hunger cues. However, you can trust other biofeedback and objective data, including weight and measurements.

Fact- There is no single reverse dieting protocol. Get that out of your heard first, and please, don't you dare compare someone else's reverse diet success to your own. How someone responds to a reverse diet is largely individualized. Some people may gain weight reversing, others may lose weight, others may maintain! How quickly someone can increase their food or decrease their cardio is also individualized. What matters is reversing and listening to your own biofeedback. To have a successful reverse, you should be looking at changes in your body weight, measurements, mood, sleep, digestion, motivation levels, and workout recovery.

Reverse dieting requires consistency, adherence, and tracking (for best accuracy). It's not for the faint of heart or for those that struggle with disordered eating. It requires carefully monitoring and tracking your macronutrients and/or calories or portion sizes. It can be stressful, hard, and require lots of planning ahead, however just like any goal, there are benefits and drawbacks. I hope if you choose to reverse, you no what you are getting into and are ready to commit to the process, and yourself!

What rate of reversing is best? If you go too quickly adding food- you may gain more weight than you would like. If you go snail slow, you may continue to live with negative symptoms and may delay improvements in your health (and happiness!).

As a general rule, you want to move as quickly as you can getting food up and cardio down while maintaining overall bodyweight to help alleviate symptoms, refuel your metabolism, and mitigate excess body fat. In general, a successful reverse will allow you to add from 250-750 calories to your day, while maintaining your bodyweight (or even losing weight!) within 1-10 lbs.

I suggest following these 3 tips to get started reverse dieting:

1. Establish your maintenance calories. If you were dieting, up your foot right away to an estimated maintenance (a good 100-250 calories up is a good start). If you were undereating, you may have to bump this even to 500 more calories. Find what caloric and macro intake you can maintain for 2 weeks without adjustments. Portion sizing with your hands may be used if you don't track, however this is not best for accuracy.
2. Bump your food first by about 50-100 calories and wait till you maintain for a full week to add more. I suggest not changing your protein intake if you can- instead, add carbs or fat!
3. Track your progress with a coach, app, or spreadsheet. Look at your biofeedback and symptoms, your measurements, bodyweight, and physique photos. If you are like me an overthink things, have someone there to be your second eye. Don't get stuck in the "spinning your wheels" part of reversing due to fear of increasing too quickly or too slowly. Ask for help!

When to go faster or slower with your reverse?

Faster	Slower
You are losing weight	You are gaining weight too quickly
You are maintaining weight well with the current changes	Your weight does not stabilize after adjustments when changes are not made in a 2 week time frame
Your hunger is up or you are food focused	You have poor consistency and adherence
Your workout recovery is poor	You have a sluggish metabolism or hypothyroidism
You have a higher NEAT level	You are in peri menopause or menopause (with heightened insulin resistance)
You don't have a significant history of dieting	You have a history of chronic dieting or yo-yo dieting

Below is an example of a protocol for reverse dieting.

Start: 45F/140C/140P – 5 days of LISS cardio at 30 min

Week 1: 45F/155C/140P- 5 days of LISS cardio at 30 min

Week 2: 50F/160C/140P- 5 days of LISS cardio at 30 min

Week 3: 50F/160C/140P- 4 days of LISS cardio at 30 min

Week 4: 50F/175C/140P- 3 days of LISS cardio at 30 min

Week 5: 50F/175C/140P- 3 days of LISS cardio at 30 min

Week 6: 50F/185C/140P- 3 days of LISS cardio at 25 min

Week 7: 50F/200C/140P- 3 days of LISS cardio at 25 min

Week 8: 53F/200C/140P- 3 days of LISS cardio at 20 min

Week 9: 55F/210C/140P- 3 days of LISS cardio at 15 min

Week 10: 55F/220C/140P- 3 days of LISS cardio at 15 min

There is largely no rhyme or reason for your choice or increasing fat or carbohydrate or pattern/cardio adjustments made. In working with my clients, I always pay close attention to not only how their physique looks and responds, weight changes, but also what they are preferring to change. Someone may want to lower cardio one week vs add in food. Another may want to add more food. When it comes down to what macro component to add, the most important things to address are:

1. State of insulin sensitivity- the more insulin resistant someone is, the more fat you should increase vs carbohydrates
2. History of dieting- if someone has a history of undereating or having lower fats, then the first step should be to bring these back to a healthier level to support healthy hormones

3. Training type and intensity- higher volume and more intense training relies on glucose vs fatty acids for fuel. Increasing carbohydrates will help to fuel workouts and replenish muscle glycogen. The increase of carbohydrates will also be likely less stored as body fat, as long as insulin resistance is not present

4. Personal preference- some people may want more fats in their diet vs carbohydrates. What someone can stick to with a reverse should come first, as sustainability in a reverse diet and consistency is key to success!

When reversing, try not freak out if you gain a few pounds in a week with adding food or decreasing calories. If you do after following your change for that week, wait another week. If you continue to gain weight after that week, then don't make an adjustment. Stay steady. If you lost that weight and fall back into your previous weight, then think of adding another food bump or lowering cardio even more. Expect weight fluctuations with reversing, especially since adding food increases glycogen levels with adding carbohydrates (which hold on to water). In addition, your body will natural ebb and flow in weight with changes in sleep, stress levels, salt or fiber intake, changes to digestion (hello constipation weight gain from poop babies!), or throughout your menstrual cycle.

The most important part of reverse dieting is adherence. The end goal should be: feeling strong, fed, and nourished, optimized hormones, a normal menstrual cycle, stable week for 3-4 weeks, and a ballpark of at least 1800 calories eaten during the day.

There is no limit on how high you can go reversing as long as you feel comfortable and confident continuing. However, you will find that you will reach a "set point" where any food further may lead to strictly fat gain. This (or the development of insulin resistance), is a sign to stop! From there, you can focus on maintaining your current plan or choose to dive into another weight loss phase when you're ready.

For Gaining Muscle or Weight

When it comes down to gaining muscle, you first have to make sure you are:

1. Training intensely with a progressive overload-focused resistance training program
2. Eating sufficiently for muscle growth (most need at least a small caloric surplus)
3. Optimizing recovery from workouts (as growth can't occur if recovery doesn't occur)

Your ability to gain muscle will depend on your ability to progress in the gym (or at home)! You don't need fancy equipment or even dumbbells, but to maximize your weight training and muscle gain, a combination of dumbbells, barbells, and cables or band-work is best. If you want a comprehensive weight training program, you can directly download one for beginners or advanced training on my website for free! The program will also dive into the fundamentals of resistance training and how to ensure progressive overload. Need or want a custom training program? Feel free to email me or reach out to me and my team directly through my website.

So, you need resistance training of some sort to build muscle- but what about calories? How fast should you gain weight and how many calories should you increase? There are a couple scenarios here to keep in mind. These largely depend on your training experience or "training age," BMR, and diet history.

If your goal is to maximize your muscle gains and minimize fat gains, the most important thing to remember is that the faster you gain weight, the more fat gain you may potentially add. Just like fat loss, slow and steady is the way to go! It is very easy to add excess body fat overall (unless you struggle with a very high metabolism, hyperthyroidism, or malabsorption issues). My suggestion for how many calories to increase and how quickly to gain weight largely depends on your training level or "training age." These suggestions have been adapted based on *The Muscle and Strength Pyramids* by Eric Helms.

TRAINING LEVEL OR "AGE"	DEFINITION	RATE OF MONTHLY WEIGHT GAIN
Beginner	New to weight training in the first year- able to progress most training loads in the gym on a week-to-week basis	1 to 1.5% of body weight
Intermediate	Have lifted for 2-3 years- able to progress most training loads in the gym on a month-to-month basis	0.5 to 1% of body weight
Advanced	Have lifted for 3+ years- able to progress in weights month-to-month or every few months depending on training regimen and training cycle	Up to 0.5% of body weight

*Chart from Helms E, Morgan A, Valdez A. The Muscle & Strength Pyramid: Nutrition. San Bernardino, CA: Muscle and Strength Pyramids; 2019.

The calories that you need in order to match this rate of gain largely depend on your TDEE, diet history, and hormonal health status. Summed up in the next chart are my general recommendations based on training age to gain muscle and minimize fat gain. Keep in mind that this will be largely individual, and just like fat loss, and one person may need a significantly larger amount of calories to gain muscle (or weight) than another.

Make sure to stay away from the mindset of the 3500 calorie rule. 500 extra calories a day x 7 days a week does not mean you will gain 1 lb of muscle per week when eating in a surplus. It also doesn't mean you only need to add 250 calories per day to gain only 0.5 lb muscle per week. Again, this rule doesn't take into account your individual needs, training, metabolism, or hormones. Stick to assessing your overall body composition markers and strength improvements to ensure muscle is being built. Notice your weight climbing too quickly? Drop your calories a bit, add some NEAT such as an extra 1,000 steps a day, or add a fun 10-20 min cardio session. Adjust in baby steps. The next chart includes my recommendations for a slow, lean muscle gain.

For example- if you are a 150 lb female and a beginner to weight training, your estimated maintenance may be 1750 calories. To gain lean muscle, you would then add 150-250 calories per day. If advanced, you may decide to add 100 calories per day. Keep in mind, any changes in your activity levels, NEAT, or hormones may change your calorie needs.

Experience Level:	Calories Above Maintenance for Lean Muscle Gain
Beginner	1–1.5%/month = about 150–250 kcals/day
Intermediate	0.5–1%/month = about 100–200 kcals/day
Advanced	Very slight increase up to 100 kcals/day

*Chart from Helms E, Morgan A, Valdez A. The Muscle & Strength Pyramid: Nutrition. San Bernardino, CA: Muscle and Strength Pyramids; 2019. *

If you are a nerd like me, you are probably wondering, WHY? Why can beginners eat more food and gain more muscle and less fat than advanced trainees? This is because as you advance in your training career, your ability to gain muscle falls due to lower muscle protein synthesis and a lower anabolic (muscle building) response to training. Essentially, your body becomes more efficient at recovering and your anabolic response to weight training diminishes.

Rises in muscle protein synthesis, aka MPS, are what is required to build muscle! Not only that, but in your "newbie" days, your body is hyper-responsive to a stimulus and less adaptive to recovering. You require less overload, tension, and "trauma" to muscle to make it grow. This is because when you train, your muscle cells develop myonuclei, which are like energy boxes. These energy boxes help you progressively overload your muscles, becoming bigger and stronger.

However, as you continue to train, these muscle cells become more resistant to muscle damage and have to work even harder to stimulate what are called satellite cells. These satellite cells help your muscle energy boxes to heal, repair, and grow! Less satellite cell recruitment means less muscle growth. Your muscles have to work harder in order to stimulate them. This is only one piece of the muscle building puzzle, but it serves as one reason why advanced training programs are more intense and include different techniques variables compared to a simple beginner program. Beginners don't need as much intensity to produce growth. They have the advantage of their MPS spikes and satellite cells.

The changes in MPS from a beginner to an advanced trainee change from elevations for up to 72 hours, to elevations for a mere 12-24 hours. This essentially means that as you advance in training, you develop fewer opportunities to build muscle tissue within your MPS window post-exercise. In addition, your training requirements for building muscle increase as your body becomes more efficient at adapting to training. This is when the "repeated bout effect" comes into play.

The repeated bout effect essentially means that your body becomes accustomed to a set training load and intensity, and is no longer stimulated by it. Think about it- those 20 lb dumbbells may be difficult to press at the beginning and produce new muscle gains, but as time goes by and they become easier to press, your body no longer has to work as hard to recover from the movement and your muscles are less stimulated and less "damaged" by your training. Lack of stimulation means lack of adaptation. Lack of adaptation, and you don't have muscle growth! This is where progressive overload comes into play to ensure that a stimulus continues to be placed on your body to enforce adaptation.

Progressive overload with intensity will always be the crucial aspect, along with sufficient calories for producing muscle growth. You just become more efficient at recovering from overload and less efficient at stimulating MPS as you train over the years. Overall- you become more efficient in the gym, less efficient at growing.

Want to be a little more aggressive and ensure you are building muscle and not worried about fat gain? That's where you can add more food into your life! Keep in mind, however, gaining weight faster doesn't mean gaining muscle faster. If you gain too much fat while attempting to gain muscle, you can also push yourself into insulin resistance. No bueno! You'll learn more about this later.

Experience Level:	Calories Above Maintenance for Lean Muscle Gain
Beginner	1–1.5%/month = about 150–250 kcals/day
Intermediate	0.5–1%/month = about 100–200 kcals/day
Advanced	Very slight increase up to 100 kcals/day

*Chart from Helms E, Morgan A, Valdez A. The Muscle & Strength Pyramid: Nutrition. San Bernardino, CA: Muscle and Strength Pyramids; 2019. *

Overall, focus on increasing your calories slowly and steadily. What macronutrients should you increase to minimize fat gain? What an excellent question and the answer to which everyone wants to know! We will cover more about this in the macronutrient section.

For Body Recomposition

Who can achieve body recomposition? In the beginning stages of weight training or after a long time off of weight training (4 months to years), the "beginner gains" or "muscle memory gains" can occur. During this time, you may be able to gain muscle more quickly with less body fat gain at the same calories compared to an advantaged "aged" trainee. You may even be able to build muscle and lose fat at the same time- known as body recomposition! The magic of body recomposition lies in a combination of nutrition at maintenance, a mild deficit or slight surplus, a high protein intake, and the proper progressive overload resistance training program.

The ability to "recomp" your body also depends on your ability to manage sleep, stress, and your nutrition quality! You CAN lose fat and gain muscle at the same time, but this "recomp" requires dedication, consistency, and hard work. Scenarios that set you up for being more likely to recomp include: being a beginner to weight training, obese individuals, those coming off a training hiatus or time off, those on anabolic steroids (10/10 don't recommend), and meticulous advanced trainers on a progressive overload plan with nutrition on point.

Calorie needs? Aim for a 50-100 calorie deficit or maintenance. Watch closely for strength improvements in the gym, changes in your body measurements, and monitor your weight and how your clothes fit. Body recomposition, in my experience, is the hardest to measure and the hardest to do, therefore I suggest having a second eye, whether it's a dietitian, online coach, or even a friend to help keep you objective. Let's be real- we all have glasses on and don't see ourselves the way we should- we tend to be our worst critics!

For Maintenance

Though it may seem straightforward, your maintenance calories can and will change! Just because you can maintain your body weight and physique at one caloric intake does not mean that you will be able to in the future. Especially as you age or go through additional dieting phases. Sad truth- the older you get, the slower your metabolism becomes, and naturally, the lower your maintenance calories will be. Another sad truth- the more you diet and yo-yo back and forth between a calorie deficit and surplus, the more adaptive your metabolism can become (and the more your hormones can take a negative hit!). Sometimes changes in your maintenance levels can be as simple as changes in your physical activity or NEAT levels. Maybe you started a higher intensity training program or went on many walks on vacation. Sometimes the changes are outside of your control, such as a boost in metabolism from being sick with a fever or having an injury. Your body is not stagnant and your metabolism will never be either. Just like you are constantly aging (dayum, that truth is real), your metabolism is constantly changing.

If your goal is to maintain your body weight or physique, I suggest weighing yourself at least once every few weeks and monitoring how your clothes are fitting. Gaining weight or clothes becoming tighter? Your maintenance may be lower. Losing weight and clothes becoming looser? Your maintenance may be higher. These changes may be from choices you made that affected your TDEE, or they may be due to alterations in hormones that are out of your control!

I commonly hear, "I used to be able to eat X amount and not gain any weight" or "I haven't changed my diet at all, but now I am rapidly gaining weight!" These changes can happen due to shifts in your metabolic rate, NEAT levels, or both! Your weight gain could be as simple as aging and decreasing your metabolic rate, or it could be something more- such as hypothyroidism, estrogen dominance, or insulin resistance contributing to changes in your total energy balance. Your random weight loss may be stress-induced, caused by illness, or from a condition such as hyperthy-roidism, a tumor, or malabsorption of your food. Either way, you can't rely on your maintenance being the same forever. It will change. Just like you change! If you notice random weight gain or loss without changes in your lifestyle, activity, or diet, I highly recommend seeking out a registered dietitian (like me!) or another healthcare professional. Better safe than sorry- and you deserve to feel in control of your own body!!

Why You Need Maintenance Periods?

I'm a HUGE fan of using maintenance periods with my clients & find they are the true game changers for maximizing the metabolism and helping in rebalancing hormones.

· · ·

I use maintenance periods for clients to:

1. Help establish a new "set point" for those building lean muscle to prevent unnecessary fat gain (I also use mini cuts for this). Building for too long can decrease insulin sensitivity & lead to too much fat gain over muscle gain.
2. Prevent metabolic adaptation that occurs during weight loss. What happens? BMR, NEAT, Leptin, reproductive & thyroid hormones go down while cortisol & ghrelin (your hunger hormone) go up). NOT GOOD FOR HORMONES. With maintenance periods- the focus is on maintaining your progress while getting calories & energy up. If find this is the PERFECT scenario when rebalancing hormones & helping with hormonal chaos or digestive distress. (Some coaches may use "diet breaks" for preventing adaptation - a maintenance period lasts a few months- not a week or two like a diet break.)
3. Prime for a building phase after a fat loss phase. This prevents fat overshooting that can occur after a fat loss period if you jump calories up too quickly. Enforcing maintenance also helps to regulate hormone & hunger levels! Dieting can heavily unregulate hunger cues- which if not controlled via tracking- can cause one to overshoot calories & regain fat they lost.
4. Give the mind a break from tracking & allow increased flexibility. For some clients-a caloric goal is set vs macros with a focus on maintaining & listening to the body over a macro goal
5. Allow the HPA (hypothalamic pituitary axis) time to regulate after a period of chronic stress or during a digestive treatment protocol. Overfeeding or underfeeding with a cortisol or gut imbalance is a recipe for continued or worsened issues.

What is important when doing maintenance periods? At first-tracking consistently & weighing a few times a week to ensure maintenance is important. After that, I find reducing weigh ins & focusing on how you look and feel overall with special attention to biofeedback is crucial.

As you are in maintenance, if you notice drops in energy & strength, sleep issues, or worsening periods, you may need more food or more time for recovery! Feeling good & photos looking the same? Average weight steady? No need to change a thing. Or, can slightly bump up food if your long term goal is building your metabolic capacity!

Why You Plateau?

Plateaus are a natural response to dieting and are largely due to metabolic adaptation. With dieting, decreases in BMR, NEAT, and PA lead to decreases in TDEE, taking you out of a negative energy balance or caloric deficit. Not only that, but you have several hormonal adaptations that contribute to your plateau as well. These include drops in thyroid hormones, sex hormones, leptin, and increases in ghrelin and cortisol.

These hormonal adaptations are actually what is most responsible for the downregulation of your BMR when dieting.

You may be asking- what is leptin? Leptin is the hormone made in your fat cells that functions as a thermostat to maintain your body weight and body fat levels. It essentially tells your body what your energy balance looks like, as well as creates a feeling of fullness after eating, and assists in glucose regulation and fatty acid utilization. When you diet and body fat decreases, leptin levels also decrease. This can lead to increased hunger, but also tells the body that energy availability is low.

What happens? Your body's leptin levels drop, and your thermostat tells your body that there is low food availability. Cue a plateau!

Decreases In:	Increases In:
Leptin (Metabolic Thermostat)	Ghrelin (Hunger hormone)
Thyroid Hormone	Cortisol
Sex Hormones (estrogen, progesterone, testosterone)	
NEAT	
Insulin	
TDEE	

Breaking a Plateau- Refeeds:

If you are dieting but not using refeeds strategically, you're missing out! A refeed is a strategic period of feeding, aimed at eliciting a hormonal response to help mitigate metabolic adaptation when dieting. A refeed involves specifically increasing your carbohydrate intake within a period of 1-3 days, while staying roughly at or slightly above maintenance calories. A refeed is best done consecutively during a 48 hour to 72-hour period (a total of 2-3 days). One-day refeeds may not elicit this same response (though it can be psychologically beneficial)- so please keep this in mind.

Why carbohydrates? It appears that leptin responds mostly to carbohydrate intake, and not with the increase and overfeeding of fat or protein. Carbohydrates not only help leptin in this case, but they also assist with the conversion of your T4 to T3!

A refeed is essentially an aid for dieting and helps "prime" for continued progress. There is very little data on refeeds, but I have found them to be game-changers for helping to prevent plateaus and mitigate the metabolic adaptation response to dieting. Whether you need a refeed or not depends on how you look (flat, depleted), feel (sluggish, fatigued), and how long you've been dieting! Remember to not use the scale as your sole indicator of progress- you also need to assess how you look and feel. The scale does not indicate any changes in body composition.

You do not need a refeed if you just started dieting or if you are in a gaining phase. Additionally, refeeds are NOT cheat meals or untracked meals. They are planned and strategic. Want an untracked meal? Do it. However I don't believe in cheat meals. Eating food is never "cheating." Food is fuel.

Refeed General Guidelines:

- Keep calories at maintenance
- Aim for 1.5-2x your daily carbohydrate intake
- Plan one every 3-4 weeks or when you see or notice plateaus or have significant increases in water retention, fatigue, and trouble sleeping

Refeeds will not always work. If your hormones have taken such a hit that your body refuses to lose weight or lose body fat, then you need to stop dieting and put your health over your physique goals. Trashing your hormones is never worth it.

Macros 101

The calories in your food come from their building blocks of varying macronutrients, or "macros" as many call them- aka protein, fat, and carbohydrates! Each macronutrient contains a set amount of calories listed below:

- Protein: 4 calories per gram
- Carbohydrates: 4 calories per gram
- Fat: 9 calories per gram
- Alcohol: 7 calories per gram

All the foods that you eat on a daily basis have differing amounts, as well as ratios, of macronutrients. Some people count their daily calories or macros consumed each day as a way to lose weight, gain muscle, or maintain their physique. This has been deemed as "flexible dieting," and allows for one to better control their intake of energy to control their metabolism or body composition.

Tracking macros can allow for furthered individualization of the diet, as some people, such as those with insulin resistance, may benefit from a lowered carbohydrate intake and this higher fat to carbohydrate macro ratio. More on insulin resistance later!

I personally love and track macronutrients myself, however "macro tracking" is not for everyone and 100% not needed to maintain a healthy body! In fact, tracking for some can become an obsessive habit and lead to disordered patterns of eating. Again, this is where individualization of not only what you eat but also how you plan what you eat, matters! Remember your calorie budget? You can set a "macro budget" as well, that allows you to be even more precise and in control of your energy intake. That's as long as tracking and budgeting doesn't cause you any mental or emotional distress.

Let's dive deeper into what the macronutrients are and what they do in the body! Whether you choose to track them or not- it's up to you, but it is essential to know what they are.

Carbohydrates:

Carbohydrates (aka carbs) are your body's preferred fuel source! They are found in a variety of foods such as grains, starches, potatoes, vegetables, fruits, and even within fat sources such as almonds and peanut butter. Carbs get a bad reputation, especially by low carb dieters, and are often demonized for being the "cause of the obesity epidemic," however the true cause of obesity or weight gain lies in the shift of calorie balance itself, not simply the consumption of carbohydrate! No matter whether you are for or against carbs, their roles in the body cannot be forgotten.

Carbs play a critical role in blood sugar regulation, metabolism, and energy production. Though not technically essential (which means the body cannot produce it and it must be consumed through the diet), they still are a macronutrient that you don't want to miss. Carbohydrates provide your body with energy in the form of glucose, which is used to make ATP. They fuel our brain and muscles and are a critical preferred source for fueling physical activity. They are also protein-sparing, meaning they prevent protein from being broken down for energy, which allows protein to be better used for tissue, as well as DNA repair! Though not technically "essential" to the body, as the body is able to produce glucose from other fuel sources such as amino acids, carbohydrates are a very important nutrient that provide energy for our bodies, as well as energy for our gut bacteria, in the form of prebiotics!

The carbs consumed in your diet can be used for energy, or can be stored to be used for energy at a later time. If your body has enough glucose to meet its needs, excess glucose (aka carbohydrates) can be stored within your liver or muscles as glycogen, or as body fat. How and when does the body determine where to store? Great question!

Carbohydrate metabolism is controlled by three hormones: insulin, glucagon, and epinephrine. If the concentration of glucose in the blood is too high (for example, you had a high carbohydrate meal such as pasta and chicken), insulin (one of your metabolic hormones) is secreted by the beta cells of your pancreas. This insulin acts like a key, allowing glucose to enter into the cells of the body, including the liver and muscles. This glucose can then either be used by the cells of your body for energy, or converted into glycogen, through a process called glycogenesis. Think "glycogen creation." This is an anabolic process, meaning energy is required (anabolism)! Which essentially means it cannot happen without enough energy and fuel from the calories that you eat. If glucose is not used for energy, and both your liver and muscle glycogen levels are capped, glucose can then be converted into triglycerides, and stored as fat, through a process called lipogenesis.

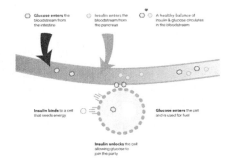

When blood glucose levels are low (as in the case of long periods of fasting, or several hours since eating), glucagon (another metabolic hormone) is secreted by the alpha cells of the pancreas to do the opposite of insulin's job. It stimulates the conversion of your glycogen into glucose. This process is called glycogenolysis and releases energy as a catabolic process (catabolism), which means that this process happens to create energy, and does not require it. Your liver is the first organ to release its glucose stores. In fact, your liver can hold around 100 g of glycogen at a time, and serves as your body's reservoir of glucose after hours since eating, or in the morning before eating breakfast. Though the muscle stores glycogen, it does not release it when your blood glucose levels drop. Therefore, when your blood glucose drops, thank your liver!

Glucose that is stored as glycogen within the muscle is actually unable to be used for energy, as the muscle does not have the enzyme called glucose-6-phosphatase, which is required for the conversion. Instead, to help bring blood glucose levels up and provide energy to the body when blood glucose is low, another catabolic process called gluconeogenesis occurs. During gluconeogenesis, glucose is then created from non-carbohydrate sources such as glycerol from fatty acids or amino acids (aka your protein stores in muscle!). This is why carbohydrates are truly not essential to consume in the diet! You can create them from fat and protein. It is also another reason why carbohydrates are so important for helping with muscle building and preservation, as they spare muscle protein and amino acids from being broken down to make glucose for energy.

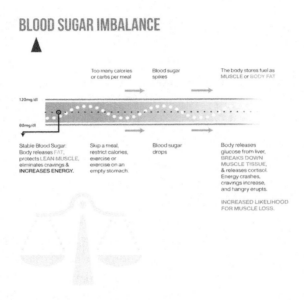

BLOOD SUGAR IMBALANCE

Too many calories or carbs per meal | Blood sugar spikes | The body stores fuel as MUSCLE or BODY FAT

120mg/dl

80mg/dl

Stable Blood Sugar: Body releases FAT, protects LEAN MUSCLE, eliminates cravings & **INCREASES ENERGY.**

Skip a meal, restrict calories, exercise or exercise on an empty stomach.

Blood sugar drops

Body releases glucose from liver, BREAKS DOWN MUSCLE TISSUE, & releases cortisol. Energy crashes, cravings increase, and hangry erupts.

INCREASED LIKELIHOOD FOR MUSCLE LOSS.

Overview of Hormones that Impact Your Carbohydrate Metabolism

Hormone	Impact
Insulin	-Increases uptake of glucose into fat and muscle cells -Increases storage of glycogen in liver and muscle -Increases fat storage (fatty acid synthesis) -Decreases fat breakdown from fat cells (lipolysis) -Stimulated by: glucose, amino acids, fatty acids, ketones, gut hormones
Glucagon	-Increases breakdown of glycogen from the liver tissue -Increases creation of glucose in liver (gluconeogenesis) -Increases fat breakdown from fat cells -Stimulated by: amino acids, gastrin, cortisol, growth hormone, exercise, low glucose levels, gut hormones, exercise, stress, infection, low blood glucose levels, fasting
Epinephrine	-Increases breakdown of glycogen in liver and muscle tissue -Increases fat breakdown from fat cells
Cortisol	-Increases muscle protein breakdown for glucose production -Enhances liver glycogen breakdown in early fasting -Increases fat breakdown from fat cells

The Cortisol Carbohydrate Connection (And Epinephrine):

Though glucagon is the hormone that most are aware of that helps to release stored carbohydrates in times of fasting or low energy, cortisol and epinephrine also play a role. Epinephrine is essentially adrenaline, one of your flight-or-fight hormones. In times of stress or extended fasting, epinephrine helps break down glycogen to release glucose for energy use. However, it does this from your muscle glycogen rather than liver glycogen. The glucose released doesn't actually enter your bloodstream like liver glycogen does. Your muscles are selfish!

Instead, the glucose released (along with fatty acids) is used primarily by your skeletal muscles for fuel. In turn, your skeleton muscles produce lactate, which can then be converted into glucose by your liver. So your body doesn't use your muscle glycogen to pull into the bloodstream here- your muscles alone specifically use this glucose. Meaning, your brain has to get glucose in another way! Cortisol helps with this. This is why in periods of fasting or periods without sufficient glucose, you can have the "brain fog" effect. Your muscles may be getting what they need, but your brain isn't.

Cortisol has a connection with carbohydrate metabolism as well. The output of cortisol from your adrenal glands (which can come from any stressor or even inflammation), helps your muscles break down their glycogen stores to release glucose for energy. It also enhances protein breakdown by breaking apart protein into its component amino acids in your skeletal muscle. These amino acids can be shuttled and transformed into glucose to be used through gluconeogenesis. In the short term, net protein balance is not affected and your hard-earned muscle won't waste away, but with chronically elevated cortisol, your muscle and your body take a negative hit.

This is where cortisol can be a demon for contributing to muscle loss. If cortisol remains elevated for a long period of time, whether due to chronic stress, extended fasting, inflammation, illness, or infection, it can cause your protein stores to start to whittle away. Remember- your body wants glucose. It will find a way to make it! By breaking down protein and amino acids, cortisol helps your body to combat stress, infection, or illness. This is part of the inflammatory response, however when it becomes chronic, issues can and will develop. More about cortisol and its importance, as well as what can go wrong, in a later chapter!

What About the Carbohydrate Insulin Theory?

The carbohydrate insulin theory states that insulin, a "fat storing" hormone, is responsible for driving fat gain and obesity, as high insulin in the body prevents lipolysis (a fancy word for fat loss) from happening. Now, we know that insulin does help drive the deposition of fat. However, this requires an energy surplus.

Carbohydrates in excess can and will contribute to fat gain in the presence of insulin. However, just because insulin is present does not mean that you will gain body fat. Again, you need a caloric surplus. You cannot gain fat or store fat without a surplus, regardless of insulin levels. In fact, insulin is not just driven by carbohydrates. It's also driven by protein! Whey protein actually stimulates insulin levels to rise more than a slice of bread! We can debunk the carbohydrate insulin theory here. Truth: carbohydrates + insulin + caloric surplus = fat gain. Enough said.

In fact, the contribution of glucose and carbohydrates to body fat relies on a process called de novo lipogenesis (DNL). However, the activity of this process is very low in animals and humans! DNL has a very small contribution to the storage of body fat. Your body will store as many carbohydrates as it can into your liver and glycogen tissues in your muscles first. Any excess in a caloric surplus can then, of course, become body fat.

How does this happen if DNL is low in animals? A couple things here play a role. First, the presence of insulin and carbohydrates help to spare fat oxidation (aka using fat for energy). This means that fat ingested is then more readily stored rather than used for energy. Now I know what you are now thinking. No, this doesn't mean eating carbs with fat makes you fat. You need a calorie surplus for this! Secondly, we know the law of thermodynamics, which states that "energy is neither created nor destroyed in an isolated system." Meaning, energy and calories that you eat have to do something. You have to consume less to lose weight or consume more to gain weight.

The law of thermodynamics doesn't mean all calories are created equal, as the body's response to the calories that you eat and the energy that you extract from them depend on digestibility, absorption, as well as the thermic effect of the calorie. For example- when digesting and metabolizing each macronutrient that you consume, you burn a different amount of calories in order to utilize them for energy. This is called the thermic effect of food, or TEF, which contributes to your diet-induced thermogenesis, aka the amount of fat you burn eating and digesting.

Thermic of Effect of Food by Macronutrient:
Protein: 20-30% burned
Carbohydrates: 5-10% burned
Fats: 0-3% burned

These are general numbers, because if you can't digest a food due to low digestive enzymes or malabsorption, you can't go through the full metabolization process either. Essentially, you burn more calories to digest a protein than you do to digest carbohydrates or fat. This is another reason for a higher protein intake- the extra protein calories are less likely to be stored as body fat. Additionally, protein increases thermogenesis AND enhances satiety! More on this in the protein section.

What Carbs are Best?

There are many types of carbohydrates that we can love and enjoy. The two main subtypes of carbohydrates can be divided into two groups based on their chemical structures- simple and complex. Essentially, all carbs are made up of various carbon, hydrogen, and oxygen molecules that link together to form different types of molecules- monosaccharides, disaccharides, oligosaccharides, and polysaccharides. The structure and number of molecules determines whether a carbohydrate is a "simple" or "complex" carb. Simple carbohydrates include mono- and disac-charides, while complex carbohydrates include any carbohydrate with three or more monosaccharides bound together, including oligo- and polysaccharides.

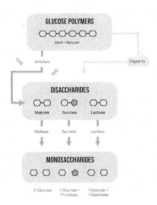

Monosaccharides are the most simple form of carbohydrate and are what all forms of carbohydrates break down to upon diges-tion! The 3 main monosaccharides within foods include: glucose, fructose, and galactose. They do not need further breakdown upon digestion themselves, and for the most part are easily digested and absorbed into the bloodstream (though fructose can be absorbed more slowly).

Disaccharides are made by the joining of two monosaccharides bound together. The 3 naturally occurring ones in your food include:

- Sucrose (glucose + fructose): the primary carbohydrate within plants (sucrose = table sugar)
- Lactose (glucose + galactose): the primary carbohydrate within dairy and milk products
- Maltose (glucose + glucose): the primary carbohydrate within seeds and alcohol

There is also high fructose corn syrup (HFCS), which is a manmade disaccharide, created by the hydrolysis of corn, which is fructose + fructose. Many people will classify the monosaccharides and disaccharides into "sugars." Knowing this, you can see that "sugars" are then naturally occurring in your food! Many food products contain different amounts of sugars, both naturally occurring (such as using fruit sugar to sweeten a product), or added sugar (such as using chemically made sucrose to sweeten a product).

How do these different sugar types affect your body? We will dive deeper into this when talking about blood sugar, but for now, just know that you don't need to worry about natural sugars. It's added sugars in your diet (such as in cakes, cookies, and candies), that you want to keep in moderation and lower in your diet. Why? Natural sugars contain vitamins and minerals, and added sugars do not!

Let's go back to complex carbohydrates. Oligosaccharides and polysaccharides make up the complex carbohydrates that you are probably more familiar with when thinking about carbohydrates, such as breads, cereals, rice, potatoes, and various different starches. They also make up the fiber found within your food and the carbohydrates found within fruits and vegetables!

During digestion of carbs, all forms of carbohydrates are broken down into the three main monosaccharides, glucose, fructose, and galactose, which are then absorbed by the gut and released into the bloodstream. All in all, complex carbohydrates are digested more slowly, are more satiating (more filling), produce a slower rise in blood glucose overall (more on this later!), and pack in more micronutrients, while simple carbohydrates are more easily digested, less satiating, and produce a faster rise in blood glucose.

The definition of "dietary fiber" and what food or food components meet this definition continues to evolve. In order to be listed as a dietary fiber on the Nutrition Facts Label, as determined by the FDA, a "fiber" must be a "non-digestible soluble or insoluble carbohydrate (with three or more monomeric units) and lignins that are intrinsic and intact in plants (aka found within the plant itself) OR isolated or synthetic non-digestible carbohydrates (with three or more monomeric units) determined by FDA to have physiological effects that are beneficial to human health. Some physiological benefits that may allow for a fiber label include: lowering of blood glucose, cholesterol, and blood pressure, increase in bowel frequency or bowel movements, or increase mineral absorption in the GI tract, and reduction of energy intake (for example- due to feeling of fullness).

Common fibers that currently meet the FDA's definition as of 2020 include: beta-glucan soluble fiber, psyllium husk, cellulose, guar gum, pectin, locust bean gum, and hydroxypropyl methylcellulose. Additional fibers that pend review for the definition include mixed plant cell wall fibers, arabinoxylan, alginate, inulin and inulin-type fructans, high amylose starch (resistant starch 2), galactooligosaccharide, polydextrose and resistant maltodextrin/dextrin. To add to the confusion of fiber, the FDA has also classified isolated fiber as "functional fiber."

Why is this important about fiber? Well, because not all fibers have the same benefits! I want you to understand that when people say to "eat more fiber" for health, it's not only about the fiber itself, but the type and the amount!

There are two main types of fiber that each exert different effects on your body! Most foods have a combination of different types of fiber. Soluble fiber, found within foods such as oatmeal, barley, chicory root, bananas, psyllium husk, legumes, and many fruits and vegetables, acts by drawing water into your GI tract, forming a gel like substance that slows down your digestion. This can help to soften your stool, slow down digestion, increase satiety (keep you full), reduce your blood sugar response to a meal, and aid in binding excess cholesterol, bile acids, and estrogen in your gut. These benefits may help in lowering your risk for cardiovascular disease, diabetes, and estrogen dominance! It has been shown that the intake of soluble fiber can help to lower A1C levels in type 2 diabetics, reduce blood sugar response to meals, and lower LDL (aka bad) cholesterol levels in the blood. Soluble fiber is also mostly highly fermentable, aka gas producing. This is why "too much fiber" can cause you to be gassy and bloated, as the fiber contributes to fermentation and gas production in your GI tract! This fermentation actually contributes to your daily energy intake, as well as produces B vitamins and vitamin K. If someone has lack of fiber or has a gastrointestinal disease or illness- this can lead to potential deficiencies! Soluble fiber is the type that is mostly suggested for diarrhea, as it helps to slow down transit time.

Soluble fiber also serves as a prebiotic fuel for your good gut bugs. Note- not all fibers are prebiotics, but many fibers can be prebiotics. Prebiotics, unlike fibers, are mostly carbohydrate polymers (aka molecules) that are not digested or absorbed within the gut. Prebiotics can also come from noncarbohydrate components as well. A prebiotic can be defined as "a substrate that is selectively utilized by the host microorganisms conferring a health benefit." In easy terms, they help you or your gut upon ingestion in some way.

The classification of a food ingredient or food component as a prebiotic requires that the food/ingredient:

- Resists gastric acidity, hydrolysis by mammalian enzymes, and absorption in the upper gastrointestinal tract;
- Is fermented by the intestinal microflora;
- Selectively stimulates the growth and/or activity of intestinal bacteria potentially associated with health and well-being

Prebiotics play a critical role in influencing your gut microbiota abundancy, diversity, and metabolism. They may help to increase the microbial diversity within your gut (especially increasing Lactobacillus and Bifidobacterium levels), support the production of SCFAs (short-chain fatty acids), as well as protect the gut from pathogens by influencing the gut lining integrity and pH levels. The production of SCFAs, including lactic acid, butyric acid, and propionic acid, can then influence multiple organs and metabolic pathways in your body, as they can diffuse through your gut cells (called enterocytes), and directly enter your bloodstream, influencing both the health of your gut lining, and your overall metabolism, hunger levels, nervous system, and immune system. They also help to enhance absorption of calcium and other minerals and regulate sodium and water absorption within your body.

Fun facts- the fermentation of prebiotics and SCFA production help to fuel the colonocytes within your gut, helping to maintain the gut lining integrity, as well as helping to inhibit pathogenic organisms and bacteria by reducing colonic pH. SCFAs also play a critical role in mucus production, inflammation, bile acid metabolism, and cholesterol metabolism. They can even affect your brain by inducing the secretion of the hormones GLP-1 (glucagon-like peptide 1), PYY (peptide YY), GABA (y-aminobutyric acid), and serotonin. Therefore, SCFAs play an integral role in emotion, satiety, cognition, mood, and brain health.

It is has been shown that prebiotics can help reduce the risk of colorectal cancer, aid in the management and remission of

Crohn's disease, reduce inflammatory cytokines (which may help improve immunity), and even play a role in regulating the neural brain pathways involved in mood, memory, and cognition. Benefits may also be seen in skin conditions, cardiovascular health, weight loss, and blood glucose regulation.

The most common prebiotics include fructo-oligosaccharides (FOS), galacto-oligosaccharides (GOS), resistant starch, inulin, pectin, lactulose, and fructans. Many foods contain natural prebiotics, such as asparagus, chicory root, onions, jerusalem artichoke, wheat, jicama, banana, barley, peas, leeks, and beans. Other natural prebiotic foods include egg plant, chia seeds, sweet potatoes, yacon root, barley, kefir, fruit, green tea, garlic, onions, and plantains.

The second type of fiber is insoluble fiber. Insoluble fiber is found in whole wheat products, nuts, beans, brown rice, nuts, and various different vegetables such as cauliflower, green peas, leafy greens, and prunes. Unlike its sister fiber, it does not dissolve in water, hence "insoluble"- not soluble in water. Instead of slowing down digestion and drawing water into the stool, insoluble fiber works by adding bulk to the stool, allowing for faster transit time and helping to prevent and treat constipation. It has little effect on satiety markers (feeling of fullness) and most forms are poorly fermented, however this is not always the case (and keep this in mind!).

The two main fibers, soluble and insoluble fiber, have different caloric values listed on the Nutrition Facts Label. This is regulated by the FDA. Soluble fiber is listed as "4 calories per gram" while insoluble fiber is listed as "0 calories per gram." This is based on the knowledge that soluble fibers ferment and contribute to caloric intake in the diet, while insoluble fibers do not and may pass through the GI tract mostly undigested. Because most foods contain both fiber types, I always suggest tracking your total fiber intake and accounting for all fibers in your caloric intake as well. The human GI tract and microbiome is quite complex, and the amount of fermentation and caloric extraction from fiber in each person may be completely different. If trying to control your caloric intake, especially if tracking macronutrients, it is best to track *all* fiber.

Fibers differentiate in their health benefits, solubility, and fermentation capability. Overall, most soluble fibers help to slow digestion and serve as a way to increase satiety, decrease blood cholesterol, blood pressure, and the blood glucose response to a meal, and also soften stools to make them easier to pass. However, most soluble fibers ferment and can produce gas and bloating. Insoluble fibers are less fermentable, helping to increase stool bulk and aid in constipation. When choosing a fiber for a specific purpose, say to help soften your stools or prevent diarrhea or constipation, make sure to look at the type of fiber along with its viscosity and fermentability, and if choosing foods, understand that most whole foods will have a combination of both!

Now that we've talked about fiber, you will better understand refined versus whole grains! Both can be listed as complex carbohydrates, as they contain more than 3 monosaccharide molecules or "sugars" linked together. Though both can be classified as a complex carbohydrate, refined and whole grains have different effects on your health, satiety, and digestion.

All forms of grains originally start as whole grain in their natural state. A whole grain contains three parts of the grain molecule:

1. The germ - which is part of the seed of the plant
2. The endosperm - which is the inner portion of the grain, mostly made of starch
3. The bran - which is the outer portion of the grain that is largely made up of fiber. The bran is the outermost layer that protects the whole grain, while the germ is the innermost component.

Whole grains contain all three components of the grain, while refined grains lose the germ and bran. This is bad news bears for getting the most bang for your buck when trying to maximize your micronutrients! The germ and bran are where the powerhouse of nutrition lies within whole grains, as this is where fiber, vitamins, minerals, and fatty acids are found. Though the endosperm in the refined grain also is nutritious, it does not contain the fiber from the bran or the fatty acids from the germ! You will not get the same micronutrients or blood sugar balancing benefits from refined grains that you will get from whole.

Essentially what this means for you is that you should be focusing on consuming most of the grains that you eat as whole grains. Make sure to read labels and don't fall for marketing gimmicks of "made with whole grain" or "multigrain." The food industry will prey on your confusion. Stick to 100% whole grain products and if wanting to avoid pesticides, organic whole grains would be your best bet.

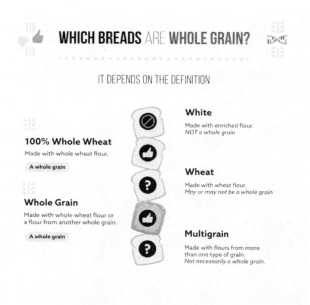

WHICH BREADS ARE WHOLE GRAIN?

IT DEPENDS ON THE DEFINITION

100% Whole Wheat
Made with whole wheat flour.
A whole grain

Whole Grain
Made with whole wheat flour or a flour from another whole grain.
A whole grain

White
Made with enriched flour.
NOT a whole grain

Wheat
Made with wheat flour.
May or may not be a whole grain

Multigrain
Made with flours from more than one type of grain.
Not necessarily a whole grain.

So what carbohydrates are best?

The best carbohydrates for your health will be ones that:

- Digest well
- Make you feel good
- Power up your micronutrients
- Help you achieve your daily fiber intake

Aim for consuming almost all your carbohydrates in the form of complex carbohydrates or in the simple carbohydrate form of fruit. My favorite carbohydrates include: potatoes (red, purple, sweet, yellow, russet), fruits and vegetables, rice (brown, wild, white, black, yellow, red), beans and legumes, low sugar whole grain cereal, oatmeal, quinoa, barley, teff, cream of rice, cream of wheat, 100% whole wheat breads and tortillas, 100% whole grain pasta or lentil based pastas, and organic corn.

What about the Glycemic Index (GI)?

Unless you have prediabetes or diabetes, there is no need to worry about the "glycemic index" (aka GI) here. The glycemic index essentially measures the rise of glucose that occurs after consuming a specific carbohydrate. Why? Well, we don't eat carbohydrates alone (or at least we shouldn't!), the blood glucose response to a carbohydrate-containing meal varies more based on the total meal intake, and our response to a food is very person-by-person dependent. What matters most is the overall quality of your diet! Typically, most simple carbs are high GI, which means they rapidly increase your blood sugar. On the other hand, complex carbs are low GI, meaning they provide a slow release of blood sugar. Focus on consuming whole grains, smart snacks, and making sure your meals are balanced with healthy proteins, carbohydrates, fats, fruits, and vegetables- and your blood sugar will be happy.

3 Main Issues with the GI:

1. Each individual responds differently to different foods
2. Serving sizes change the response
3. Meal components change the response

If you have been diagnosed with prediabetes or diabetes, this is where you will want to pay attention to your blood glucose levels, especially your postprandial glucose levels. You may find that your insulin needs are heavily increased when consuming higher GI foods and you may need less with low GI foods. If you have blood sugar issues, working with a health professional to find what carbohydrates help you manage your blood sugar best is key. As your insulin needs will change and your response to different carbohydrates will change based on the type and total meal or snack components.

Carbohydrate Digestion

Carbohydrate digestion starts in your mouth with the help of salivary amylase mixed with your saliva. The rest of their digestion occurs in your small intestine with the help of your pancreatic enzymes, specifically pancreatic amylase. Remember, carbohydrate digestion doesn't occur in your stomach due to it's high acidity.

Starch and carbohydrate molecules are then broken down into their monosaccharides: glucose, fructose, and galactose. Each molecule is absorbed into your bloodstream via various transporters, all which require sodium, water, and potassium to work. Once transported, they enter your bloodstream and can be used for energy by your body. The absorption of all carbohydrates (except fructose) requires energy in the form of ATP and uses several of the same transporters for absorption. Fructose does not require this and does not compete for absorption. This means the rate of glucose absorption is not inhibited by the addition of fructose and the addition of fructose to glucose increases absorption rate.

What does this mean for you? If you are a weight training or endurance athlete, consuming fructose with glucose can be a helpful strategy to increase the carbohydrate content of your meal and facilitate additional glycogen storage without minimizing transporters.

Fructose - The Devil?

Fructose is a naturally occurring sugar found in fruits, vegetables, honey, agave, and molasses. It can also be found in highly processed foods in the form of high fructose corn syrup (HFCS), which is commonly found in breakfast cereals, pastries, fruit juices, and sugary drinks. HFCS is commonly blamed for contributing to obesity, weight gain, diabetes, cancer, etc. It's quite frequently victimized, and for what reason? Being a chemical?

I hope you know and understand that all fruit-based fructose is a healthy addition to your diet and should not be feared, or removed (unless you have an inborn error of metabolism and can't digest fructose- yes that is a thing). In fact, studies show that consuming fruit before a meal may lessen the blood glucose rise (aka glycemic response) from a meal.

Here are the facts about HFCS. HFCS in simple terms is a chemically made syrup containing fructose and glucose molecules. It has about 1.7x more sweetness than sucrose itself (aka table sugar), allowing food manufacturers to sweeten their products with less sugar, thus saving them money and actually saving you calories. No organism or body can distinguish where the molecules of fructose, sucrose, or glucose, or carbohydrates in general come from when ingested. Biologically, they will metabolize the same exact way.

So why is it demonized then? Well, fructose bypasses your tightly wound insulin levels. When you consume glucose, insulin is signaled and glucose can enter into your bloodstream where it can be used or stored into liver or muscle glycogen. On the other hand, fructose does not stimulate insulin and does not go straight into the bloodstream. Instead, it goes to your liver. There, your liver can convert the fructose into glucose and THEN release it into the blood, or it can take it and store it as glycogen, or store as body fat. In addition, fructose bypasses an enzyme in your liver called phosphofructokinase (PFK), which essentially helps to blunt the conversion of glucose to body fat. Fructose skips this step. This is where the debacle lies.

Physiologically, this means that fructose has the ability to be more readily converted into fat to be stored. If in an energy surplus, this could be bad. Excess fructose in an energy surplus will contribute to the formation of body fat, and can also cause the development of fat around your organs, leading to diseases like fatty liver or NAFLD (nonalcoholic fatty liver disease). However, in caloric maintenance or a caloric deficit, this won't happen! The fate of fructose depends on the body's fuel needs and energy status.

HFCS gets a bad reputation because the foods that contain it (or contained it), are highly processed, and easy to consume in large quantities, leading to energy surpluses, and indeed, fat accumulation. However, if replacing with any other form of sugar, the same energy surplus and fat accumulation can occur!

I hope this gives you clarity on fructose. You don't need to avoid it, especially when it comes down to whole food sources. However, it would be best, especially if you are trying to maximize your health and metabolism, to consume less or minimize your consumption of foods with HFCS. You will get way more bang for your buck consuming fruit packed with vitamins and minerals.

The Gluten Conundrum?

Gluten has been called the devil by many. The rise in gluten-free products, though incredible for those with gluten allergies, sensitivities, or Celiac disease, has 100% taken hold of this growing fear of gluten, and become what I think is a terrible marketing strategy to push "health" on a product. Don't get me wrong, the rise in Celiac disease (an autoimmune disease triggered by the consumption of gluten) and gluten sensitivities is indeed occurring, but we have to ask- why?

Most people don't understand what gluten really is or why it can cause health concerns. I am sure some of y'all think gluten is a carbohydrate. Let's get the facts straight here. Gluten is a protein found in many grain products such as wheat, barley, and rye. The gluten protein contains prolamins, a kind of protein, that can make them resistant to digestion, increasing the prevalence of their numbers in the small intestine when ingested. Some claim that "gluten is toxic" and that these undigested particles can contribute to a heightened immune system response. But what determines if these undigested gluten particles actually create a problem or not?

Your reaction to gluten depends on the health of your intestinal barrier, immune system, and inflammatory responses. If you have a healthy intestinal wall, aka lack of intestinal permeability, and no food allergy or immune response, gluten shouldn't be an issue. However, if you have intestinal permeability or a poor functioning immune system, the gluten can then trigger an immune response, causing you problems. Problems that may be gut-specific such as gas, bloating, constipation, diarrhea, or may include symptoms without gut problems such as increased joint pain, muscle aches, headaches, hives, rashes, acne, and brain fog.

It is my own thinking that gluten is not an issue in the general population. However, it becomes an issue if someone is immuno-compromised, lacks a healthy gut lining, or is experiencing an upregulation of their immune system. In practice, I have seen gluten sensitivities occur due to infections and dysbiosis, such as SIBO (small intestinal bacterial overgrowth), Candida, H. Pylori, and even parasites. When the immune system is calmed down, infections or overgrowths removed, and the gut lining is supported, these people have been able to add gluten back into their diet without problems!

There are some hypotheses and guesses to why gluten sensitivity and Celiac Disease is increasing in the US. Some think it's due to shifts in the microbiome, either from how someone is raised along with their environment, their early life exposure to gluten, impact of environmental toxins, or the rise and use of antibiotics. Others believe it's due to the use of glyphosate and herbicides on wheat based products or affected by gut infections and increased intestinal permeability. What we don't know is why the rise has occurred. We can only speculate.

Think you may have a gluten problem? Celiac disease can be diagnosed by your doctor with an assessment of antibodies to a gluten challenge and intestinal wall biopsy. A gluten sensitivity or "intolerance" is harder to pinpoint. Most people self-diagnose these and can tell by changes in symptoms and health status with the removal of gluten. However, I find this sets someone up for food fears. Also, the benefits of removing gluten from their diet are not always due to the actual gluten, but instead are due to the change in the overall quality of their diet.

Other people try to rely on food sensitivity testing, which assesses immune response to foods. Here's the catch though...**food intolerance testing is a waste of money. I said what I said (and I mean it).**

You probably have seen people posting about their experiences with food intolerance testing using tests such as the Pinner Test or

EverlyWell. These are commonly used to assess for not only gluten sensitivity but also other food sensitivities that people think they may or may not have.

Essentially, these tests measure your immune system IgG reactivity to foods. Not only is this **NOT** an accurate marker of testing, but it doesn't give you a reason WHY a food could be an intolerance or issue in the first place! I get frustrated when people are given these to diagnose "allergies." **You can't diagnose an allergy with an IgG response**.

"Food allergies" can be due to:

- An IgE-mediated food immune reaction that produces a life-threatening allergic response called anaphylaxis
- Symptoms are commonly associated with hives swelling, dizziness, itching, and anaphylaxis that may require emergency medical care
- The top 9 food allergens include: milk, wheat, tree nuts, eggs, soy, fish, shellfish, peanuts, and sesame

ADVERSE FOOD REACTIONS

"Food intolerances" can be due to:

- An actual immune response, as in the case for gluten in Celiac disease
- Non-immune response due to lack of digestive enzymes, high histamine levels, sensitivity to a food additive or preservative, or even simply due to stress
- A "pseudo-food intolerance," as in the case for low gut immune function (Sec IgA levels), or underlying overgrowth, pathogen, or parasite
- Fear of a food, which is commonly seen in those with past disordered eating
- Symptoms are commonly associated with gas, bloating, cramping, nausea, joint pain, or change in bowel movements

Therefore, there is a distinct difference between an allergy and an intolerance. What does science say about this food intolerance IgG based testing? Right now, the evidence is lacking to support the use of these tests in diagnosing reactions to foods. Results have shown that these tests are not a clinically relevant or valid strategy to address food intolerances and are unreliable as they show both false positive and false-negative results.

Remember, it is super important to realize that the production of IgG antibodies is a normal part of your immune system! When you eat a certain food, your body naturally increases the presence of IgG antibodies to that food. This is considered a harmless immune response to food and explains why the foods that you eat most frequently show up in food sensitivity testing as foods you are most sensitive to.

The sad truth- following the "results" from these tests can lead to food fears, nutrient deficiencies, and unnecessary restriction. This doesn't mean that your symptoms are not valid - just that the testing isn't. The gold standard for food intolerances is an elimination diet with reintroduction done under the supervision of a professional, most recommended, a registered dietitian. Don't waste your money on a test that could restrict you for no reason, cause food fears, and leave you still not feeling your best!

If you suspect a gluten sensitivity or intolerance, or issues with any specific food, work with a registered dietitian like me to do a proper elimination diet and reintroduction to see if gluten is indeed a supervillain for you, or not. Don't get me wrong, people have issues with gluten. I am one of them. I don't get gut distress, but I have increased joint pains, muscle aches, and brain fog. In my case, I then remove gluten. I also have hypothyroidism, which serves as an additional reason to remove it (see the thyroid chapter for more details!). Remove it if you need to. Don't remove it just because Karen tells you to.

One last thing about gluten and going gluten-free. In order to see a true difference with going gluten-free, you must completely remove it for at least 4 weeks. Additionally, you must remove potential cross-reactivity in your environment and with dining out. Foods and grains that have gluten cross-reactivity include: millet, barley, kamut, spelt, malt, corn, oats, and rye. Foods with gluten that you may miss include: salad dressings, soy sauces, soups, energy bars, beer, candy, brown rice syrup, thickeners, and seasoned meats.

Gluten is a sneaky little demon and as you can see, it can be hidden in sauces, condiments, drink powders, dietary supplements, and even toothpaste! If you are going to try going gluten-free, you need to focus in on label reading.

The Great Grain Debate

One of the biggest controversies regarding carbohydrates lies within the power of grains. Are they good for you, or are they bad for you? The great debate divides the opponents into opposite sides, from the paleo community to the flexible dieting community. Both stand their ground, picking and choosing their scientific evidence based on their opinions. This is where our answer lies, for science never lies.

This conundrum is just like with gluten. I truly think people can have sensitivities, as well as have allergies, to grains. However the grain itself is not a demon for your health. Remember, you want to limit refined grains due to their differing nutrient profile and blood glucose response compared to whole grains, but the grain itself should not be avoided. The grain itself is not the issue. It's specific food intolerances you may have, a gut infection or overgrowth, heightened intestinal permeability, or a heightened immune response that causes issues. Most people, just like with gluten, can consume grains just fine if they are healthy.

Remember, grain quality matters! Whole grains and refined grains metabolize and digest quite differently in your body. For example, the fiber within the bran of whole grains helps to slow the digestion of starch into glucose, helping to maintain steady blood sugar levels and create a steady rise, whereas refined grains produce a rapid spike in blood glucose (and can produce a rapid drop as well). The fiber also helps to lower blood cholesterol and remove waste within the digestive tract, including excreting excess estrogen from the body.

Another case against grains lies in insulin resistance, food allergies, and inflammation. However, this is in relation to more than just grains, but also total carbohydrate and insulin levels in the body! The great grain debate tends to be "go grains!" or "no grains!" Instead of focusing on limiting grains, the focus should be on overall carbohydrate quality in the diet. If you then have a specific grain sensitivity or intolerance, limit them. If not- spare yourself the struggle. Grains taste great.

Insulin Resistance & Carbohydrates

If you have insulin resistance, your body is not adequately able to lower its blood sugar levels in response to eating carbohydrates. This can occur because of a lack of insulin to bring glucose into the cell for energy use (due to a pancreatic beta cell dysfunction), increased liver glucose production, or cellular resistance to insulin. Remember- think of insulin like a key allowing glucose to enter into the cell for energy. When the cells are resistant, the key can't open the lock, and the glucose can't enter the cell. Instead, it remains in the blood!

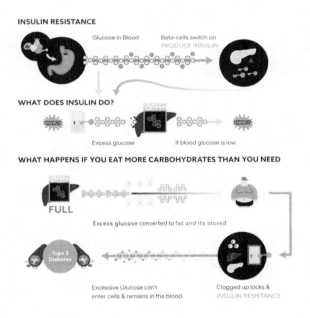

Unless there is sufficient insulin to lower blood glucose back to normal, your blood glucose levels remain elevated. This glucose causes your blood to become "sticky" like honey. You don't want sticky blood. You want it flowing like a river! "Stickiness" causes your blood to flow less freely, heightening the pressure against your blood vessels and capillaries. Cue kidney issues leading to possible chronic kidney disease, retinopathy (eye damage), and neuropathy (nerve damage to your legs and feet) once your insulin resistance leads to Type 2 Diabetes.

To avoid insulin resistance and enhance insulin sensitivity, you should consume a balance of healthy, whole grains or complex carbohydrates, avoid constantly spiking your insulin (aka no snacking all day), and focus on lifestyle and exercise techniques such as incorporating resistance training, cardio, and your NEAT levels in order to enhance insulin sensitivity.

Please keep this in mind- it is not the carbohydrate alone that causes insulin resistance but a variety of genetic, lifestyle, and overall dietary factors including a sedentary lifestyle, poor diet, and chronic inflammation. Maintaining a healthy body weight, staying active, fueling your body right, and getting proper sleep are important steps to lower your risk for insulin resistance and improve your overall health.

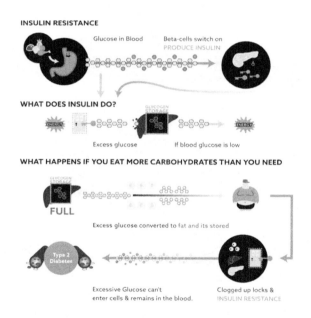

What About Glyphosate Use On Grains?

Glyphosate is an herbicide, aka weed killer, known as "Round Up" produced by Bayer (owned by Monsanto). Monsanto created it largely to be used on GMO (genetically modified organisms) crops that were created with a resistance to glyphosate, meaning that the crop wouldn't be harmed with its use, but the surrounding weeds and pests would.

Here's the thing about glyphosate. There are studies to show that it can serve as an endocrine disruptor and the WHO (World Health Organization), part of the IARC (International Agency for Research on Cancer), has concluded that it is "probably carcinogenic to humans," meaning it may increase your risk of developing cancer. Some studies show that it has carcinogenic potential both to DNA cells in vitro (aka when only cells are studied outside of a living organism), within mice, and correlations have been made within observational human studies. However, other studies show no association of increased risk. So what is the truth?

The truth is we don't know the safety just yet. We know that glyphosate does not easily pass through the skin, and that it is ingested, absorbed, and eliminated quickly in the body. How it affects the body depends on exposure and amount. Toxicity also depends on who is being exposed. Humans aren't cells and they aren't mice.

Glyphosate is a newer chemical, and long term safety studies have yet to be done. Just because it can cause cancer, doesn't mean that it will. To me, a potential carcinogen is one to be avoided if possible. We could go on and on about how studies are done, who is doing the funding, and how the WHO classifies something as carcinogenic (remember- alcohol is too!). However to save this from becoming a long winded rant, avoid it if you want. I will.

Proteins

Protein is an essential nutrient that is required for the synthesis, repair, and rebuilding of almost all the organs and tissues within your body. Not only do you need it for growth and repair of your muscles, bone, ligaments, and connective issues (including your skin, hair, and nails), but you also require it to make your hormones, neurotransmitters, enzymes, cell transporters, and the foundations of your immune system. Protein is required to maintain life and is marked as an essential nutrient!

The ingestion of protein stimulates muscle protein synthesis, which turns your body on an anabolic, recovery mode. Anabolic essentially just means "building," whereas catabolism means "breaking down." During weight training and workouts or between means, you become catabolic. The ingestion of food and especially sufficient dietary protein is what helps you become anabolic. Remember- you grow muscle by recovering from training, not by training alone. The combination of resistance training plus adequate protein intake help to stimulate muscle protein synthesis to grow and maintain muscle. Sufficient dietary protein also helps ensures the growth of your other tissues, creation of sex hormones, neurotransmitters, and enzymes.

Protein is also your best friend when it comes down to meal satiety (or fullness) and balancing your blood sugar. It also has the highest TEF (your thermic effect of food), about 30% compared to carbohydrates (5-10%), and fat (about 1-3%). It requires the most amount of energy to digest and is the one macronutrient that is least likely to contribute to body fat gain when consumed in excess. What does this mean? Consuming a higher protein intake shouldn't be a concern when it comes down to building muscle and limiting fat gain. In addition, a high protein diet has been shown to be more helpful in aiding weight loss than a low protein diet, largely due to its ability to help maintain fullness and preserve lean body mass.

Proteins are made up of building blocks called amino acids. Out of the 20 amino acids that can make up a protein, 9 are essential to your body, as your body cannot produce them on its own. You are required to ingest them from the foods that you eat! Some amino acids have specific and beneficial functions within your body. Here are a few examples:

- Tryptophan: a precursor to serotonin and epinephrine-low amounts can affect mood and increase risk of depression. If low, sleep may also be hindered.
- Tyrosine: a precursor to dopamine, norepinephrine, and epinephrine and is required for the creation of thyroid hormone. Too little tyrosine can lead to hypothyroidism or cause adrenal imbalances and an insufficient stress response. Dopamine helps to control memory, thought, and emotions and is heavily linked to the reward systems in your brain. Low tyrosine and low dopamine can increase risk of Parkinson's disease.
- Arginine: forms nitric oxide and citrulline in the body which is required for the maintenance of your blood pressure, inhibition of platelet aggregation, and vasoconstriction and dilation of your smooth muscle cells. Arginine is a common amino acid consumed by bodybuilders or weight training to help increase cellular swelling, producing a "pump" in the gym.
- Glutamine: the most abundant amino acid that serves as a metabolic fuel for your immune cells and gut cells. Glutamine supplementation can be beneficial for enhancing recovery from an injury or poor gut health, as it helps to maintain a healthy gut lining.
- Glutamate: an excitatory amino acid and major brain neurotransmitter that is important for brain development and memory. It serves as a precursor to GABA in the body. GABA is an inhibitory neurotransmitter that plays major roles in brain cell communication, cognition, the stress response, and fear/anxiety.

You need more than just sufficient protein- you need sufficient amino acids, especially the essential ones! Essential amino acids cannot be made or synthesized by your body and require consumption via the diet. Nonessential amino acids can be created from precursors such as glucose or other amino acids. This means that you can make one nonessential amino acid from another amino acid. Some call these "interchangeable" amino acids. Conditionally essential amino acids are amino acids that become essential during specific disease or metabolically stressed states such as in infection, illness, or burns.

What Proteins Are Best?

The anabolic effect of a protein appears to be largely controlled by: total amino acid content, leucine content, and protein digestibility. In order to stimulate muscle protein synthesis (MPS), all amino acids are required. However, it appears that leucine has its own "magic" MPS ability. Leucine helps to stimulate a complex called mTOR (mammalian target of rapamycin), that acts as a significant "push" for stimulated MPS. In the short term, leucine supplementation alone may increase MPS, however to maximize MPS, all amino acids should be present along with sufficient levels of insulin.

In general, you want to focus on consuming protein that has:

- A high biological value- essentially, this marker reflects how readily a consumed protein can be used for protein synthesis.
- High protein digestibility- aka the protein is able to be digested, broken down into amino acids, and used. If you can't digest it- you can't use it! Animal-based proteins have the highest digestibility (90-99%), with plant sources falling short (60-80% depending on type). This is because plants contain fiber and "anti-nutrients" such as phytates and tannins that can inhibit digestion and absorption. Good news – cooking can help reduce these anti-nutrients, however it doesn't fully eliminate them

and doesn't impact the fiber content. Plant-based protein powders tend to have a higher digestibility in relation to the whole food based plant protein itself, as the anti-nutrients are mostly removed. For example, pea and brown rice blend protein can stimulate MPS just as much as whey protein!

- All needed amino acids. Though you can simulate MPS and get protein from vegan or vegetarian sources that may not have all amino acids, ensuring to get multiple sources throughout the day to ensure daily consumption of all amino acids is important. Why? If your body needs an amino acid and can't get it from the diet, it will take it from the organs and tissues in your body. This means you break down body tissue to make new proteins. This is where consuming multiple sources of protein with vegan or vegetarian diets becomes even more crucial.

Meat eaters or pescatarians, you are pretty safe when it comes to getting adequate protein intake and ensuring that your proteins are higher in biological value, digestibility, and contain a variety of amino acids. Minus collagen and bone broth, which are limited in tryptophan, most animal based proteins are "complete proteins," meaning they contain all the amino acids you need!

However, if you are a vegan or vegetarian, and your goal is to maximize muscle mass or muscle retention, you may need to pay a little more attention to your protein sources. As previously indicated, plant proteins are lower in both biological value, digestibility, and amino acids variety. Most plant proteins are "incomplete proteins," meaning that they do not contain all the needed amino acids. For example, lysine is the lower amino acid within cereal grains, while methionine is the lowest in soy. Plant proteins tend to be much lower in leucine as well, and therefore if wanting to maximize MPS, consuming multiple sources of plant proteins in one meal may be needed to maximize MPS and ensure all amino acids are consumed.

A great way to ensure you are consuming all essential amino acids with a vegan or vegetarian diet is to use complementary proteins. These do not have to be consumed in one meal together (though that would be optimal for muscle growth!). As long as they are consumed over the course of your day, your body will get what it needs. You can use complementary proteins by matching up two different types of incomplete proteins. Try combining one plant protein that is limited in a specific amino acid with another protein that contains more of that limited amino acid.

For example, you can pair:

- Nuts or seeds with rice
- Soy with leafy greens
- Grains with legumes or peas

I have not seen any issues of protein deficiency in vegetarian or vegan clients as long as they get variety in their diet. Gaining muscle and strength is not an issue either, as long as one ensures to optimize their amino acid intake, focus on leucine content within their protein choices, and of course provides sufficient calories for growth. Worried? Fear not, most people have no issues consuming all required amino acids with plant-based diets- as long as they focus on variety!

How is Protein Metabolized by the Body?

Protein metabolism is controlled by a combination of amino acid entry, exit, degradation, and hormone stimulation. Essentially, it is controlled by the protein you eat (amino acid concentration), your fuel availability (energy balance - fed, fasted, deficit, or surplus), and the hormones in your body. These hormones can either increase/stimulate protein synthesis, or stimulate degradation and breakdown. Together, it's the combination of what and how much you eat, your overall health status, and what you do that impacts your protein metabolism.

- **Hormones that increase protein synthesis**: insulin, growth hormone, and testosterone
- **Hormones that decrease or halt protein synthesis:** glucagon, catecholamines (including cortisol), glucocorticoids, thyroid hormone

Just like your metabolism, protein metabolism is never static. However, it can be easier to simplify protein metabolism into either catabolism or anabolism to better understand how it is built or degraded in the body.

In a positive energy balance with the ingestion of food and stimulation of protein synthesis, the protein (broken down into amino acids in your intestines) you eat can have a few different fates. It can be thrown into the amino acid pool to form new proteins, shunted into what's called the TCA cycle to become glucose via gluconeogenesis, oxidized to create energy to be used by your body, or used to produce new fatty acid or triacylglycerol (TAG) that can be used for fuel or deposited as body fat.

When breaking down protein in a catabolic state with a negative energy balance (such as during a workout, between meals, or fasting), there are potential fates for the amino acids and protein in your body. The nitrogen that is attached to the amino acids you ingest are removed via ammonia or urine and the carbon skeleton from the protein can be used to produce energy, new glucose, fatty acids, enzymes, or neurotransmitters. What about the amino acids? They can be used for energy via gluconeogenesis.

Your catabolic state fates change based on time without sufficient food intake and fuel availability. Short term fasting, such as between meals, stimulates gluconeogenesis, which allows for the breakdown of your protein sources to be used to synthesize and make new glucose for energy. Remember your carbohydrate metabolism? Your body has no insulin and higher glucagon levels. Along with the release of glucose from your liver and muscle glycogen levels, gluconeogenesis is attempting to provide your body with its preferred method of fuel- carbohydrates- to ensure you have energy! In the short term, there are typically no consequences to this, minus potential low blood sugar.

Long term fasting or starvation causes your body to deplete its liver and muscle glycogen stores and causes a blunt in gluconeogenesis. Instead of breaking down protein for glucose, the body shifts to preserve protein for daily life processes and instead relies on what are called ketone bodies for fuel. Your body shifts to mobilize fat (or triacylglycerol) from fat cells for energy production. This breakdown forms an acetyl-CoA molecule that can be used to produce ketones.

This ketone creation and protein breakdown adaptation is a safety response to low carbohydrate intake, ketogenic dieting, or starvation. The body will rely on ketones for fuel from adipose tissue or dietary fat to preserve muscle and protein stores. This is where ketogenic dieting has potential benefits when dieting, as the body shifts to preserve lean muscle mass and in addition relies more on fat oxidation for energy than body glucose stores. Over time, once adipose stores are depleted or without sufficient ketone production, your body will then go back to breaking down protein (and muscle tissue) for energy.

However- just because you are using fat of energy and oxidizing fat, doesn't mean that you are losing body fat! Rule of thumb- energy deficit is king. Metabolic ward studies show that when calories and protein are matched, there is no benefit to ketogenic dieting overall for weight loss than a higher carbohydrate diet. More on ketogenic diets later!

Something to be aware of- during hypermetabolic disease states such as hyperthyroidism, cancer, and AIDS or with burns, infection, or severe injury, the adaptation to muscle and protein preservation does not occur. Instead, the body relies on gluconeogenesis and protein breakdown for fuel. This is why a high protein intake as well as sufficient caloric intake is essential for these cases to prevent muscle loss and detrimental healing and health outcomes (such as unintentional weight loss).

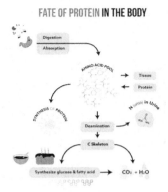

FATE OF PROTEIN **IN THE BODY**

Fun fact- protein metabolism accounts for 15-20% of resting energy expenditure within your BMR in your body!

The Common Conundrum- More Protein Does Not Mean More Muscle!

This is an issue I see quite frequently. People think eating more protein means gaining more muscle. Not the case. You don't want more protein. You want optimized protein, and an optimized metabolism and "fuel furnace." Remember, extra protein in the diet may not contribute to body fat gain, however, it takes more calories for your body to use that protein as energy. Not optimal if you want to gain muscle or grow. The extra protein has to convert into glucose or a fatty acid in order to be used. And now it won't just be "peed" out with excess. The nitrogen atom will, but not the amino acid and carbon skeleton. What you eat and digest, you will absorb and use somehow- so use your macronutrients wisely. Optimize your protein intake based on your goal and what you need and then use the rest of your calories wisely to optimize energy and your metabolism! Looking at you 140 lb woman pounding down 170g protein a day. Stop that.

What About Protein Safety?

Extra protein (up to 3.0 g per kg of body weight in healthy people) is not likely to harm you or your kidneys, regardless of what the media or Karen from work says. You should worry about protein intake if you have kidney disease, however if your kidney is like a spring chicken and working the way it should, you should be far from concerned about protein's safety. Do make sure to increase your water intake with a higher protein diet, as the extra nitrogen load needs some love to excrete. I suggest consuming at least 1 gallon a day.

Protein & Cancer (And Anti- Cancer Nutrition in General!)

You may have also heard that "protein feeds cancer." This stems from the "fact" that cancer can be stimulated by mTOR (mammalian target of rapamycin) and IGF-1 (insulin-like growth factor 1), which are both stimulated by protein intake. However, exercise also stimulates IGF-1. Exercise has been proven to reduce the risk of cancer. Would you stop exercising to lower IGF-1? Nope! The benefits outweigh the risks.

Just like exercise, protein can also be protective against cancer. Adequate protein intake can ensure sufficient dietary amino acids to help regulate the immune system, fight off infections, and plays a critical role in DNA creation and repair. DNA damage and oxidative stress can contribute to cancer proliferation. Don't skimp on your protein- skimp on the lies the media tells you.

Another lie about cancer while we are at it- sugar does not feed cancer either. Many diets high in sugar, are low in fiber and nutrients and contribute to inflammation, weight gain, and malnutrition- all of which can increase the risk of cancer. The truth is- anything can potentially feed cancer. Cancer can shift fuel sources. It's smarter than we give it credit for. You also can't just starve cancer. It will mutate. The worst thing you can do if you HAVE cancer is not eat enough. You can't fight it without fuel.

My research and experiences at MD Anderson showed me that the true power of nutrition in cancer prevention and treatment lies in consuming sufficient calories, more plants, and getting color and variety in the diet. The best "anti-cancer diet" is low in processed foods and meats, high in plants and fiber, and jam packed with nutrient quality. But preventing cancer is more than diet alone- it's also lifestyle, genetics, and environment.

To lower your risk for cancer, focus on minimizing stress, staying active, and reducing your environmental toxin load. Regarding proteins- focus on the quality of your proteins and consume at least half of your proteins as plant proteins. Avoid the intake of processed proteins/meats, refined carbohydrates, alcohol, and other known chemical carcinogens. Limit your red meat intake to 6 oz per day (or 18 oz per week) and pack up the punch in your diet with phytochemicals and antioxidants. Aim for at least 5 portions of vegetables and fruits per day- but the more the merrier.

See the appendix for a nutrient, antioxidant, and phytochemical chart! I would argue that safety should be a concern with the type of proteins ingested based on the protein's saturated fat content. More on this in the fat section! In the end, most proteins are safe for you as long as you aren't allergic or sensitive to them (as in the case for some with eggs, shellfish, or dairy products).

Fats

Fat is the most energy-dense of your macronutrients, providing a whopping 9 calories per gram vs carbohydrate and protein's 4 calories per gram. This is where "fat makes you fat" comes from. Fat doesn't really make you fat. Fat is very calorically dense (and delicious), and too much fat can add more calories to your diet per gram than your other macronutrients!

Fat is an essential nutrient, just like protein, and is required for the creation of your hormones, maintenance of cell membranes, regulation of cholesterol levels, protection of your organs, regulation of body temperature, absorption of fat-soluble vitamins (A, D, E, and K) and minerals, and serves as an energy reserve for your body. We need fat to survive, both in our diets, and on our bodies! Additional benefits of fat include blood sugar stabilization after meals, increased meal satiety, and maintenance of cognition.

There are many types of fats in your body that each play essential roles and functions in different bodily tissues. All the fats that you eat are made up of chains of fatty acids. When ingested, these chains are broken and the fatty acids are reassembled and packaged into chylomicrons (lipoproteins, aka fat + protein) that can then be sent throughout your body for use. The fate of this breakdown depends on your body's fuel needs and caloric balance.

If energy is needed or in a fasting state (including a few hours after a meal), fats are used for energy. If energy is not needed or there is a surplus of fuel or calories, fats are stored as body fat. This body fat can be later used for fuel when needed. Dietary fat won't make you fat in this way though. Just because you consume a lot of peanut butter before bed does not mean that you will gain weight and body fat! Too much fat and in a caloric surplus, you will. Otherwise, the fat storage is only temporary, and these stored fats will be used, and weight maintained, as long as energy balance is neutral.

Fat Storage vs Fat Usage

Dietary fats are metabolized in the body with the help of your digestive enzymes, liver, and gallbladder! Upon the ingestion of a fat, fats are largely broken down in your small intestine by enzymes called lipases. Large particles of fat are mixed or emulsified with bile salts (produced in your liver and stored in your gallbladder), creating micelles. These micelles are "attacked" by your lipase enzymes and broken down further into fatty acids and glycerol molecules.

Once broken down, these micelles get absorbed into your intestine in the form of chylomicrons, which then pass into your lymphatic system and then the bloodstream to be shuttled for energy storage or use. Why can't they just be absorbed directly? Fat molecules are too large for that! They must go through a "Cinderella story" of transformation to be made small enough to be absorbed.

Your absorbed and transported chylomicrons can be stored into muscle or fat tissue, or used for energy. Fats are stored as triglycerides in your fat cells (aka adipocytes). Triglycerides are essentially three fatty acids attached to a glycerol molecule. When fats need to be used for energy after storage, these triglycerides are broken down and oxidized. This allows the fat to be shuttled from adipose tissue and into your bloodstream for energy use.

The regulation of fat release vs usage is largely dependent on energy needs and the presence of insulin. After a meal with sufficient calories and energy, your hormone insulin helps to shuttle fatty acids for energy use or storage, as well as helps to keep fatty acids inside your adipocytes/fat cells.

After a few hours without eating, during periods of fasting (including sleeping), or during low intensity exercise, insulin levels drop and calorie and energy availability is low. This allows for hormones such as epinephrine (and cortisol) to help mobilize the fatty acids from adipocytes, and for the release of an enzyme called hormone sensitive lipase, resulting in lipolysis. Lipolysis is just a fancy term for the fatty acids being broken apart from their glycerol molecule backbone.

After lipolysis, these fatty acids and the glycerol molecule leave your fat cells and enter your bloodstream to be used for energy, traveling attaching to a protein called albumin.

If used for energy, fatty acids can be transported into either your cells for energy, or muscles. The glycerol component can be used to create glucose through gluconeogenesis, which largely is performed in the liver and kidney. The release of fatty acids and the glycerol molecule act as substrates to provide the body with fuel when energy stores are low, helping to maintain blood glucose levels.

Note that the fatty acids from lipolysis can not become glucose-they have a separate fate. If energy is needed, the fatty acids are shuttled to your mitochondria to produce ATP. I am sure you remember the phrase "the mitochondria is the powerhouse of the cell." It forever reigns true. A handful of complex biochemical reactions occur in your mitochondria, allowing you to make ATP and energy from the foods that you eat- including all your macronutrients!

During exercise, fats are your primary energy source during low-intensity activities or when your heart rate is approximately less than 70%. However again, just because you use fat, does not mean that you will lose fat. Fat loss requires a caloric deficit. Refer to my cardio talk for more details here.

Types of Fat

Not all fats in your diet are the same. Knowing the differences can help you determine which to include the most of in your diet, and which to proceed with caution with. There are four main types of fats that differ based on their molecular structure. These structures, as well as the food's vitamin/mineral content, are what determines whether they are more or less beneficial for your health. I will not label any fats as "bad," except for the case of trans fat. I truly believe that when it comes down to bad vs good fats- it's about moderation and fat balance.

- Polyunsaturated Fats: These contain two or more double bonds in their structure and are traditionally liquid at room temperature. Their structure and bonds are "unsaturated" with carbons, and therefore the structure produces multiple kinks. These kinks allow polyunsaturated fats to stack less easily on top of issue when stored in the tissues of your body.

Polyunsaturated fats include two essential fatty acids that are required by your body- Omega-3s and Omega-6s.

Omega-3 fats help to reduce inflammation, support healthy hormones, and maintain cell membrane integrity. They have been shown to help reduce pain, aid in recovery, and even reduce symptoms of PMS and arthritis. Omega-3s help produce anti-inflammatory prostaglandins (PGE1) that can help to combat inflammation in your body! This is why they can be highly beneficial in chronic inflammatory conditions and diseases.

The 3 types of Omega-3 fatty acids include:

- ALA (alpha linolenic acid)- found in plant-based foods such as flaxseed, chia seeds, hemp seeds, walnuts. ALA can convert to EPA and DHA in the body.
- EPA (eicosapentaenoic acid) and DHA (docosahexaenoic acid)- found in fish oil and fatty fish such as salmon, anchovies, sardines, mackerel, and herring

These omega-3s (as well as omega-6s) are essential to your body. You have to consume them in your diet or your health will take a hit. Cue PMS problems, chronic pain, and increased risk of illness and infection. Vegans and vegetarians need to be super careful here, as the conversion of ALA to EPA or DHA is limited.

Omega-6 fats also help to support your hormones and regulate inflammation. However, not all omega-6 fats are created equal. Highly refined processed vegetable oil and omega-6 based fats can easily become rancid and oxidize in your body, leading to chronic inflammation and tissue damage. Unlike omega-3s, they produce proinflammatory prostaglandins (PGE2). Chronic inflammation greatly increases your risk of chronic diseases such as cardiovascular disease (CVD), diabetes, fibromyalgia, and cancer. Chronic inflammation also spells a recipe for disaster on your hormones, mood, and pain levels.

Does this mean avoid all omega-6s? No! I recommend avoiding or limiting the processed vegetable oil sources of omega-6s, and otherwise- aiming to consume at least a 2:1 ratio of omega-6 to omega-3s in your diet. The greater focus on omega-3s, the better!

Examples of omega-6s to avoid include: corn, soybean, safflower, cottonseed, grapeseed and sunflower oils- they are commonly used by restaurants to cook (as they are cheap!) and within packaged foods.

Omega-6s to include: coconut, pistachios, pumpkin seeds, sunflower seeds, evening primrose oil, and borage oil.

Polyunsaturated fats can be omega-6 or omega-3 based.

Monounsaturated fats: These contain one double bond in their structure. Examples include: olive oil, avocado, nuts, seeds, and olives. Monounsaturated fats may help to decrease your risk of cardiovascular disease (CVD), as they can help to increase good HDL cholesterol levels.

Saturated Fats: These contain no double bonds in their structure and are solid at room temperature. Their skeletal carbon chains are "saturated" with hydrogens, allowing them to easily stack on top of each other in your tissues. Examples include: animal meats, egg yolks, coconut oil, dairy products, lard, and palm oil.

Saturated Fats, Diet, & CVD

Saturated fats get a bad reputation for being one of the many causes of cardiovascular disease, as in excess, they may raise both good HDL and bad LDL cholesterol. The "diet-heart" hypothesis is what holds saturated fat accountable to increased CVD risk. It states that increased levels of LDL and decreased levels of HDL, as well as particle size (specifically small apolipoprotein B), are large contributing factors to CVD risk. However, dietary fat is not the only thing that impacts these markers and CVD risk.

CVD is multifactorial so dietary fat should not be the sole blame. Total diet quality, including intake and type of carbohydrates and fruit/vegetable intake play critical roles. In addition, it is not just cholesterol that increases your risk of CVD. Other markers such as blood triglycerides and the presence of hypertension, diabetes, overweight/obesity, and lifestyle choices such as lack of physical activity and smoking also play a role. The cause of cardiovascular disease being due to either low HDL, high LDL, or instead, due to lipoprotein molecule size continues to be up for debate. However, in general, high LDL cholesterol and low HDL cholesterol may increase your risk for developing cardiovascular disease, and that is where saturated fats become demonized.

So- avoid saturated fats? No! Saturated fats can be filled with beneficial fat-soluble vitamins and minerals and they play a crucial role in the health of your cell membranes, immunity, production of hormones, as well as aid in liver function. They also can have antimicrobial properties, protecting against harmful pathogens in your gut. Saturated fats aren't the demon the media tries to make them out to be.

Research shows from both observational and clinical control studies that replacing saturated fats with refined carbohydrates in the diet produces no beneficial risk reduction for CVD, and might even increase the risk even more. However, research also shows that replacing saturated fats with polyunsaturated fat may help to reduce your risk of heart disease. This reduction risk is low, though may be clinically significant if one is at risk. Read again the types of polyunsaturated fats- as replacing them with processed vegetable oils would not be the smart choice to make. This saturated fat debacle and CVD causes remain hot topics. Researchers and medical doctors (even dietitians) continue to fight back and forth on the matter.

My conclusion- get a variety of dietary fats, limit or avoid processed vegetable oils, consume mostly omega-3 polyunsaturated fats, and incorporate saturated fats in moderation. If you want to avoid or reduce your risk of CVD, decrease your consumption of alcohol and refined grains, focus on eating half of your proteins as plants, be active for 30 minutes a day, and monitor your blood levels of cholesterol and triglycerides yearly. If they start climbing up, changes need to be made! Your overall dietary pattern and types of foods chosen are far more important than micro-analyzing saturated fat.

Trans fats: Though no longer in most food products, as they have not been fully phased out although required to be removed by the FDA, trans fats are chemically made from polyunsaturated fats to help increase shelf life and food product stability. They are produced through a method called "hydrogenation" that essentially turns previous fat oils into solids to be incorporated into food products. The byproduct of this process is a "partially hydrogenated oil," or "trans fat," for short.

Trans fats are the worst of the fats. They are well known for increasing bad LDL cholesterol and increasing risk of heart disease and inflammation in the body. Trans fats can sometimes still be found in: fried foods, packaged foods including chips, crackers, pastries, cookies, or wraps, nut butters, and pie/pizza crusts.

Legally, food companies can label any food as "trans fat-free" as long as it has less than 0.5 g per serving. Not good- 0.5 g per serving can add up! Take, for example, a whipped topping with a 1 tbsp serving size. Who eats 1 serving? Not me!! Trans fats can add up and cause harm. Avoid these like the plague and look at your nutrition labels for the words "partially hydrogenated" in the ingredients.

How Do You Lose or Burn Fat?

Not like you expect! Remember your law of thermodynamics. Matter, or energy, is neither created nor destroyed. When you lose fat, the energy stored in your fat cells have to go somewhere. The fatty acids and glycerol can be removed from your fat cells and adipocytes and used by the cells of your body for energy, but the process has to eliminate energy as well. What happens? Upon breakdown, your body fat generates heat (which is used to control your body temperature) and ultimately produces CO_2 (carbon dioxide) and water.

Thus, when you lose body fat, the fat is actually exhaled as you breathe and the water is lost in urine, sweat, or your breath. Isn't that cool? You literally lose fat by breathing, sweating, and peeing!

This is where some people notice that they may not lose weight for a week, and then all of a sudden, they have a "whoosh" effect of weight loss. Contrary to what some people say, this is not because your body fat cells "fill-up with water first" before shrinking and losing fat. Fat cells are lipophilic and hydrophobic. They won't just grab water and bring it into the fat cell. Instead, what happens is you retain water, possibly due to stress, lack of sleep, inflammation, or a heavy workout, and when this stress goes away, cortisol drops, allowing for the water you retained to be lost. WHOOSH goes the weight!

Where Keto Diets Seem Promising- At First...

When you start a ketogenic diet, you drastically drop the carbohydrates in your diet. As you do this, your body starts to deplete its liver and muscle glycogen stores, utilizing as many carbs for energy as it can, until your stores are depleted and the body can adapt to produce ketones for energy. As you drop those carbohydrates, and your body's glycogen storages drop, so does your total body water content! This is why ketogenic diets at first can produce a large amount of weight loss. For every gram of glycogen that you lose, you also lose 2-3 grams of water! Water weight is lost with the loss of muscle and liver glycogen. So yes, one may lose a lot of weight at the start of a ketogenic diet, but is that body fat? Maybe. Maybe not. A caloric deficit will dictate that.

So What Should Your Macros Look Like?

This largely depends on your goals, insulin sensitivity, diet history, and training intensity. It also can depend on personal preference! Just like trial and error to find your maintenance calories, you also need trial and error to find your macronutrient needs. Don't want to track them? You can skip this section!

I largely believe "diets" fail because people have not found the best "diet" for them. By "diet"- I just mean way of eating. Your nutrition and diet should be mostly easy and enjoyable for you. Yeah, in some cases you may not like the fruits and vegetables you need and have to force-feed yourself, but if you are like me and adore carbohydrates, then a low-carb or ketogenic diet and high-fat macronutrient ratio may not work for you!

The most important thing with planning out your macros is finding out what you can stick to. Sustainability is key. Remember, when calories are equated (without insulin resistance or metabolic or hormone dysfunction), it doesn't really matter the macro ratio you choose, as long as protein and calories match.

Lower fat vs lower carb diets or specific macronutrient ratios each have their own benefits and drawbacks. Some researchers or doctors may claim that "carbs cause insulin resistance" and suggest a low-carb or ketogenic diet, while others will claim that "fat causes insulin resistance" and preach a low-fat, higher carbohydrate diet. I could go on for days about the "obesity cause" or "contributors to cardiovascular disease." I refuse to make one single claim or take sides. My "diet dogma" lies in what works for you.

When programming out and choosing your macros and macro ratios- I say find what makes YOU feel best, what keeps you satisfied, and what is sustainable for your lifestyle. Find what optimizes your health and happiness. Some people find higher carbohydrate dieting to be more sustainable, provide more energy, and be more satisfying and enjoyable. Others may find that a higher fat intake helps keep their hunger at bay and allows them to enjoy their foods more. Be willing to experiment with yourself and look less at the "scientific data" and more at your own unique body.

There are some instances, such as in metabolic or hormonal imbalances or insulin resistance, in which one diet or macronutrient ratio may be more helpful or beneficial than another. This is where a registered dietitian like me can come into play to help you individually! However, diet quality is key. With all diets, the quality of your diet matters just as much as the quantity.

Time to calculate!

Remember:

- 9 calories are in each gram of fat
- 4 calories are in each gram of carbohydrate
- 4 calories are in each gram of protein

Step 1- Set Your Protein Needs.

For Sedentary Individuals	1.2-2.0 g/kg
For Weight trainers or resistance athletes	1.6-3.0 g/kg
For Endurance athletes	1.2-2.5 g/kg
For Dieters	1.5-2.5 g/kg
For Pregnancy	1.6-2.0 g/kg
For Seniors or Older Adults	1.2-2.0 g/kg

228 | THE WOMEN'S GUIDE TO HORMONAL HARMONY

For math purposes- there are 2.2 lbs in 1 kg. To convert your bodyweight to kilograms or kg, divide your weight in pounds by 2.2. For a 150 lb woman, her weight in kilograms would equal 68.2 (68.18 rounded to the nearest decimal).

Let's stick to the 150 lb woman. Let's name her Laura. If Laura's goal is to gain muscle and she weight-trains, her protein needs are set at 1.6-3.0 g/kg. Typically, I keep people in my "sweet spot" of 2.0 g/kg within this range. For Laura, this would equate to:

$$68.2 \times 2.0 = 136 \text{ g protein per day.}$$

136 g protein x 4 calories per gram of protein would then mean that 544 of her daily calories would come from protein. If Laura was 150 lbs and had a daily TDEE from her Mifflin-St Jeor equation of 1780 calories, that would mean that she would be consuming 30.5% of her calories from protein and have 1,236 calories left to use for her carbohydrates and fats.

The more you weigh however, the less these protein recommendations hold true. If you are over 170 lbs, it would be best to use your lean body mass to calculate your protein needs or ideal body weight.

Your lean body mass (LBM) is equal to your total weight minus fat mass and includes your: organs, tissues, bones, skin, muscle tissue, and body water. You can estimate your lean body mass, or have a scan such as a DEXA, InBody, or BodPod done to estimate. DEXA scans are gold standard and the most accurate markers, however using an InBody or BodPod could give you a good starting estimate.

How to calculate your ideal body weight (IBW):

IBW for men= 50 kg + 2.3 kg for each inch over 5 feet

IBW for women= 45.5 kg + 2.3 kg for each inch over 5 feet

Why focus on lean mass or IBW?

If Laura weighed 200 lbs and had approximately 130 lbs of lean body mass- her protein needs would be 118 g if she stuck to my 2.0 g/kg sweet spot. If instead, Laura decided to use her IBW at a height of 5'3" her IBW would be calculated as: 45.5 kg + (2.3 kg x 3) = 52.4 kg. Her protein needs would then (at my sweet spot), be 105 g of protein.

Notice these large differences! In reality, the extra protein using the lean body calculation would not harm Laura. She could consume more protein if she would like, or use the lower end calculation. However, based on the science and benefits behind higher protein diets, I would recommend the higher calculation.

Step 2- Set Your Fat Intake

In general, I suggest starting with 25-35% of your intake from fat. If you know you have insulin resistance, then you may want to start on the higher end at 35-45% fat. I suggest trying to never let your fat drop below 0.2 5g/lb or 0.55 g/kg. Remember, you need fat for healthy hormones, skin, cell fluidity, and brain function! Keeping your fat higher may be beneficial to maintain healthy hormone levels, especially while dieting.

For Laura, she has 1,236 calories left for fat or carbohydrates. If she wishes to set her fat intake at 30%, then her calculation for fat would be 1780 x 0.30 = 534 calories for fat. Since there are 9 calories per gram of fat, 534 calories divided by 9 calories per gram would equal to about 59 g fat.

This leaves Laura with 705 calories left for carbohydrates: 1780 calories − (531 calories from fat + 544 calories from protein) = 705 calories

Step 3- Set Your Carbohydrate Intake

Laura now has 705 calories left. She can now divide these calories by 4 calories (as carbohydrates have 4 calories per gram), and her carbohydrate intake will be set at 176 g carbohydrates per day.

Overall:

Macronutrient Recommendations	Protein	Fat	Carbohydrate
General Start	1.2-2.5g/kg bodyweight	25–35% of total calories	Remaining calories to meet daily intake

*Chart from Helms E, Morgan A, Valdez A. The Muscle & Strength Pyramid: Nutrition. San Bernardino, CA: Muscle and Strength Pyramids; 2019. *

Determining Meal Timing

In order to maximize your health, energy, and metabolism, when you eat does matter!

While meal timing may only have a small impact on your physique, it can have a big impact on your energy levels, gym performance, and blood sugar regulation. Meal timing is of upmost importance when it comes down to training performance, especially in the case for endurance training and team sports. However, since most of the people reading this book are not marathon runners or football players, I am going to focus on practical meal timing strategies for the every day person.

Poor meal timing can leave you with imbalanced blood sugar, low energy levels, poor adherence due to insatiable hunger, and increase your risk of overeating and binge eating. The goal is to provide a steady source of fuel for your body and brain throughout the day, optimize muscle protein synthesis for building or preserving muscle, and preventing rapid spikes and dips in your blood sugar, which can influence your hormonal and adrenal health.

The easiest way to determine meal timing for you is to ask yourself: "How many times a day is a sustainable eating pattern for me?". Some people prefer larger, less frequent meals, while others prefer smaller, more frequent meals. Pay attention to what makes you feel your best!

The easiest way to structure your meals is to divide the total macronutrients that you consume throughout the day and divide that by the number of meals you plan to have.

For example:

4 meals a day- 25% of daily carbohydrates, protein, and fat per meal

5 meals a day- 20% of daily carbohydrates, protein, and fat per meal

For a macronutrient goal of 50g fat, 200g carbohydrates, and 130g protein per day at 4 meals a day, that would be per meal: 12g fat, 50g carbs, and 33g protein.

This is an easy way to spread your macronutrients and food intake throughout the day. There are adjustments you can then make to better optimize pre or post workout nutrition, and you can shift some of the macros from one meal to the next meal based on that alteration.

Pre and Post workout meals- What is Best?

Multiple factors exist here- What are your goals? When was your last meal? (and what was it?) What type of training do you do? How insulin sensitive are you? What's your post workout meal like and when do you have it? I will try and make this as simple as possible for you based on common lifting scenarios:

1. If you plan to eat within 1-2 hours before lifting, a mixed meal is adequate as long as it's not too high in fat and fiber to inhibit your digestion and performance (individual variances here). You may benefit from a small carbohydrate snack prior to lifting for addition energy if you ate 2 hours prior to your workout (15-30g carbs suggested). **Suggestion if eating 1-2 hours before lifting: 5-20g F, 20-60g C, 25-40g P**

2. If you plan to eat an hour to 30 minutes prior to lifting, a quick digesting or mix of slow and quick digesting carbohydrates and a protein source with low fat and low fiber may be optimal to help give you energy and not screw up your digestion during your lift. **Suggestion if eating 30 minutes prior to lifting: 20-30g carbs, 10-30g protein**

3. It you're insulin resistant, dividing up at least 4-50% of your daily carbs between pre and post workout may be beneficial as you are most insulin sensitive during these times. **Suggestion if insulin resistance- consume half of your daily carbohydrates pre and post workout**

4. If you're training fasted, either lift fasted and have a low fat, high carbohydrate and protein meal post workout, or consume an essential amino acid or protein shake during your workout. The drink would be more important for those in a contest prep or diet phase who don't want to lose muscle. If you're just a regular "gym goer" don't worry about it! Training fasted is not recommended with any hormonal or adrenal imbalance. **Suggestion if training fasted- consume a low fat, normal meal post workout 10-20g F, 20-60g C, 25-40g P**.

Remember these facts when planning out pre and post workout meals:

- If you eat within a few hours pre workout- muscle protein synthesis is STILL elevated right when you finish, so getting in your protein immediately post workout isn't necessary. You won't lose your gains.
- Your pre workout meal may just be a pre workout snack, and that's okay! Your pre workout helps to fuel for energy, stabilize your blood sugar, and preserve your muscles. Find a meal or snack that you enjoy, that digests well, and helps you feel your best when training.
- Protein's goal: spike muscle protein synthesis, aid in growth and recovery, preserve lean muscle tissue and build new muscle tissue
- Carb's goal: immediate energy for training, fills glycogen stores (which are not fully depleted post workout if you're just lifting- they are for endurance training!), cause insulin spike, help to reduce cortisol
- Fat's goal: slower digesting form of energy; helps to stabilize and prevent the blood sugar response to a carbohydrate; slows digestion when added to a protein or carbohydrate (which may or may not impact your digestion in a pre workout meal)

Macro Adjustments for Fat Loss or Muscle Gain

Remember, a calorie deficit is king to lose weight. Protein is the most important macronutrient to keep stable to help preserve lean muscle tissue and aid in hunger and satiety, therefore adjust your fats and carbohydrates in order to further your deficit. I suggest keeping your protein level between 1.5-2.5g/kg of bodyweight.

1. Muscle Gain or Reverse Dieting:

Adding Calories via Fat

Pros	Cons
-Easy to add & more concentrated per volume of food -May help digestion	-May be more readily deposited as body fat -Less anabolic than carbohydrates -May hinder protein synthesis if high pre or post workout -Does not fill depleted glycogen stores -Response to type of fat may influence adiposity in building phase

Adding Calories via Carbohydrates

Pros	Cons
-Refills depleted glycogen stores -Preferred source of energy in the body -Less stored as body fat -More anabolic than fat	-May require higher volumes to get more calories -Less common to find low fat, carbohydrate choices -Insulin resistance may be worsened by addition of carbohydrates

2. Fat Loss

Decreasing Calories via Fat:

Pros	Cons
-May allow for better fat mobilization -May help decrease intake highly processed, less filling foods	-May increase hunger levels more than decreasing carbs -May negatively impact hormones in the long term if inadequate -May slow digestion if under 45g

Decreasing Calories via Carbohydrates

Pros	Cons
-May better support hormone production -Helps to reduce insulin resistance	-May negatively impact performance -If under 130g may greatly reduce cognitive function -May negatively impact the gut microbiome if fiber is not met

8

THYROID 101

"The Thyroid is the powerhouse of your metabolism."

J ust like how the mitochondria is the powerhouse of the cell, your thyroid is the powerhouse of your metabolism! It plays critical functions in regulating your metabolism, body weight, and energy levels. It also plays important roles in regulating your heart rate, blood pressure, body temperature, appetite, blood cholesterol and lipid metabolism, digestion, carbohydrate metabolism, growth and repair, cognition, musculoskeletal health, reproduction, nervous system, and more!

Why does this matter? Anything that causes abnormal function of your thyroid itself, or causes abnormal thyroid levels in your blood, can greatly influence almost every single cell and tissue in your body! Thyroid trouble can create further hormone, adrenal, or gut imbalances, can progress autoimmune diseases, as well as wreak havoc on your energy and body composition. Want to optimize your health, energy, and metabolism? Well- you need to optimize your thyroid!

Your thyroid is a butterfly-shaped gland found at the base of your neck, just below the larynx. It is in charge "fueling" almost every cell function in your body, from metabolism, mood, cognition, hormones, heart rate, to growth and repair. Your thyroid is what can "decide" if you lose weight, have energy, are fatigued, have a normal menstrual cycle, feel depressed or anxious, or can focus (or not) on day-to-day work tasks. Basically, your thyroid is the ultimate queen in your body, so it's important to respect it, honor it, and make sure it's optimized!

Thyroid physiology can get quite complex, so let's break it down piece by piece, starting with thyroid hormones, what thyroid disorders exist, and how thyroid hormones are produced and converted. See the below definitions as a general basis to start:

Key components of your thyroid:

- T4 (Thyroxine)- the inactive form of thyroid hormone can convert to either T3 or RT3
- T3 (Triiodothyronine)- the active form of your thyroid hormone that is responsible for thyroid hormone's work and actions in the body
- RT3 (Reverse Triiodothyronine)- the inactive form of thyroid hormone produced from T4 mainly due to stress, infection, cortisol dysregulation, or nutrient deficiencies
- TRH (Thyrotropin-releasing hormone)- a hormone produced by your hypothalamus that stimulates the release of TSH from your pituitary gland. It is regulated by T4 and T3 blood levels.
- TSH (Thyrotropin-stimulating hormone)- a hormone produced by your pituitary gland that stimulates your thyroid to produce T4 and T3
- TPO (thyroid peroxidase)- an enzyme found in your thyroid gland that is involved in the production of T3 and T4. Thyroid peroxidase converts iodide into iodine in the body, which is required to attach to tyrosine in a

thyroglobulin molecule to create thyroid hormone.
Elevated TPO antibodies are found in Hashimoto's
which causes autoimmune attack of the thyroid and
lowers the production of thyroid hormone produced

- Calcitonin: secreted by the thyroid when high calcium
levels are found in the blood and inhibits calcium release
from the bone

Truth is- most conventional doctors do not do a full thyroid panel
and many women go about their lives in a hypothyroid state,
STRUGGLING for years. I was there. I know I struggled until I
took matters into my own hands and did testing myself.

Does this sound familiar? Dry or thinning hair, hair loss, fatigue,
depression, brain fog or reduced mental clarity, hoarseness of
voice, goiter, enlarged thyroid gland, dry skin, low perspiration,
muscle loss, muscle aches or weakness, joint pain, constipation,
weight gain or trouble losing weight, bradycardia (low resting
heart rate, usually below 60 bpm), hypertension, elevated LDL,
infertility, abnormal sex hormones, peripheral neuropathy, cold
intolerance, cold hands and feet, an irregular menstrual cycle.

If you said yes too many of those symptoms, you need to check
your thyroid! If you don't fully assess your thyroid, you aren't fully
assessing your health. Don't worry, later in this chapter I will give
you the exact labs to ask for, and what to do if your doctor won't
test them.

How Your Thyroid Works

Your thyroid produces four types of thyroid hormones, T1, T2,
T3, and T4, as well as calcitonin. T4 (thyroxine) is the main
hormone produced (about 80-93% of thyroid production) and is
required to be converted into T3 in order to do its job. T3 (triiodothyronine) is produced in much smaller quantities (about 7-
20% of production), however is the main thyroid hormone that
doesn't require conversion to do work. Your thyroid also produces

small amounts of T1, T2, and calcitonin. T4 and T3 are the major thyroid hormones involved and created by your thyroid gland. They are what do most of the metabolic work in your body.

Quick Facts:

1. Only about 20% of the T3 (your active thyroid hormone) in your body is directly produced by your thyroid gland.
2. T4 must convert to T3 in order to do its job.
3. The conversion process of T4 to T3 occurs within multiple tissues throughout your body. Approximately 20% of your thyroid conversion occurs in your gut.
4. There are many factors that can increase or decrease the conversion of T4 to T3. If T3 isn't made, you will have hypothyroid symptoms.

How is your thyroid controlled? It's a beautiful and intricate, complex process! In a normal, healthy individual, your thyroid is controlled through a negative feedback loop, in which circulating T4 and T3 levels stimulate your hypothalamus to secrete TRH (thyrotropin-releasing hormone). TRH then stimulates TSH (thyroid-stimulating hormone) to be released by your pituitary gland. TSH then stimulates your thyroid gland to either increase or decrease the production of your thyroid hormone. Overall, low levels of thyroid hormones then feedback to TRH, which increases TSH and tells your body to make more thyroid hormone. If thyroid hormone levels are high, then TSH goes down, and your thyroid produces less thyroid hormones. Notice how there are multiple organs, not just your thyroid involved. This intricate feedback loop controlling your thyroid involves your hypothalamic-pituitary-thyroid axis (HPT axis).

Let's recap. Your pituitary is controlled by your hypothalamus, which produces TRH. TRH stimulates TSH, a pituitary hormone, that signals to your thyroid to increase or decrease thyroid hormone production based on current levels of circulating thyroid hormones. Thyroid hormones are then released by your thyroid and converted into active thyroid hormone (T3) or inactive thyroid hormone (RT3- more on this later) within your body's tissues. This is done through a feedback loop that acts like a "metabolic thermostat" in your body.

The Thyroid Thermostat:

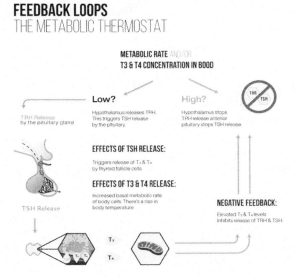

Typically, when T4 and T3 levels are low, as in the case of hypothyroidism, TRH tells your pituitary to produce more TSH, which signals to the thyroid to produce more T4 and T3. When T4 and T3 levels are high, as in hyperthyroidism, TRH then tells your pituitary to produce less TSH, which then decreases the amount of thyroid hormones produced by your thyroid.

Essentially, the thyroid and pituitary work together to control thyroid levels in the body like a thermostat. If it gets "too cold" and thyroid hormones are low, TSH will go up. If it gets "too hot" and thyroid hormones are high, TSH will go down. This is how the body tries to stabilize your thyroid hormones within the body, as you don't want too much or too little thyroid hormone.

To summarize:

- When your thermostat reads T4 and T3 as being low, TSH creeps up, indicating hypothyroidism
- When your thermostat reads T4 and T3 as being high, TSH drops down, indicating hyperthyroidism

I don't want to confuse you, but there are multiple reasons why your thermostat may have issues "reading" properly. For example, TSH may be normal, and yet your T4 and/or T3 may be low. This is commonly seen in subclinical and cellular hypothyroidism, as well as euthyroid sick syndrome. It also occurs in the beginning stages of Hashimoto's, in an inflammatory state, or in the presence of a hypothalamus or pituitary malfunction. I know, it's complex.

Here's a step by step of overall how the thyroid should work:

Step 1: Hypothalamus secretes TRH- thyrotropin-releasing hormone
Step 2: Pituitary responds to TRH and releases TSH-thyroid-stimulating hormone
Step 3: Thyroid responds to TSH, signals for creation and secretion of thyroid hormones (mostly T4 with little T3)
Step 4: Thyroid hormones attach to TBG (thyroxine-binding globulin) to travel to various tissues in the blood
Step 5: Thyroid hormones are converted by peripheral tissues with the help of adding enzymes. T4 becomes T3 or RT3.
Step 6: Thyroid hormone can enter the cells of the tissues.

Step 7: Serum T4 and T3 levels provide feedback to TRH to restart the cycle.

Now that you have a good basis for how the thyroid works- let's dive into what can happen with the thyroid and the conditions that can arise with the lack of, or too much, thyroid hormone.

The Top 6 Conditions Associated with Thyroid Dysfunction:

- Hypothyroidism: decreased activity of the thyroid gland, resulting in low thyroid hormones
- Hashimoto's Thyroiditis: decreased activity of the thyroid gland due to autoimmune attack of thyroid antibodies to the thyroid
- Hyperthyroidism: increased activity of the thyroid gland, resulting in elevated thyroid hormones
- Grave's Disease: increased activity of the thyroid gland due to autoimmune attack of the thyroid
- Thyrotoxicosis: excess circulating thyroid hormone, can be short term or related to a "thyroid storm"
- Thyroiditis: inflammation of the thyroid, causing short term hyperthyroidism (for a period of 3-6 months)

Hypothyroidism:

Hypothyroidism is defined as decreased activity of the thyroid gland, which can affect your metabolism, reproductive, cardiovascular, mental, and physical health. Your thyroid can affect almost every cell and organ in your body! Hypothyroidism affects 1 in 10 women, with a 5-8x higher likelihood for women to have thyroid problems over men! It is estimated that 12% of the US population will develop a thyroid condition sometime during their lifetime.

There are three main types of hypothyroidism. Primary hypothyroidism involves damage or malfunction of the thyroid gland itself, while secondary hypothyroidism involves a disease or malfunction of other organs or tissues that then affect thyroid function, such as pituitary or hypothalamus-related issues. Subclinical hypothyroidism occurs when thyroid levels may be slightly low with a normal or slightly elevated TSH.

It is estimated that 2-7% of adults in the US have subclinical hypothyroidism. Many times this goes undiagnosed, leaving someone struggling with hypothyroid symptoms sometimes for years! How does this happen? Their doctor doesn't do a full thyroid panel! I got you- we will dive into this soon.

Hypothyroidism can be immune or non immune-related. Immune-related hypothyroidism is called Hashimoto's Thyroiditis, and affects women 10x more than men. In the United States, Hashimoto's is the most common type and cause of hypothyroidism. This autoimmune disease can lay "dormant" in many people, however once triggered, it creates attack on the thyroid, resulting in hypothyroidism and potential irreversible damage to the thyroid. For many cases, the thyroid swells, creating a goiter from the thyroid's attempt to produce more thyroid hormone. If caught early, Hashimoto's patients can prevent severe damage to their thyroid and are able to manage their disease without the use of medications and exogenous thyroid hormone. However, if not caught in time, thyroid destruction can result in inadequate thyroid hormone production with irreversible thyroid gland damage. In this case, the lifelong use of exogenous thyroid hormone medication is required.

Active Hashimoto's can be distinguished by antibody presence, through TPOab (thyroid peroxidase) antibodies, and TgAB (antithyroglobulin) antibodies. During active Hashimoto's, these antibodies attack thyroid tissue, thinking that it is a foreign invader. The TPO antibody attacks thyroid peroxidase (the enzymes involved in T4 to T3 conversion), while TgAB antibody attacks thyroglobulin (a key component of thyroid hormone). This results in the depletion of thyroid hormones, prevents adequate thyroid conversion, and prevents the body from getting the active thyroid it needs! Again, Hashimoto's, if left untreated or not caught, can result in irreversible thyroid damage, resulting in the need for exogenous thyroid hormone to maintain adequate thyroid hormone for the rest of someone's life. However, when caught early and managed, one can likely maintain thyroid function without the use of medication. I am reiterating this so that you understand the importance of getting a full thyroid panel when you notice thyroid-related symptoms. You may have the ability to save your thyroid!

Hashimoto's often presents with an enlarged thyroid gland (goiter), however, this is not seen in all cases. In the beginning stages of Hashimoto's, thyroid hormone levels and TSH may actually be normal! This is where Hashimoto's can be a sneaky thyroid thief- as any present antibodies will continue to attack the thyroid without the person even knowing (reminder again to always get a full thyroid panel done!).

What causes the immune and thyroid attack? Molecular mimicry! In molecular mimicry, your body mistakes a normal cell for a foreign invader. This can be triggered and initiated by a virus, bacteria, stealth infections, mold toxicity, heavy metal toxicity, food intolerances such as gluten, wheat, or soy, gut infections, etc. These factors can trigger a "thyroid storm" which can then accelerate into an autoimmune attack. This can set someone right into hypothyroidism, or can set someone into a short term hyperthyroid state followed by hypothyroidism, known as thyrotoxicosis. Genetic risk factors to Hashimoto's include having the MTHFR enzyme (more information found in the gut health chapter) and additional autoimmune diseases such as Celiac or Lupus.

Unfortunately, Hashimoto's is an autoimmune disease. In an autoimmune disease, any stressor can be a potential trigger. Think of autoimmunity like a car race. There is a trigger that leads to damage of your thyroid cells. Let's pretend the trigger (aka a thief) takes away money from the bank and the bank (your thyroid!) is destroyed. The "bank" sends out a signal to the police (hypothalamus) that something is wrong. Immune cells, aka the cops, come in and strive to save the bank. The bank can either be continued to be destroyed by other thieves, stay in signal mode as the cops don't know what's going on, OR can be resolved when the cops catch the thief. However, the damage done to the bank may be irreversible.

The Car Race Tends to Follow This Pattern:

1. A combination of a trigger, genetic predisposition, and intestinal permeability or low immune function sets up a storm
2. Thyroid cells start to get attacked and antibodies develop.
3. 3. The thyroid sends a signal for help as thyroid levels drop. TSH goes up.
4. The immune system sends an attempt to save the thyroid gland from attack. They mistake thyroid tissue for a foreign invader.
5. The thyroid gland continues to be attacked and damaged by the body's own lymphocytes (white blood cells).
6. Thyroid hormone creation diminishes and the thyroid can no longer produce enough thyroid hormone for the body's needs.

It's a nightmare for people.

Regardless of the type of hypothyroidism, having a low thyroid can result in a host of havoc to the body. Signs and symptoms of hypothyroidism include (but are not limited to): Weight gain, hair loss, chronic fatigue, low heart rate, dry skin, digestive problems like chronic bloating, constipation, or diarrhea, joint and muscle pain, irregular menstrual cycles (or none!), cold intolerance, depression, anxiety, dry skin, brain fog, insomnia, loss of libido, swelling of the face, loss of eyebrow hair, cold hands and feet, elevated cholesterol levels, and swollen thyroid or a goiter. It's important to also note that these are signs and symptoms of other conditions, so it is very important to always test and not guess to determine the true root cause and condition. In addition, not all hypothyroid cases result in the same or all symptoms.

People with Hashimoto's may experience the confusing roller-coasters of going hypothyroid and hyperthyroid all within the same week. Postpartum hypothyroidism can also create this experience, in which one goes hyperthyroid briefly, and then has a resulting hypothyroid state. The upswings of hyperthyroidism with Hashimoto's is called thyrotoxicosis and can be life threatening. That is why it's essential to be in tune with your body and that you understand the different signs and symptoms associated with abnormal thyroid levels.

Hyperthyroidism

Hyperthyroidism is defined as having an overactive thyroid, in which too much thyroid hormone is produced.

There are many forms of hyperthyroidism including thyrotoxicosis, thyroiditis, and Grave's disease. The development of hyperthyroidism, just like hypothyroidism, can be related to genetics, as is the case for autoimmune Grave's disease, or a side effect of a tumor, thyroid nodules, medications, high iodine levels, or infection.

In Grave's disease, TSH receptor antibodies or thyroid stimulated immunoglobulins (TSI) react with TSH receptors, causing thyroid cells to produce excess thyroid hormone. This may put someone in a chronic state of hyperthyroidism.

Hyperthyroidism caused by nodules or goiters can be referred to as toxic nodular or multinodular goiters. The goiter or nodules produce temporary increases in thyroid production, causing thyrotoxicosis. Some hypothyroid patients actually develop nodules, causing hyperthyroidism. This can be confusing, as you can swing from hypo to hyperthyroid, and then back to hypothyroid. The cause of a nodule or goiter formation may stem from diet, genetic, or environment influences. Infections or viruses may also play a role in the rise of autoimmune attack via Grave's as well as the creation or trigger of the growth of a nodule.

Thyroiditis can also occur and produce short term hyperthyroidism, as seen in the case of postpartum thyroiditis. Thyroiditis involves inflammation of the thyroid gland and may last a few weeks to months, with a potential to be followed by hypothyroidism. It is speculated that some may have a genetic predisposition to developing hyperthyroidism, and that a trigger, just like Hashimoto's and molecular mimicry, can set off a cascade of attack, creating the hyperthyroid state.

Causes of hyperthyroidism may include medications, pregnancy, virus or infection, gut infections, heavy metals, hyperemesis gravidarum, tumors, micronutrient deficiencies, excess exogenous thyroid medication, and high iodine levels. Drugs that can interfere and contribute to hyperthyroidism include lithium, interferon alpha, amiodarone, etc.

Diagnosis can be made based on TSH, free T4, and free T3 levels. In general, low TSH with high T4 and high T3 indicate a state of hyperthyroidism. Grave's disease accounts for about 70% of hyperthyroid cases, and can be distinguished by the presence of antibodies, specifically TRAbs (thyrotropin receptor antibodies) and TSI levels. Doctors often also check the thyroid via a scan to assess for nodules or goiter presence.

Symptoms of hyperthyroidism include: hair loss, shakiness, increased appetite, anxiety, increased heart beat, heart palpitations, bulging eyes, peripheral edema and swelling, insomnia, trembling of hands, heat intolerance, shortness of breath, weight loss/ loss of muscle mass, diarrhea, infertility, sweating, presence of a goiter, and fatigue.

Hyperthyroidism is commonly treated with antithyroid drugs, radioactive iodine, or surgery, and the use of beta-blockers is common to help with symptom management. Antithyroid drugs include propylthiouracil, methimazole, thiamazole, and carbimazole. Each drug has its own mechanism of action to decrease thyroid hormone production. Some work to decrease iodination of thyroglobulin by reducing the work of thyroid peroxidase, causing the lowering of thyroid levels. Remember, thyroid peroxidase is involved in the creation of thyroid hormone. It oxidizes iodide atoms to form iodine atoms that attach to tyrosine residues on a thyroglobulin molecule, producing thyroid hormone. Prevention of TPO can reduce the signal of TSH to increase thyroid production, helping to decrease excess thyroid hormone production. Sadly, it is quite common for hyperthyroid patients who are treated with antithyroid drugs to develop hypothyroidism later on. They can also increase risk of infection by lowering white blood cell count. Currently, methimazole is the first drug of choice by many doctors due to having less side effects.

Radioactive iodine ablation is also used as a method to treat hyperthyroidism. It works by damaging or destroying parts of the thyroid, which in turn decreases its production. This is a common treatment used in thyroid nodules. In this case as well, it's common for someone to develop hypothyroidism after treatment. Surgery (known as a thyroidectomy) can also partially or fully remove the thyroid or a thyroid nodule. The removal of the thyroid gland results in lifelong hypothyroidism, which requires lifelong exogenous thyroid hormone medication to treat. Surgery can also be performed when bulging eyes are present, called Grave's ophthalmopathy. Orbital decompression surgery or scar tissue removal may be performed.

Beta-blockers are commonly prescribed to help reduce the side effects of excess thyroid hormone, including heart palpitations, increased heart rate, shakiness, and nervousness. These drugs are commonly used in the treatment of high blood pressure and congestive heart failure. Their mechanism of action is not by inhibiting thyroid hormone production, however they can help alleviate symptoms prior to further treatment. Beta-blockers work by blocking the effects of your hormone epinephrine (aka adrenaline), causing your heart rate to slow with less force production, lowering blood pressure, and helping to improve blood flow.

During hyperthyroidism, high levels of T4 and T3 stimulate fat mobilization and carbohydrate metabolism in the body, which leads to increases in metabolic rate. This metabolic increase can lead to undesired weight loss and loss of muscle mass. Increases in thyroid hormone can also increase the output of stomach acid, digestive pancreatic secretions, and bile acids, which can lead to diarrhea, malabsorption, and nutrient deficiencies. These deficiencies can in turn cause fatigue, low blood sugar, and further enhance weight loss. There is increased risk of bone loss and the development of osteoporosis, as thyroid hormone has a direct catabolic (break down) effect on bone mineral homeostasis. Excess thyroid hormone can decrease free estrogen and testosterone levels by increasing sex hormone binding globulin (SHBG). This results in decreased free hormone levels (as noted in my hormone chapter), as SHBG is the carrier protein of hormones in the blood. Too much SHBG causes hormone levels to be bound, and less free hormone is available. This results in further metabolic, hormonal, and health chaos! In addition, estrogen plummeting, which participates in bone protection, causes further risk of bone loss and risk of developing osteoporosis.

Antibody Distinctions

Thyroid antibodies are seen in all forms of autoimmune thyroid disease- including Hashimoto's thyroiditis, Grave's disease, autoimmune atrophic thyroiditis, or post partum thyroiditis. If caught early, thyroid damage can be prevented, antibodies can be lowered, and thyroid health can be improved. Don't make the mistake of not testing antibodies, as they can develop (or be diminished) throughout a lifetime.

Symptoms are Messengers- Don't Kill the Messenger

Understanding the meaning behind certain signs/symptoms is important in order to understand that these symptoms aren't your body hurting and hating you, but rather are the result of your body trying to tell you it needs help and healing! Symptoms are like a fire alarm, and are your body's way of saying, "Help! There is a fire! Something is wrong!" Weight gain results from reduction in metabolism and alterations in sex hormones (as T3 is directly in charge of metabolic rate), mood changes may occur due to shifts in serotonin, neurotransmitters, hormone levels (such as high or low estrogen, testosterone, and progesterone), or nutrient deficiencies. Fatigue occurs due to lack of T3 creation, resulting in less work for the cell from less ATP and energy production. Cold intolerance occurs due to changes in thermogenesis, which can cause body temperature to drop and increases sensitivity to cold. Digestive issues can result from food intolerances, intestinal permeability, lack of hydrochloric acid or pancreatic enzyme production, or slowed gut motility. In turn, lack of stomach acid, pancreatic enzymes, and bile acid secretion can result in potential overgrowths and malabsorption.

Let's talk more about the digestive issues I mentioned. A common complaint in hypothyroidism is digestive distress- including gas, bloating, constipation, and increased food intolerances. Here's the thing- hypothyroidism can cause digestive issues, however digestive issues can also cause hypothyroidism! What happens physiologically? The body produces less stomach acid, less pancreatic enzymes, less bile, and slows down your gut motility, which happens via what is called your "migrating motor complex" (which is greatly influenced by your vagus nerve which connects your gut to your brain!). These effects can result in trouble digesting and absorbing food, early feelings of satiety, and bouts of constipation or even diarrhea! They also increase the risk of bacterial or fungal gut overgrowths and gut infections due to slowed motility, constipation, and over-fermentation of food sitting in the intestine. Additional digestive effects include:

- Decreased absorption of nutrients (creating potential deficiencies)
- Increased risk of estrogen dominance and hormonal imbalance (if estrogen is not properly metabolized and excreted, it recirculates)
- Reduced immunity and serotonin creation (hello getting sick, mood swings, anxiety, and depression)
- Inflammation- This inflammation can create autoimmune attack, further thyroid inhibition, and then cause intestinal permeability which can create "food intolerances" that really aren't intolerances- just full body inflammation!

Thyroid Requiring Nutrients

Your thyroid hormone production requires nutrients such as iron, iodine, tyrosine, zinc, selenium, vitamin E, B2, B6, vitamin C, and vitamin D. These nutrients are required to be able to make your thyroid hormones! Think of each nutrient as part of a recipe for your favorite cookie (which I hope is not oatmeal raisin because they are trash). Each part of your recipe is critical to the final, delicious product made! If you are low in salt, sugar, butter, eggs, or you have too much of anything, you can screw up your cookies! Same goes for your thyroid. You need each component in optimal amounts for the creation of adequate thyroid hormones.

FACTORS THAT AFFECT **THYROID FUNCTION**

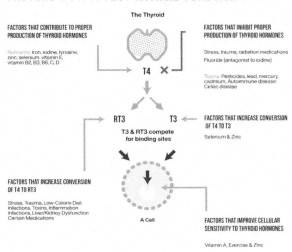

The Thyroid

FACTORS THAT CONTRIBUTE TO PROPER
PRODUCTION OF THYROID HORMONES

Nutrients: Iron, iodine, tyrosine,
zinc, selenium, vitamin E,
vitamin B2, B3, B6, C, D

FACTORS THAT INHIBIT PROPER
PRODUCTION OF THYROID HORMONES

Stress, trauma, radiation medications
Fluoride (antagonist to iodine)

Toxins: Pesticides, lead, mercury,
cadmium, Autoimmune disease:
Celiac disease

T4 ✗

RT3   T3 ←

FACTORS THAT INCREASE CONVERSION
OF T4 TO T3

T3 & RT3 compete
for binding sites

Selenium & Zinc

FACTORS THAT INCREASE CONVERSION
OF T4 TO RT3

Stress, Trauma, Low-Calorie Diet
Infections, Toxins, Inflammation
Infections, Liver/Kidney Dysfunction
Certain Medications

A Cell

FACTORS THAT IMPROVE CELLULAR
SENSITIVITY TO THYROID HORMONES

Vitamin A, Exercise & Zinc

It's not just about the nutrients involved, however. There are also factors that can inhibit your thyroid hormone production which include: thyroid or pituitary damage, chronic stress and high cortisol levels, infections, trauma, chemotherapy or radiation therapy, specific medications such as birth control, fluoride (which is an antagonist to iodine), heavy metals, environmental toxins, and elevations in antibodies in autoimmune disease (in which antibodies such as TPO can prevent production). Other factors that can inhibit production include pesticides, food intolerances, leaky gut (in which lipopolysaccharides decrease deiodinase activity), adrenal dysfunction, excess iodine or l-carnitine, and alcohol. Why is this important? Remember, your thyroid is the powerhouse of your metabolism! Any of these factors that affect your thyroid function can also affect your overall health and happiness.

Your thyroid hormones are made up of iodine molecules and an amino acid called tyrosine, which are attached together to a thyroglobulin molecule and are created and stored inside your thyroid. Your main thyroid hormones get their names based on the number of iodine residues attached to a thyroglobulin. T4 has

4 iodine atoms attached to a thyroglobulin and is the inactive version of your thyroid hormone. This is the storage form of your thyroid hormone that is then released into the blood, then converted to T3 when needed based on tissue or organ needs. T3 on the other hand has 3 iodine atoms attached to its thyroglobulin molecule and is the active form of your thyroid hormone. Your thyroid can produce small amounts of active T3 hormone, but most of your active thyroid hormone is produced through thyroid conversion in your body's tissues. These tissues convert T4 to T3 at different rates based on their individual needs.

Nutrient	Why You Need It	How to Get It
Iodine *too much can increase thyroid antibodies and cause hypothyroidism as well*	Building block for thyroid hormone	Iodized salt Kelp Saltwater fish Supplement or Multivitamin
Selenium	T4 to T3 Conversion	Liver Animal proteins Supplement Brazil Nuts (1= 96 μg of selenium!)
B Vitamins	T4 to T3 Conversion, energy, immunity, coenzymes	Leafy Greens Beets Liver Animal Products Whole Grains Nuts/Seeds Supplement
Zinc *too much can deplete copper levels*	T4 to T3 Conversion, immunity, carbohydrate metabolism, wound healing	Liver Animal Products Spinach Supplement

Nutrient	Why You Need It	How to Get It
Iron *Vitamin C increases absorption, Calcium decreases*	T4 to T3 conversion, iodide to iodine conversion, component of hemoglobin to transport oxygen through the body	Leafy greens Fruits Whole Grains Animal Products Liver Nuts/Seeds Supplement
Tyrosine	Building block for thyroid hormone, stress relief	Animal products Kelp or seaweed Supplement
Omega-3 Fatty Acids	Essential for EPA & DHA, hormone production, cell membrane function/integrity, combat inflammation	Fatty Fish Nuts/Seeds Animal Products (organic higher in Omega-3 than conventional) Fish/Krill/Cod Liver Oil Supplements

Nutrient	Why You Need It	How to Get It
Vitamin D	Immunity, reproduction, cardiovascular health, wound healing, bone health, insulin regulation, thyroid absorption	Sunlight Fatty Fish Eggs (Omega 3 fortified based-organic has higher levels than conventional) Liver Dairy Supplements
Vitamin A	Immunity, thyroid absorption, skin & eye health	Liver Spinach, Kale Carrots Sweet Potatoes Eggs Orange Fruits & Vegetables Supplement
Protein *Intake based on needs and activity*	Growth & repair, enzyme production, cellular structures, hormone production, storage & transport	Meats Dairy Nuts/Seeds Tofu & Soy Whole Grains Eggs Legumes & Peas

Thyroid Hormone Conversion

The amounts of inactive vs active thyroid hormone are what set the stage for your metabolism. What do I mean by inactive vs active? In order for thyroid hormone to do work in your body, they must convert to T3! T4 is not metabolically active and must convert to T3 in order to do its job. Remember that most of your thyroid hormone produced is in the form of inactive T4. This means that conversion of your thyroid hormone is the critical component to ensuring that you have the thyroid hormone that you need for actual work in the body: T3!

T4 to T3 conversion is powered by deiodinase enzymes. These enzymes, labeled as DIO1 to DIO3, are membrane-bound seleno-cysteine enzymes that work to either activate or deactivate thyroid hormone based on tissue needs. Their activity is heavily influenced by inflammation, nutrient deficiencies, endocrine disruptors, heavy metals, insulin levels, cortisol, and the availability of necessary cofactor nutrients. There are various deiodinases found within your body. DIO1 is found in cell plasma membranes mostly in the liver, kidneys, thyroid, and pituitary. It is involved in the conversion from T4 to T3 to a smaller extent. DIO2 is found in the cell endoplasmic reticulum within the thyroid, central nervous system, pituitary, and skeletal muscle. It is involved in the converse from T4 to T3, RT3 to T2, as well as plays a critical role in your body's thermogenesis and in the T4 mediated negative feedback look between your tissue thyroid levels and HPA axis. DIO2 is the most prevalent deiodinase. DIO3 is found within plasma membranes mostly in the central nervous system, skin, and regenerating tissues including the brain, making it extremely important during fetal development. It also is involved in the inactivation of T3, in which its importance in fetal development lies in protection from high maternal T3 and T4 levels.

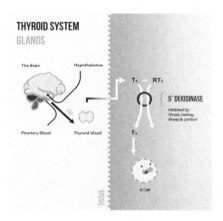

These deiodinases require nutrients such as iodine, selenium, zinc, iron, B-vitamins, protein, vitamin A, vitamin D, tyrosine, dietary carbohydrates, and cortisol. In a healthy individual, your thyroid has no issues converting T4 to T3, but in the presence of stress, trauma, infection, nutrient deficiencies, inflammation, high insulin levels, environmental toxins, liver or kidney dysfunction, heavy metal toxicity, medications, or low-calorie dieting, T4 can covert away from the active form of T3, and instead, produced an inactive thyroid hormone, reverse T3 (RT3). This conversion issue can be created through the direct competition of RT3 and T3 for the thyroid hormone receptor in the cell, or due to factors that inhibit T4 to T3 direct conversion. Again, we need your thyroid hormones to convert from T4 to T3 in order for your thyroid hormone to do its job. RT3 will prevent that from happening. This conversion shift is really a safety mechanism for your body. It sees lack of nutrients and oxidative stress via inflammation, infection, or toxins as a warning to conserve the body's cellular function and go into survival mode. RT3 is not what you want to happen, but it serves as a marker of "chaos" in the body for you to look for within lab work.

Your RT3 is like the reverse function in your car. Thyroid hormone can only move forward and do its job if it's moving forward! You want and need adequate T3 in your body to proceed with the creation of ATP for energy. Low T3 can hinder growth and development (causing decreased workout recovery or muscle growth), decrease metabolic rate (causing weight gain or struggles with weight loss), lower fat mobilization and carb metabolism (further hindering your metabolism), slow gut motility (causing constipation, gas, and bloating), decrease protein synthesis (contributing to muscle loss), decrease mental clarity (causing forgetfulness or brain fog), lower reproductive hormones (contributing to PMS problems, infertility, or endometriosis), and lower body temperature and heart rate (causing bradycardia and impaired exercise tolerance). High T3 can result in the complete opposite of low T3!

Now, just because there is proper conversion of T4 to T3 does not mean that T3 can enter and be used in the cell. T3 not only needs to be created from T4, but it also has to go from the bloodstream and into the cell in order to do its job. Within your bloodstream, your thyroid hormones travel with a buddy called thyroxine binding globulin (TBG). Think of TBG like a boot on a car. Your thyroid hormone is like a car trying to leave to its destination once it gets to the cell- but when bound with TBG, it has a boot on it. With the protein and boot, thyroid hormone can't be used. This is where having HIGH TBG can decrease levels of free thyroid hormone, causing hypothyroidism, and LOW TBG can cause increased levels, causing hyperthyroidism. Many factors can influence TBG, but one of the most common culprits is high estrogen levels. This can be due to birth control usage, environmental toxins, gut disorders/bacterial overgrowths, heavy metals, etc. See Chapter 4 for more details on estrogen dominance! High TBG can also be caused by certain medications or corticosteroids.

Cellular Hypothyroidism

Your thyroid hormones travel with TBG in the blood, and this is why measuring FREE thyroid hormones is essential to adequately measure thyroid function. Testing total thyroid may give you a small picture of the amount of thyroid hormone in your blood, however it doesn't tell you how much thyroid hormone is available to be used! There's one more caveat here. Just because thyroid hormone is free to be used, doesn't mean it can enter the cell to do its job. This is called cellular hypothyroidism and is a culprit for many that continue to struggle with hypothyroid symptoms, despite having "normal" lab values.

In cellular hypothyroidism, blood values of your thyroid can look normal, however you still exhibit crippling signs of hypothyroid symptoms! What can cause this? Many times, cortisol is the demon here. You need enough cortisol for thyroid hormone to enter the cell, but high cortisol can also inhibit entry, as well as convert your T4 into RT3, lowering T3 availability. Therefore, it's important to maintain normal cortisol levels for thyroid hormone absorption to be optimized. High or low cortisol levels can be seen in chronic stress, over-exercising, and adrenal or pituitary disorders. Two well known adrenal disorders altering cortisol levels include Cushing's Disease (high cortisol) and Addison's Disease (low cortisol). These can be diagnosed clinically by various adrenal markers by your doctor, however you do not need a clinical diagnosis to have an adrenal imbalance that can hinder your thyroid! See Chapter 9 for more information on managing cortisol and the cortisol connection.

Other factors that can cause cellular hypothyroidism include genetic thyroid hormone resistance, high insulin levels, and inflammation. Having poor cell membrane stability can also affect thyroid absorption. Strong, healthy cell membranes are vital to allow for your cells to take in needed nutrients and to keep out toxins & bacteria. They provide your body's cell components (including your mitochondria!) with structure, stability, and protection. Think of your cell walls like a gate around your yard. You need your gate to be firm and solid, not bending and breaking. You can help maintain health cell walls by reducing inflammation in your body, ensuring adequate micronutrients, and eating healthy amounts of dietary fat! This is because dietary fat is what makes up the building blocks of your cell walls. Make sure you give your cell gates the building blocks they need to support cell structure. You can also help improve cellular sensitivity to thyroid hormone by ensuring adequate micronutrient intake, eating an anti-inflammatory diet, managing stress, exercising in a way that makes you feel good, and balancing your blood sugar!

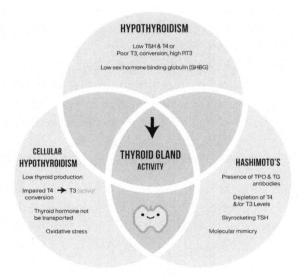

The Thyroid "Breakfast Club"

Your thyroid and your hormones are BFFs. They like to do things together. Kinda like with the Breakfast Club. If one starts to function sub-optimally, the other one likes to follow suit. I like to think of the classic case of peer pressure. Your thyroid and hormones are very good at bullying each other to cause further havoc in your body! "When the thyroid jumps off the cliff- so can your hormones!" Hypothyroidism can cause estrogen dominance, low estrogen, low progesterone, high testosterone, and even low testosterone. Read that again- it can increase AND/OR decrease sex hormones. This is why a personalized care treatment is imperative with proper testing and you shouldn't just supplement based on your own guesses.

What can happen to cause these issues physiologically? Hypothyroidism decreases sex hormone binding globulin (SHBG), which is a protein that transports testosterone and estrogen throughout the body. SHGB is made in the liver, so any problem with your liver, as well as hypothyroidism itself, can influence SHBG levels. SHBG binds hormones in the blood to transport them in the tissues of your body, but when they are high or low, this can cause high or low hormone levels. Just like your thyroid, your hormones have to be free in order to do their work. High levels of SHBG can decrease free estrogen or testosterone, directly leading to low hormone levels. Low SHBG can increase free estrogen or testosterone, leading to high levels. Progesterone also likes to jump off the cliff with thyroid abnormalities, which can result in heavy PMS, irregular menstrual cycle, or infertility.

Estrogen dominance additionally can decrease the conversion of T4 to T3, due to suppression of the sodium iodine transporter and increased thyroid binding globulin, which can reduce the thyroid hormone available. High estrogen can also reduce bile acid and pancreatic secretion. Beyond digestion distress and increasing the risk of overgrowth, a buildup of bile acids can impact overall metabolism and inflammation.

Common Root Causes of Hypothyroidism:

There many factors that can cause or contribute to hypothyroidism, whether that is related to damaging the thyroid itself through molecular mimicry, reducing or altering thyroid production or conversion, or inhibiting thyroid absorption at the cellular level. Common root causes can be seen below:

1	**Nutrient deficiencies** (Specifically selenium, iodine, B vitamins, Vitamin D, iron, thiamine, zinc, magnesium, omega 3's)
2	**Nutrient excess** *(too much zinc can induce a copper deficiency, too much iron can cause hemochromatosis (iron overload), too much B6 can cause peripheral neuropathy, and too much iodine can increase TPO antibodies)*
3	**Environmental toxins** *(BPA, heavy metals, xenoestrogens, parabens)*
4	**Gut infections** *(SIBO - 'Small Intestine Bacterial Overgrowth', candida, fungal overgrowths, parasites)*
5	**Food Intolerances** or **Intestinal permeability** *(aka leaky gut)* ; low stomach acid
6	**Chronic infections** *(EBV being common)*
7	**Hormone dysfunction** *(Estrogen dominance, low progesterone, low or high testosterone)*
8	**Adrenal dysfunction** *(High Cortisol or Low Cortisol both can happen!)* or pituitary dysfunction *(Pituitary tumor or post brain/head injury)*
9	**Medications** including: Lithium *(used in psychiatric treatment)* , anti-seizure medications, Amiodarone *(used to treat heart arrhythmias)* , Sulfonylureas *(used in type 2 diabetes)* , Gastric acid reducers
10	*(PPIs used in reflux)* , H2 receptor antagonists *(taken commonly as allergy medications to decrease histamine levels)*
11	**Radioactive iodine treatment**
12	**Medications** *(birth control, beta-blockers, glucocorticoids, antiepileptic drugs)*
13	**Pregnancy** *(postpartum hypothyroidism)*
14	**Thyroid tissue damage**
15	**Tumor growth**
16	**Genetics** *(such as the HLA-DR3 gene)*
17	Severe **Caloric Restriction** & **Undereating**

Here's a review of what can happen to create havoc with your thyroid:

- Inadequate thyroid hormone production- too much or too little made

- Thyroid immune attack- causing too much or too little thyroid hormone to be made
- Poor thyroid hormone conversion- causing too little T3 or too much RT3
- Poor thyroid hormone absorption- not allowing T3 to be used
- High or low TBG- lowering the amount of thyroid hormone available to be used
- Pituitary has defect in signal to your thyroid
- Hypothalamus has defect in signal to your pituitary

Thyroid Testing:

Thyroid healing should be about treating you, the patient, not treating the labs. Labs should be used to guide your treatment, however true care should address you as the full person. You are not your labs! This is very important to remember. So many doctors go off of blood work alone, and this is such a disservice to you as a patient and person, because not only are you not a number, but your symptoms and feelings are 100% valid and should be addressed, despite "normal" lab values. In fact, just because a lab may look "normal" for your thyroid does not mean that your thyroid may not need some love! Remember my discussion on cellular hypothyroidism? Some doctors are not aware of this condition, and many overlook subclinical levels as well. This is where you have to step in, address your symptoms, and be the advocate of your own health! Remember, your doctor works for you. If your doctor makes you feel bad about asking questions, is unwilling to do testing, or dismisses you or your symptoms, you have every right to fire your doctor and get a new one.

As of now, conventional medicine mostly uses TSH as the end-all-be-all marker of thyroid function. It blows me away! Doctors, including endocrinologists, are trained to use TSH as a "valid marker of hypothyroidism." They are taught to diagnose hypothyroidism with a TSH of 5.0 or greater and taught to only test antibodies if TSH is greater than or equal to 10.0. The trouble is, as you now know- TSH is only a pituitary marker! It says nothing about what thyroid levels look like in the bloodstream! In addition to the problem with TSH, doctors do not always check for free thyroid hormone levels. Some only check "total" or "indexed" thyroid, which may give you some information, but still does not tell you what your active thyroid hormones levels are. Remember, serum and blood thyroid levels say nothing about what is free and able to be absorbed and used by your cells. Total thyroid, just like total hormone levels, only tells you what MAY make it to the target destination, not what IS getting to its destination.

It is imperative that you understand this, that way you can ensure you are getting a complete thyroid panel when you've requested a "thyroid check." A full thyroid panel should, at a minimum, consist of TSH, Free T4, Free T3, TPO antibodies, and TgAB antibodies. There are many other important and significant tests that are also recommended, however minimally, those are the five tests to perform to assess thyroid function.

Recommended Thyroid Function Tests with Reference Ranges:

- TSH-: 0.3-4.2 mIU/L
- Free T4: 0.9-1.7 ng/dL
- Free T3: 2.8-4.4 pg/mL
- Serum rT3: 10-24 ng/dL
- TPO and TgAB Antibodies: less than 4 IU/mL

There is a difference between "normal" and "optimal" thyroid hormone levels. Just like a "normal" amount of creamer in your coffee vs your optimal amount. Your optimal may not be someone else's optimal. Someone may need a bit more T3 in their body to feel good. Someone else may need less. This is where working with a good clinician is imperative to ensure you are being treated not to just match a lab value, but to also find what levels make you feel your best. Clinicians should also not be chasing labs alone- but instead work to address and get rid of the root cause of your thyroid troubles.

Why do most doctors stick to TSH? Why don't they do a full panel?

Current conventional hypothyroid treatment includes the following:

- Diagnosis of hypothyroidism based on TSH
- Assessment of thyroid antibodies if TSH is at or equal to 10
- Starting dose of T4 only (levothyroxine or Synthroid) if persistent hypothyroid symptoms or high TSH, with a starting dose of 25 mcg evaluated every 2-3 months
- Medication adjustments based on TSH and T4 levels
- "According to the current model, normalizing serum TSH is generally considered the target of therapy, and serum T3 is typically not measured or monitored"

Endocrinologists and medical doctors follow these standards in their care guidelines. It's not that they are not following science. They just aren't always aware of the more detailed physiology of the thyroid. Why is this conventional treatment problematic? Not only does it not take into account your total thyroid lab assessment (meaning you could go misdiagnosed), but it also does not address individual genetics, root causes, thyroid conversion, medical and diet related history, environmental, or lifestyle influences. This can result in a host of medical issues if someone is started on the wrong medication or is left at a low or too high dose for a long period of time. I can't say this enough- you have to be your own health advocate!

Misdiagnosis

Unfortunately, if you do not get a full thyroid panel done or get a full blood work panel in general, you are at risk for a misdiagnosis. Many thyroid-related and hormonal symptoms are non specific, meaning they look the same. Some patients may go years with unfound Hashimoto's disease, not being diagnosed until it's too late and their thyroid gland is destroyed. Others may have symptoms of depression or anxiety that the doctor throws an antidepressant at.

It's imperative that you become your own health advocate and if your doctor won't do a full panel, that you find someone who will or order once yourself.

Additional labs that may indicate hypothyroidism: elevated LDL cholesterol, hyponatremia (low blood sodium), hyperprolactinemia (high prolactin), anemia (can be low B12, folate, or iron), high CRP, altered liver values, high BUN (blood urea nitrogen), abnormal sex hormones.

Symptoms of hypothyroidism include: dry or thinning hair, hair loss, fatigue, depression, brain fog or reduced mental clarity, hoarseness of voice, goiter, enlarged thyroid gland, dry skin, low perspiration, muscle loss, muscle aches or weakness, joint pain, constipation, weight gain or trouble losing weight, bradycardia, hypertension, elevated LDL, infertility, abnormal sex hormones, peripheral neuropathy, cold intolerance, cold hands and feet, and an irregular menstrual cycle.

The Ferritin & Iron Connection

Low iron levels can be a contributing cause to hypothyroidism and can lie hidden as an underlying, unaddressed reason as to why medication may not be helping to alleviate symptoms. The symptoms of iron deficiency can mimic hypothyroidism, including fatigue, weakness, muscle and joint pain, low sex drive, brain fog, feeling cold, anxiety, depression, and shortness of breath. This is why I suggest always completing a full thyroid panel with iron levels when first addressing any thyroid trouble, or if one has symptoms of iron deficiency. Low iron can be caused by insufficient dietary intake, poor hydrochloric acid in the stomach, medications, or genetic defaults in blood cell shape or metabolism (such as polycythemia vera or Thalassemia). Ferritin is the storage form of iron, and will be the last to be depleted in the body. Therefore, assessing serum iron may give a more current level of iron intake, which % iron saturation and TIBC (total iron binding capacity) will assess for the % of iron bound in the blood. TIBC will go up with iron deficiency.

Iron levels to assess: Ferritin, Serum Iron, % Saturation, TIBC

Copper, Iron, and Vitamin A- Is It Really Iron?

It's not just iron that is involved in the regulation of your iron levels. The status of your copper (in the form of ceruloplasmin) and Vitamin A levels also play a role. If you are struggling with bringing up your iron or ferritin levels (ferritin being your storage form of iron), then you may have an additional deficiency in copper or Vitamin A.

Vitamin A specifically aids in mobilizing the iron stored in your cells (called erythrocytes). Copper also helps to mobilize your iron. If copper levels are low, iron is stored in your tissues & not free in the blood to be utilized. Since iron carries oxygen, this can result in devastating health consequences, with the last stage of iron deficiency and anemia resulting in both low ferritin and low hemoglobin levels. This will result in major fatigue, shortness of breathe, dizziness, hair loss, and weakness. A copper deficiency also can lead to a thyroid hormone deficiency, not only through reducing iron utilization, but by directly depleting free t4 levels. Copper is a required nutrient for the creation of thyroid hormones!

Micronutrients and minerals need a balance, just like your hormones. Too much iron can cause a copper deficiency, while too little copper can contribute to an iron deficiency. In addition, too much copper can contribute to a zinc deficiency (or worsen estrogen dominance), and too much zinc can induce a copper defiance. Zinc is needed for the conversion of T4 to T3 (inactive to active thyroid hormone). If you have low Zinc, you may have normal T4, but low T3 levels.

Balance is what we want. To confuse you even more, too much Vitamin A can induce a Vitamin D defieicny, as Vitamin A and Vitamin D compete for each other. A deficiency of both can trigger hypothyroidism. This is why it's important to have a variety of food in your diet, as well as test before adding in a high dose single supplement of any vitamin or mineral. Too much is not a good thing. Balance is key!

Additional Labs to Assess with Thyroid Disorders:

- CBC (Complete Blood Panel) and CMP (Complete Metabolic Panel)
- Vitamin D
- Vitamin B12
- Ferritin, Serum Iron, % Saturation, TIBC
- Serum copper and ceruloplasmin
- RBC Vitamin A, Zinc, and Magnesium
- 4 Point Cortisol Test
- Sex hormones: estradiol, free testosterone, progesterone

Thyroid Medications in Hypothyroidism:

Finding and treating the root cause of your thyroid troubles is essential in order to take your health and happiness back into your own hands! Thyroid medications can be a crucial component of a treatment protocol, helping you to achieve and maintain adequate thyroid levels as well as reduce or get rid of your hypothyroid symptoms. However, taking exogenous thyroid hormone will not always fix the root of your troubles, and can even mask them or make things worse! You have to make sure you are your own advocate of your health and instill it in yourself to listen to your symptoms and invest in proper testing that may help you in getting to the root cause of your hypothyroidism. For some people with hypothyroidism, medications are required, as is the case for Hashimoto's patients with thyroid damage, insufficient thyroid hormone production, or post-thyroidectomy. In other cases, medications can be useful to help briefly bring your thyroid levels up back to normal and alleviate symptoms while the root cause of your hypothyroid state is addressed, such as a gut infection, viral infection, or hormonal disorder. Either way, make sure to use medications as a tool, not a crutch, in treatment.

It's important to point out that if taken when unnecessary, such as in the case of under eating, over exercising, or chronic dieting, medications may simply mask the underfed state causing low thyroid. This may potentially cause downregulation of thyroid hormone production and enforce you to rely on exogenous thyroid in order to maintain sufficient hormones throughout your lifetime. This is another reason I am very passionate about proper testing and assessment! Exogenous thyroid can be quite expensive, and there is no need to take medication if you can resolve the issue through diet, lifestyle, and supplementation alone.

There are four different main types of thyroid hormone medications: T4 only, T3 only, compounded thyroid, and desiccated thyroid. Each has their own benefits, risks, and effects on the body and comes in different forms and dosages. Finding the thyroid medication that you feel best on and that optimizes your thyroid levels may be tricky and can take for some, trying a few different brands. Don't lose hope, and again, remember to address your root cause. Medications won't do their job if the root cause of the thyroid trouble is not addressed. If you feel your medication is not working for you, your dosage is wrong, or you are not receiving the proper labs you need to evaluate your health, don't hesitate to speak up to your doctor. Remember, your doctor works for you. If he/she will not listen or discuss their reasoning, or they dismiss your requests and feelings, don't be afraid to self order your labs, tests, and get a new doctor.

T4 only-

T4, thyroxine, is the inactive form of thyroid hormone. T4-only medications include Synthroid (name brand), Levoxyl, Thyroxine, Tirosint, and Levothyroxine (generic form). Each medication has different ingredients and fillers, which may be a hit or miss dependent on the patient. For example, levothyroxine contains lactose, gluten, and corn, while Tirosint is free of them, as well as free of additional fillers and dyes. This is important to keep in mind and look into, as taking a medication with a filler or ingredient that you are intolerant or sensitive to can induce worsened, or new, symptoms. T4 medications have a half life of 7-10 days. This means that it takes 7-10 days for the concentration of the medication to reduce in your bloodstream by 50%. This helps T4 medications provide a lower risk of inducing hyperthyroidism.

T4 medications are currently the first line of treatment for hypothyroidism and are started at a typical 25 mcg dose. Many doctors will then see patients every 8-12 weeks to assess labs and make dosage changes, bumping typically by 25 mcg at a time. I highly suggest checking labs every month if possible when just starting on medications, checking labs until stable. Checking every three months is far from optimal, because if the dose is too much or too little, this may leave you in distress with a host of crippling symptoms for weeks!!

For some patients, T4 medications do just fine! However, not everyone does well on T4-only medications. Why is this? Remember, T4 is not your active thyroid hormone. Taking T4-only medications requires you to have sufficient thyroid hormone conversion in order to receive sufficient active thyroid hormone (T3). Common conditions that T4 medications may not be helpful to alleviate symptoms and provide sufficient T3 include: Hashimoto's, cortisol dysregulation, nutrient deficiencies or infections that suppress thyroid hormone conversion, and post hyperthyroid treatment.

T3 only-

Some patients may use T4 medications along with T3, or solely use T3 in treatment. T3 medications commonly prescribed include Cytomel (brand name), liothyronine (generic), or may be compounded within a compounding pharmacy with T4. T3 exists in fast release, as well as slow release forms and peaks in the blood about 2-3 hours after ingestion. Because it has a peak serum rise of 4-6 hours (with a 2.5 day half life), it may be beneficial to some patients to multi-dose throughout the day, which prevents a large dump of T3 earlier in the day, creating a crash later in the evening. Multi-dosing allows for a more steady rate of T3. Slow release forms also can help to decrease the T3 dump and ensure a more steady T3 release into the bloodstream. To best explain this, think of T4 as the gas in the tank of a car. Your gas tank holds on to the storage form of your thyroid hormone, with a longer half life. T3 is the energy you get from pushing the gas pedal. If you floor your pedal all at once, you risk overwhelming your car with gas (cue hyperthyroid symptoms), however if you press on the gas at a more steady rate, you may find that you are better able to manage your energy levels and prevent the side effects of T3 swings.

Side effects of T3 supplementation include increased anxiety, heart palpitations, increased heart rate, anxiety, tremors, and shortness of breath. Some of these side effects can be common when just starting a T3 medication, as the body is not used to the thyroid hormone yet. However, too much T3 and continued symptoms can put you into a hyperthyroid state. The goal with medications is to stabilize thyroid levels, not provide the body with more than it needs.

T3 medications are typically added to T4 after months of T4 medication adjustments not improving labs or symptoms. They can be added alone, or compounded along with T4 in a compounding pharmacy. T3 medications can be extremely helpful if someone has conversion issues, however, if taken with T4 medications, the conversion issue may result in excess RT3 creation, making your hypothyroid symptoms worse. This is common in the case of high cortisol levels, inflammation, or low iron (low ferritin, the storage form or iron). If you take a combination of T4 and T3, and have worsening symptoms or do not feel better, you may want to talk to your doctor about adjusting your dose, looking further into nutrient deficiencies or cortisol dysregulation, or trying a different medication. Please note that T3 supplementation may increase levels of SHBG, leading to decreased testosterone and estrogen levels. Ensure to keep notice of your hormones and SHBG levels when starting T3 or desiccated thyroid hormone, which contains T3.

Desiccated Thyroid hormone:

Desiccated thyroid hormones contain a combination of T4, T3, T2, and T1. There are a variety of different forms that exist, and the amounts of each thyroid hormone differs based on the brand. Most brands contain approximately a 4:1 ratio of T4 to T3, providing approximately 38 mg of T4 and 9 mg T3 per grain (desiccated hormone is measured based on a "grain" value). This grain equivalent can be compared to T4 only and T3 medications by mg or mcg of thyroid hormone. See the thyroid conversion chart provided for more details. In general, 50 mg of T4 only medication equates to ½ grain of desiccated thyroid hormone, which provides 32.5 mg T4. 100 mg of T4-only medication can also equate to 1 grain of desiccated thyroid hormone (which then provides 65 mg of T4 and 25 mcg of T3).

Brand names of popular desiccated thyroid include: Armour, WP Thyroid, Westhroid, NP thyroid, Nature Thyroid, and Thyroid USP. Just like T4-only medications, each person's reactions to a medication may be different based on fillers and ingredients. I like to think of finding your optimal thyroid hormone and dosage like finding Cinderella's glass slipper. It may not be a good fit using one, but you just have to keep trying until you find your proper form and dose! Do remember, exogenous thyroid hormone won't do its proper job unless the root cause of the thyroid problem is revealed and removed (if possible). Desiccated thyroid medications are most helpful for anyone with conversion issues, as they reduce the conversion needed and provide active thyroid hormone themselves. If you struggle with cortisol dysregulation, nutrient deficiencies, inflammation, or gut health issues such as SIBO or dysbiosis, desiccated thyroid may be beneficial to you. It can also be extremely helpful for those with Hashimoto's, however if antibodies are present, you may feel worse and create further autoimmune attack. This is because in the presence of TPO and TgAb (thyroglobulin antibodies), the thyroid is under autoimmune attack. Dissociated thyroid hormone may worsen this attack.

Desiccated thyroid hormones are made from the porcine (pig) thyroid gland. The gland is frozen, minced, and dried into a fine powder, which is then created into pill form. Many conventional doctors are hesitant to suggest desiccated thyroid, as they fear lack of regulation. However, this type of medication is thoroughly regulated by the USP (United States Pharmacopeia) for quality. It's compounded T4 and T3 medications produced in compounding pharmacies that can have the most error in dosages. Compounded T4 and T3 medications involve the creation of individual compounded thyroid hormone dosage using synthetic thyroid hormone. They can be quite helpful for eliminating fillers and individualizing dosages, allowing for fast or slow release forms, however their percent of error in dosage accuracy may not be as reliable.

Thyroid (USP)	Thyroid (USP)	Thyroid (USP)	Levothyroxine *Synthroid T4*	Liothyronine *Synthetic T3*
1/4 grain (16.25 mg)	1/4 grain (16.25 mg)	1/4 grain (16.25 mg)	25 mcg	5 mcg
1/2 grain (16.25 mg)	1/4 grain (16.25 mg)	1/4 grain (16.25 mg)	50 mcg	
3/4 grain (16.25 mg)	1/4 grain (16.25 mg)		75 mcg	
			88 mcg	
1 grain (65 mg)	1 grain (65 mg)	1 grain (60 mg)	100 mcg	25 mcg
			112 mcg	
1.25 grain (81.25 mg)	1.25 grain (81.25 mg)	125 mcg		
			137 mcg	
1.5 grain (97.5 mg)	1.5 grain (97.5 mg)	1.5 grain (90 mg)	150 mcg	
1.75 g grain (113.75 mg)	1.75 g grain (113.75 mg)	175 mcg		
2 grain (130 mg)	2 grain (130 mg)	2 grain (120 mg)	200 mcg	50 mcg
2.25 grain (146.25 mg)				
2.5 grain (162.5 mg)				
3 grain (195 mg)		3 grain (180 mg)	300 mcg	
4 grain (260 mg)		4 grain (240 mcg)		
5 grain (325 mg)		5 grain (300 mcg)		

1 grain = 38 mcg of T4 & 9 mcg T3

Don't make these medication mistakes:

1. Expecting to feel better instantly. It may take a few weeks for the T4 in your thyroid medication to build up in your bloodstream. In addition, it may take a few months for your hormones, if affected by your hypothyroidism, to get back to a healthier state. Remember that your thyroid and hormones are BFFs and their health tend to go hand in hand! Therefore, be willing to give your medication some time prior to jumping into trying a new medication. Make sure you are checking your thyroid labs every 2-3 months (I suggest every 4 weeks until optimized with adequate free T4 and T3), and if you continue to feel bad despite adequate levels, look into cellular hypothyroidism being a contributing cause.

2. Using TSH as a marker for medication adequacy and adjustments. TSH is a pituitary marker. It says nothing about what amount of thyroid hormone is in your bloodstream or getting into your cells! Always ensure that you are getting free T4 and free T3 checked when assessing labs and medication dose changes.

Another thing to keep in mind is that TSH will drop on exogenous thyroid hormone. This does not necessarily mean you are hyperthyroid, as some doctors may state. On exogenous thyroid medication, as long as free T4 and free T3 are normal, it is normal for TSH to be low. This is the body telling your thyroid to not produce any more thyroid hormone because it has enough taken exogenously! However, if your TSH is low and your free T4 and/or free T4 are high or if you have signs of hyperthyroidism, your dose may be too high, putting you into a hyperthyroid state.

3. Starting too low of a dose, increasing too quickly, or waiting too long to test and adjust. There is no need to wait months to assess your thyroid labs if you continue to feel awful and symptomatic weeks into a new dose. If you do not feel better, or feel worse, don't wait! You shouldn't have to be miserable for months. Stick to the rule of thumb of 4 weeks if you don't feel better, but don't hesitate to reach out to your doctor if any adjustment makes you feel worse or gives new side effects. Staying at a too low of a dose results in decreases in TSH which then decreases your natural thyroid production, and in turn, you may produce less thyroid hormone and not be getting enough exogenous thyroid hormone, making you feel even worse. It has been reported that for many, going up by 0.25 mcg of a T4 medication or ½ grain of desiccated thyroid every 3-4 weeks helps patients to find their right dose, lower side effects, and relieve their symptoms.

4. You assume side effects are all from medication changes. A medication can only do its job if the root cause is not influencing its action. For example, low or high cortisol levels and low iron can inhibit the absorption of desiccated thyroid hormone, and inhibit the conversion of T4 to T3 with T4 medication usage. If the thyroid hormone cannot be used, as in the case

of desiccated thyroid hormone, this can cause elevations of T3 in the bloodstream, leading to hyperthyroid symptoms that are influenced by the medication, but caused by cortisol or nutritional deficiencies. In addition, adrenal issues can create a poor response to T3, as the T3 may cause a flux of adrenaline that further worsens your adrenal imbalance. Make sure to address adrenals and fellow nutrient deficiencies or excess and don't simply blame a medication for "not working".

5. You take your medication incorrectly. Your thyroid medication should be taken on an empty stomach, at least 45 minutes before any food or supplements, caffeine, or coffee/tea. Taking with food can reduce absorption, as will supplements like calcium and iron. Medications can also prevent absorption, such as in the case for hormonal birth control. Strive to take your medication away from any food or drink or other supplements/medications- giving your body 45 minutes.

6. You switch from brand name to generic or vice versa. Even if the dose is technically the same, you may react to the different fillers or dyes within the different medications.

7. Not multi-dosing if needed with T3. As I have already discussed, T3 has a half life of 4-6 hours. Taking too much T3 early during the day may result in a crash mid day, especially if you struggle with cortisol dysregulation. Multi-dosing your T3 or using a slow, sustained release form may help to prevent this crash. Some find that multi-dosing desiccated thyroid hormone when prescribed more than 1 grain a day is beneficial as well. Always speak with your doctor, however if you struggle with cortisol issues, multi-dosing may lower the burden on your adrenals.

8. Not assessing for potential formula changes. For example, Armour thyroid adjusted its ingredients by reducing the amount of dextrose, and in turn

increased methylcellulose. This caused some reactions in patients, reporting that their Armour was "no longer working" (my thoughts is that the cellulose may have caused a mild sensitivity reaction OR was harder for some people to digest and then absorb, lowering the actual thyroid hormone that was received). It's important to stay on top of changes in your medication formula, as any adjustment in ingredients, especially if you are sensitive, may cause a reaction or change the way that you feel on your dosage.

9. Not solving the root issue. Whether the root cause of your hypothyroidism stems from under eating, food intolerances, cortisol imbalances, nutrient deficiencies, estrogen dominance, or infections, the issue must be resolved or medications can not do their work. They also won't fix the root issue. If the root cause is not fixed, no amount of medication is going to bring your overall health back. Medications aren't magic!

10. Taking "thyroid boosting" supplements. This may seem like a grand idea if you are hypothyroid to help give your thyroid a "boost"- however this can do more harm than good! Not only are dietary supplements poorly regulated, but their dosage of ingredients may be harmful to your thyroid and be overdosing you on certain ingredients or micronutrients. For example- low iodine can be a cause of hypothyroidism. However, too much iodine can as well. Many thyroid boosting supplements can contain iodine, whether that is elemental or natural, in the form of kelp. Too much iodine can also induce further autoimmune attack and cause hyperthyroidism. You need a goldilocks balance with iodine. Many "thyroid boosting" blends also contain tyrosine, which is a required amino acid to create thyroid hormone. However, too much tyrosine can cause adrenaline to be overproduced, which spells a recipe for disaster if you have high cortisol levels.

How to Find Your Root Cause

This is where the digging has to be done. You will need to do a detailed and complex evaluation of your current and past health! Focus on looking at the following categories that may play a role in why your thyroid took a hit in the first place. I won't be diving into specific treatment protocols here. Why? That would be silly of me and potentially dangerous for you.

1. Diet & Digestion- assess for diet contributions, such as nutrient deficiencies, nutrient excess, or food intolerances. Start with a wide overlook at not only what you are eating but also how much. Could you be under eating and over-exercising? Could you have nutrient deficiencies that developed from medications, such as with the chronic use of allergy medications, PPIs (proton pump inhibitors), birth control or antidepressants?

Some medications can alter not only how much you absorb but also how you digest. For example, allergy medications can lead to low stomach acid. This can lead to poor protein digestion (increasing risk of gas/bloating/overgrowths) and a lack of B12, iron, magnesium, and calcium.

Medication Type	Nutrients Depleted
Birth Control	Folate, Zinc, Magnesium, B vitamins, Vitamin A, Vitamin C, Melatonin, Selenium
PPIs & Antacids	Vitamin B12, Folic Acid, Vitamin D, Calcium, Iron, Zinc
Antidepressants	Coenzyme Q10, B-vitamins
Cholesterol Drugs	Coenzyme Q10
Anticonvulsants	Vitamin D, Calcium, Folic Acid, Biotin, L-Carnitine, Vitamin B12, Vitamin B1, Vitamin K, Copper, Selenium, Zinc
Corticosteroids & Anti-inflammatories	Calcium, Vitamin D, Magnesium, Zinc, Vitamin C, Vitamin B6, Vitamin B12, Folic Acid, Selenium, Chromium
Cardiovascular Drugs	Calcium, Magnesium, Vitamin B1, Vitamin B6, Vitamin C, Zinc, Coenzyme Q10, Potassium, Sodium, Calcium, Folic Acid, Zinc
Diabetic Drugs	Vitamin B12, Folic Acid, Coenzyme Q10
Antibiotics	Calcium, B-vitamins, Folic Acid, Vitamin K *gut microflora depleted*

2. Inflammation- this can come from anywhere- gut or viral infections, under eating, over-exercising, emotional distress, trauma, heavy metals, or food intolerances- you name it, the list keeps going. Excess inflammation can blunt the production of thyroid hormone, increase production of reverse T3 (which competes with T3), and prevent thyroid absorption in the cell by causing mitochondrial dysfunction or cortisol dysregulation. TSH levels with inflammation based thyroid disease may or may not change, so a full thyroid panel is essential and testing a 4 point cortisol is suggested. Elevated C-reactive protein via blood may indicate inflammation.

3. Genetics- assess for the possibility of gene-induced nutrient deficiencies.

For example, the MTHFR gene (methylenetetrahydrofolate reductase) gene codes for the MTHFR enzyme that helps to convert one of your amino acids, homocysteine, into methionine. Lack of this conversion decreases your ability to transform synthetic vitamins into their biologically active forms. It can also lead to the build up of homocysteine in the blood, which can cause inflammation, chronic disease, and tissue damage.

50-60% of the US population has one copy of the MTHFR gene. This most likely won't inhibit methylation. However, having two copies of the gene increases your risk for nutrient deficiencies, specifically of folate, B-vitamins, Sam-E, MSM, and magnesium, and also prevents absorption of non-methylated vitamins. If you have two copies of the MTHFR gene, you can't fully process non-methylated vitamins/minerals, such as folic acid or synthetic non-methylated B vitamins. Good news- food sources all have the methylated forms already! However, if you have developed a nutrient deficiency, or plan to use a multivitamin and have an MTHFR mutation, you may need a methylated multivitamin with methylated forms such as methyl-folate, pyridoxal-5-phosphate (P5P), and methylcobalamin (B12).

Not everyone needs a methylated multivitamin though. For some people, especially those with a slow COMT (Catechol-O-methyl-transferase), too much methylation can heavily increase anxiety and depression! I tend to suggest for people to use ½ methylated and ½ non-methylated vitamins if they are unaware of their genetic status.

Another gene to be on the look out for is the VDR (vitamin D receptor) gene. This gene influences your vitamin D receptor function and a defect here can increase your risk of Vitamin D deficiency. Lack of Vitamin D can decrease your immunity and insulin sensitivity, while increasing your risk of chronic disease, illness, depression, bone loss, and the development of autoimmune diseases. Low Vitamin D will also make you extremely fatigued and feel like trash. Nobody wants to feel like trash.

Please don't replete yourself without the care of a medical professional. Please also do not fall for "genetic based diets." More on that in the FAQ chapter!

4.Overgrowths - Overgrowths of bacteria or fungi as in the case for SIBO (small intestinal bacterial overgrowth), Candida, or H pylori can trigger hypothyroidism and lead to additional symptoms and nutrient deficiencies. More about these in my gut chapter.

5. Intestinal Permeability- See my gut chapter for all the details here.

6.Viral Infections- Epstein Barr Virus (EBV), Lyme Disease (a tick-borne illness), and Bartonella (cat-scratch fever) are just 3 viral infections that can contribute to hypothyroidism, chronic fatigue, autoimmune disease, neurological disorders, arthritis, and chronic inflammation. Testing can be tough, especially for Lyme disease, in which testing may or may not catch an infection. Make sure to work with an MD if you suspect a viral infection as a cause. Antibiotics or anti-virals can help to eradicate an infection along with diet and lifestyle management.

Epstein-Barr virus, also known as "mono" or mononucleosis, is a member of the herpes virus group. In younger individuals, it's commonly called the "kissing virus" as it is spread via saliva and respiratory droplets. EBV is very contagious, and is typically passed person to person through sharing utensils, cups, or as it is nick-named, kissing.

After initial exposure, there is a period of several weeks in which EBV develops, known as the incubation period. During this time, antibodies elevate and symptoms may be felt, including fatigue, fever, sore throat, swollen lymph nodes, an enlarged spleen, and muscle weakness. Most symptoms and infections resolve within a few months. After treatment, EBV never completely goes away and lies dormant within the immune system. The viral numbers and antibodies decrease, however the virus remains in the body and has a chance to reactivate in times of stress or a compromised immune system.

Testing:

This is where it can get tricky. EBV can be acute, or chronic, and having a full EBV panel is required in order to differentiate. Commonly a "mono" test is performed, which tests for a heterophile antibody, which 25% of those with mono may or may not produce. The presence of antibodies to ECV help establish infection occurrence but must be read and interpreted with caution. Below includes a full panel with analysis insights. It is estimated that 90% of the adult population have IgG class antibodies to VCA and EBNA and that most people in the US are infected by it at some point in their lives.

1. VCA IgM- This marker will elevate in an acute infection, however will not elevate in a recurrent infection.
2. VCA IgG- This marker will elevate in an acute infection or with a history of past infection. It can not be used to measure current activation or reactivation. Once you have had EBV, this marker will remain elevated your entire life.
3. EA-D IgG- This marker is an early antigen and will be positive with a current infection or reactivation infection. It may remain elevated after an infection has been resolved.
4. EBNA IgG- This marker will elevate after 2-3 months of an initial infection and will remain elevated your entire life. It does not usually appear with an acute infection.

Possible results

Marker	Primary Infection	Recent Infection (3 months)	Past Infection	Reactivation Infection
VCA IgM	+	+/-	-	-
VCA IgG	+	+	+	+
EA-D IgG	-	+	-	+
EBNA IgG	-	+/-	+	+

Treatment of EBV may involve antibiotics or herbal therapies such as l-lysine, cat's claw, monolaurin, and olive leaf. To keep it at bay and prevent reactivation, focus on optimizing your diet quality, reducing your environmental toxic burden, supporting your immune system, and prioritizing sleep and stress reduction. EBV reactivation is more common with high stress, poor diet, and a compromised immune system. Ensure if you suspect EBV to work with a qualified health care professional.

Lyme Disease is caused by a bite from an infected tick carrying a bacteria called Borrelia burgdorferi. It is most often seen in areas with lush vegetation, such as woody, bushy and grassy areas of the northeastern United States, however infections have also been noted across the United States.

Symptoms include:

- Red dot and bull's eye rash upon immediate infection (does not always show up)
- Fever, chills, fatigue, body aches, headache, neck stiffness and swollen lymph nodes
- Later infections may result in irregular heartbeats, liver disease, rashes, impaired muscle movement, full body weakness, impaired memory, and Bell's Palsy (temporary paralysis to one side of the face)

The most common Lyme disease tests include an ELISA (Enzyme-linked immunosorbent assay) or Western Blot. These tests look for antibodies to the bacteria Borrelia, produced by an infection, and are indirect- meaning they measure for a response to an infection, and not an infection itself. Testing with these two methods are not strain specific, so false negatives may miss a diagnosis if only one strain is tested. For best testing, I suggest the IgeneX Lyme Immunoblot which tests for multiple strains and has a higher sensitivity.

7. Parasites-

Parasites are no joke & don't just come from foreign countries! According to the Centers for Disease Control (CDC), parasites affect millions of Americans, who can either live happily in unison, or suffer silently. Parasites can be a major cause of chronic health issues - including digestive issues, hormonal imbalances, skin rashes, & chronic fatigue. Truth is- if a parasite is there, you can't truly heal your body- including any gut infections, Hashimoto's, hypothyroidism, hormonal imbalances, mold exposure, heavy metals, or combat viruses such as Lyme disease. They can keep your immune system depressed & even trigger depression/anxiety.

Signs & symptoms can greatly vary in each person based on what parasite, co-infections, & additional health havoc.

Symptoms Include:

- Abdominal pain
- Bloating
- Night time abdominal cramping
- Constipation
- Diarrhea
- Insomnia
- POTS
- Adrenal imbalances
- Always hungry
- Anal itching (worsening at night)
- Random weight gain or loss
- Unexplained anemia
- Rashes, eczema, hives
- Eye floaters
- Mental disorders
- Internal vibrations
- Chronic fatigue
- Joint or muscle pain
- Multiple food intolerances
- Headaches/migraines
- Dizziness or weakness
- Teeth grinding
- Brain fog

The 3 main types of parasites include:

1. Protozoa (single-celled organisms such as Giardia, amoebas, trichomoniasis, blastocysts hominis)
2. Helminths (aka worms)
3. Ectoparasites (insects, fleas, ticks, mites)

If you struggle with chronic symptoms like these that come & go randomly may be worth potentially looking at a parasitic cause. Especially if symptoms come & go in cycles or symptoms more so in the evening (parasites are more active at night & live/breed in weekly cycles). Testing is difficult as it can be hard to diagnose parasites- but my favorite testing includes the stool testing such as the GI map (though it only tests a few), Parasitology Center, Parawellness Research, as well as endoscopy's, X-rays, MRIs, & CAT scans.

Treatment should be individualized with anti-parasitics herbals or antibiotics. The most common antibiotics include metronidazole (Flagyl), Alinia, and tetracycline. My favorite herbal treatments for parasites include wormwood, olive leaf extract, berberine containing herbs, black walnut, and mimosa pudica. CellCore Biosciences makes a full moon kit that I have found to work well for parasite "cleansing"

Common sources of infection include:

- Lakes, rivers, fresh water
- Pets
- Infected food, water, or feces
- Raw fish or sushi
- Insect bites
- Baby toys or child play areas

If worried about parasites, simple ways to reduce possible infection includes washing your hands, cooking food properly, drinking only filtered water, choosing safe sexual habits, watching and testing any pets, ensure adequate stomach acid (your first line of defense), and being careful with any fresh water swimming or abroad traveling.

Additional Causes of Hypothyroidism: These can be covered in greater detail throughout the book include:

- Hormone or Adrenal Dysfunction
- Poor detoxification
- Endocrine Disruptors

My "Thyroid Healing" Protocol: (Done WITH a Medical Professional!)

- Test don't guess- ensure you get a full thyroid panel, assess micronutrient status (such as iodine, magnesium, B12, iron, folate, and zinc)
- Focus on identifying and reducing triggers, healing the gut and intestinal permeability, supporting the immune system, and reducing inflammation
- Maximize your micronutrients through an anti-inflammatory diet and remove only what causes YOU specific issues- this may or may not include soy, gluten, wheat, nuts, eggs, shellfish, nightshades, corn. There is no best "thyroid healing" diet, though if an autoimmune disease is present, you may want to avoid gluten due to its effect on molecular mimicry. Soy may or may not inhibit thyroid function, so assess how you feel and how your levels and antibodies change if you choose to eliminate it.
- Decrease intake of: potential trigger foods, processed vegetable oils and trans fats, refined carbohydrates. Don't fear cooked cruciferous vegetables, however do try to avoid uncooked goitrogenic foods which can displace iodine and inhibit thyroid hormone conversion.

Nightshade vegetables found in tomatoes, potatoes, eggplant, peppers, and some spices can also cause trouble. I find that most people respond to specific nightshades, not the nightshade family itself. Search for your food triggers and keep as much variety in as you can.

- Reduce toxic burden and inflammation by ensuring to drink filtered water, use an air filter in your home, and remove endocrine disruptors. Though you may think your fridge water is healthy, make sure to assess your area's water quality, as regular fridge or simple Brita filter won't filter out excess heavy metals, arsenic, lead, chlorine, or fluoride, all which can in excess contribute to thyroid trouble. See more on water filters and heavy metals in Chapter 6.

- Don't rule out the potential for mold at play, which can lie hidden and leave your thyroid a wreck- see Chapter 6 for more.

- Exercise in a way to feels good versus drains you. If you have a history of overexercising- you may need months of reducing activity in order to help heal your thyroid. Stress can cause chronic cortisol issues, which can lower thyroid hormone production, conversion, and absorption.

- Help your gut and digestion by eating mindfully, chewing your food slowly, and staying away from foods that flare up your symptoms or cause inflammation. See Chapter 10 for gut healing strategies.

- Focus on stress relief and self care- choose activities that fuel up your health and happiness vs tanking it and stealing your sanity. Again, high stress levels are not nice to your thyroid.

- Support a healthy gut by eating lots of plant-based foods, including fiber to feed your healthy gut bugs and avoid the overuse of antibiotics

- Monitor your medications and supplements- many supplements and medications can have interactions and make you feel worse. Make sure to work with a health professional before starting or stopping a drug or supplement.

- Prioritize sleep! Aim for 7-8 hours a night. The more the better! For your best night's sleep- see Chapter 9.
- Assess for potential dental infections and see a biological dentist. Infected root canals, amalgam or mercury based fillings, cavitations, and periodontitis can be triggers to an underlying thyroid disease. Your mouth is the first road to your blood stream, so make sure it's healthy!
- Be kind to yourself and choose a healing vs victim mindset. Your thoughts can hinder your healing, so focus on what is in your control vs yelling at yourself for what isn't. You can hold yourself back from healing through a negative mindset. Your body can feel it!

"The Best Diets for Thyroid Diseases"

You might hate me here, but there is no single best diet for hypothyroidism or hyperthyroidism. Each person needs a different amount of food and nutrients based on their own genetics, lifestyle, history, and symptoms. What triggers one person may not trigger another! I always suggest working one on one with a dietitian if you suffer with hypothyroidism to ensure that your diet is the perfect "Cinderella slipper" fit for you. I know you may have already googled these, but let's dive into some common "diets" thrown to help thyroid disease.

There are four popular "Hashimoto's diets" you may come across in your research. These include:

- Whole 30
- Specific Carbohydrate Diet (SCD)
- Gut and Psychology Syndrome Diet (GAPS)
- Paleo/Autoimmune Paleo

The commonalities of these diets are that they include:

- Elimination of grains
- Promotion of micronutrients
- Reduction of inflammatory foods

Each one of these thyroid diets have their pros and cons, and notice, they aren't individualized! These are options for you that you may find helpful, however like I said, I recommend working with someone one on one to individualize your diet.

Guidelines for Whole 30:

- Eat whole, health-promoting foods are meat and poultry, fish and seafood, eggs, fruits, vegetables, and nuts and seeds.

This list comes with a few caveats:

- All of these foods must be unprocessed.
- None of these foods may be used to recreate recipes that mimic baked goods, junk foods, or sweet treats.
- Foods considered whole but not health-promoting are eliminated during this protocol.
- Off-limit foods include alcohol, sugar, grains, legumes, dairy, and food additives commonly used in processing. These additives are artificial sweeteners, carrageenan, MSG, and sulfites.
- No weighing yourself at any time during the 30 days.

Benefits:

Food Group Elimination

Whole30 is skillful at identifying and choosing to eliminate food groups that may worsen inflammation and damage the thyroid, like gluten. As for dairy and soy, these are tolerated on a case-by-case basis. Eliminating both will prevent guessing which one is the trigger for you specifically, but special care will need to be taken during reintroduction of foods.

Lower Inflammation

Although it is not explicitly stated, the no grains and no legumes rule does apply to oils. Grain and legume oils are corn, bran, soybean, and peanut oil. However, it is a recommendation to avoid sunflower, safflower, canola, grapeseed, and sesame oil, too. Avoiding the grains and these oils will help to reduce inflammation, the presence of which can affect proper thyroid function.

Increase Micronutrients

Diversifying your diet through lifestyle modifications that reduce processed foods and increase plant foods promote micronutrient intake.

Risks:

30 Days

The length of this protocol is 30 days, while Hashimoto's is an autoimmune disease that will not end when this program does. You will have to choose what to do yourself after the 30 days is up.

Food Morality

Foods are viewed as good or bad and allowed or not-allowed. Many of the foods on the off-limit list might not be inherently bad for your individualized body. It is up to you and your healthcare practitioner to decide which foods do and do not work for you. Proceed with caution if you have a history of disordered eating.

Cure-All Marketing

Diet, alone, will not completely eliminate your symptoms of Hashimoto's, but it can help. Thyroid disease is a complex illness that requires addressing the root cause whether that be nutrient deficiency, exposure to toxins, infections, or adrenal dysfunction.

Specific Carbohydrate Diet (SCD)

The SCD is "a treatment to induce remission of active inflammation" and is commonly used now to help alleviate Crohn's disease, a chronic inflammatory bowel disease, as well as with SIBO management (small intestinal bacterial overgrowth). While it has restrictions on sugar, lactose, and all grains, it is still a complete, nutritionally adequate diet.

The diet is supposed to starve "bad" bacteria in the gut to improve the composition of the gut microbiome while reducing symptoms of GI distress.

Guidelines for the SCD Diet:

Foods to consume:

- All unprocessed meats and eggs

- All natural cheeses (except ricotta, mozzarella, cottage cheese, cream cheese, processed, or spreadable cheeses)
- Homemade yogurt cultured over 24 hrs
- Most legumes
- Most nuts and nut flours
- All-natural peanut butter
- Most non-starchy vegetables (not canned)
- All fruits and 100% juices with no additives
- Honey
- Saccharin

Foods to avoid:

- All processed/added sugar except honey
- All grains
- Canned vegetables
- Starchy vegetables
- Some beans
- Seaweed
- Canola oil
- Commercial mayonnaise
- High lactose dairy products
- Candy
- Sweet chocolate

The focus is on low-sugar, low lactose, and the elimination of all additives and grains.

Unlike Whole30, corn oil is allowed even though it is a grain derivative.

Illegal beans include soybeans, chickpeas, bean sprouts, mung beans, fava beans, and shelled peanuts.

Benefits:

Heals the microbiome

By eliminating complex carbohydrates this reduces bacterial over-growth caused by fermentation. Simple carbohydrates are easily absorbed, so the bacteria in the intestines are not given time to feed on it.

Lowers inflammation

Similar to the Whole30 diet, elimination of gluten itself will reduce the incidence of autoimmune attacks and protect the thyroid. The dairy allowed on this diet is supposed to be organic and lactose-free, which are usually better tolerated. The fermented yogurt is also full of probiotics, which provide digestive support. I would advise to reduce saturated and seed oils and focus on healthy fats instead, although it is not specified.

Risks:

Might be too difficult to follow

The ins and outs of this diet are a lot to remember in the beginning but can be made manageable through referring to a chart or written down list of accepted foods. Some guidelines are not as black-and-white as others, namely, sugar, dairy, and beans. It may also at times feel unfamiliar and restrictive.

Time commitment

Unlike Whole30, the average length of time recommended for followers of the SCD diet is around 1 full year. Results seen after 1 year are significant changes in microbial stool composition and decreases in disease activity and inflammatory markers.

Gut and Psychology Syndrome Diet (GAPS)

GAPS is "designed to heal and seal the gut lining, rebalance the immune system, and restore the optimal bacterial ecosystem within the GI tract." It was created to treat the unique needs of patients afflicted by intestinal and neurological conditions, which are thought to result from an imbalanced microbiome ecosystem. It aims to heal leaky gut and prevent toxins from accessing the bloodstream, which would impede brain function. GAPS protocol is an adaptation of the SCD, and it restricts difficult-to-digest foods while emphasizing nutrients that directly provide digestive support.

Guidelines for the GAPS Diet

This diet works in two phases, the introductory phase and maintenance phase.

In general, here are the guidelines for the overall GAPS diet.

Foods to include:

- Broth with every meal
- Fresh eggs (if tolerated)
- Fresh meats, fish, and shellfish
- Canned fish in oil or water
- All natural cheese, homemade yogurt, ghee
- Anti-inflammatory oils
- Nuts
- Mostly cooked non-starchy vegetables
- Beets
- Winter squash

292 | THE WOMEN'S GUIDE TO HORMONAL HARMONY

- Lima beans
- Peas
- All fruit
- Honey
- Cellulose
- Fermented foods

Foods to eliminate:

- Grains
- Pasteurized dairy
- Starchy vegetables
- Simple carbohydrates

Phases of the GAPS Diet

Each phase will also include food from the previous phases.

- Homemade bone broth, soft tissues from bones used in making broth, juices from fermented vegetables, and ginger tea with honey between meals.
- Raw organic egg yolks, meat & vegetable stews, fermented fish, homemade ghee, and increased daily amount of homemade yogurt and juices from fermented vegetables.
- Ripe avocado, nut butter/egg pancakes, eggs made with animal fat, and sauerkraut/fermented vegetable solids.
- Meats (non-barbecued or charred), cold pressed olive oil, fresh pressed vegetables juices, and nut-flour based breads.
- Cooked apple puree, raw vegetables, and fresh pressed juices with fruits and vegetables.
- Raw fruit, honey, and diet-adhering cakes/sweet treats.

Supplements for the GAPS Diet

- Probiotics
- Essential fatty acids
- Cod liver oil
- Digestive enzymes

Benefits:

Elimination

- Like other "Hashimoto's Diets," GAPS eliminates known "trigger" foods such as gluten and pasteurized dairy.
- Reduces Some GI Symptoms
- Anecdotally, the GAPS diet has been shown to reduce bouts of GI upset resulting in bloating, indigestion, and general digestive irritation.

Risks:

- Lack of Neurological Research
- Absence of research is not lack of efficacy, but it does help in establishing legitimacy of a diet. The lack of research present is regarding the claims of healing autism, Tourette's, and other neurological disorders. For those able to last through the introductory phase, it is recommended to give the diet a try.
- Poor Adherence
- This diet can last anywhere from 1 to 2 years and is slightly less restrictive than the SCD diet overall. The problem of adherence lies in the beginning phases where intake is strictly controlled, but it is definitely doable.

Paleo & Autoimmune Paleo Diet (AIP)

The AIP diet "addresses underlying inflammation stemming from the gut and brings the microbiota back into balance while optimizing nutrient intake."

Autoimmune paleo takes the original paleo diet, which is marketed as being based on the diets of our ancestors, and furthers the food restrictions while increasing nutrient consumption.

Guidelines for the Paleo/AIP diet

Paleo:

Foods you can eat on the Paleo diet:

- Meat and fish
- Eggs
- Fruits
- Vegetables
- Nuts & seeds
- Anti-inflammatory fats & oils
- Foods to avoid on the Paleo diet:
- Grains
- Dairy
- Legumes
- Added sugars
- Artificial sweeteners
- Inflammatory oils
- Trans fats

AIP

Foods to include with AIP:

- Lean meats, liver

- Vegetables, excluding nightshades (tomatoes, potatoes, peppers, and eggplant)
- Restricted amounts of fruit,
- Fermented foods
- Omega-3 abundant seafood
- Anti-inflammatory oils

Foods to avoid with AIP:

- Everything not allowed on a traditional paleo diet
- Coffee
- Eggs
- Nuts & seeds
- Nightshades (tomatoes, potatoes, peppers, and eggplant)

Benefits:

Physical & Emotional Health

- In addition to a lifestyle intervention, AIP lowers inflammation and supports the immune system. Following a restrictive diet such as this may add to additional stress, but working with an RD can alleviate this problem.
- Improves Bowel Diseases
- 6-week adherence to the AIP improved Mayo clinic scores, which correspond to measures of ulcerative colitis/ bowel inflammation. These symptoms include bowel movement frequency, rectal bleeding, presence of mucus, and disease activity.

Risks:

- Not Shown to Improve Thyroid Function
- Alone, this diet will not cure thyroid disease, but none of these diets will do that alone. What it will do is address

preventable autoimmune attacks related to inflammatory food consumption.

Takeaways about the "Best Diets for Thyroid Disease"

There is no best diet. Eating and follow a specific diet pattern may help in alleviating symptoms and getting you one step closer to eating better and identifying your potential food intolerances. However, follow a specific diet protocol can be overly restrictive diet can set you up for disordered eating, and they may not improve the health of your thyroid.

It is up to you and your healthcare provider to decide which diet is best for you. Aim for a diet you can stick to long term, that reduces your symptoms, maximizes your nutrition, and allows as much flexibility and variety as possible!

My Top Supplements for Thyroid Disorders

Please remember, supplementation should be made by a clinician or health care provider and is always based on individual root cause and needs. Don't take anything without being overseen by a health professional.

Potential Supplements and Nutrients for All Types of Thyroid Disorders:

- Omega-3s: help to support the immune system, cell membrane integrity, and decrease inflammation. Omega 3's can be found in animal proteins such as chicken, red meat, fish, eggs, as well as in flax, chia, or hemp seeds, soy beans, seaweed, algae, and walnuts.
- Curcumin: helps to reduce inflammation and combat oxidative damage. Curcumin can be found in turmeric,

however the active component is most concentrated in supplement form.

- Multivitamin: acts as a micronutrient "safety net" to ensure your body has the necessary co-factors and nutrients for energy production (methylated forms needed based on genetics, such as MTHFR mutation)
- Vitamin D with K2 (based on Vitamin D levels): low levels of Vitamin D are linked to weak bones, insulin resistance, depressed immune system, low energy levels, and increased risk of auto-immune flares. K2 is required for Vitamin D metabolism and prevention of calcium loss from bone, therefore make sure to take a Vitamin D with K2 included. Natural sources include dairy, salmon, eggs, sardines, liver, fish, mushrooms, orange juice, and tofu.
- Magnesium: fights inflammation, serves as a co-factor in regulating Vitamin D levels, helps stabilize blood sugar, regulates blood pressure, and supports a healthy immune system. Magnesium is required from T4 to T3 conversion and can aid in improving Vitamin D levels and decreasing risk of renal stones caused by high calcium levels. Magnesium is also depleted with high stress, so magnesium may be warranted if cortisol dysregulation is present. Natural sources of magnesium include chocolate, spinach, avocados, tofu, nuts, and whole grains.
- Vitamin A: deficiency may increase autoimmune disease development and worsen hypothyroidism. Vitamin A is required for iodine uptake and a deficiency may be seen with or worsen iodine deficiency. Vitamin A may also aid in reversing iron deficiency as it increases iron absorption by mobilizing stored iron into erythrocytes. It also participates in the uptake of T3 in your cells. Vitamin A can be found in dairy, fatty fish, animal proteins, and is highly concentrated within liver. If deficient, a liver supplement may be necessary.
- B-vitamins: B-vitamins help in the production of thyroid

hormone, energy creation, serve as co-factors to the creation of other vitamins/minerals, and participate in the formation of red blood cells and DNA synthesis. B-vitamins, such as B12, are common deficiencies seen in hypothyroidism and may cause of exacerbate thyroid issues. B-vitamins can be found in animal proteins and plant foods such as whole grains, legumes, and dark leafy greens. B-vitamins become depleted with high cortisol and stress, therefore ensuring to check for a deficiency is suggested with any suspected thyroid or adrenal imbalance.

- Zinc: required for the creation of TSH, T4 to T3 conversion, as well as immune function, protein synthesis, and cell growth and division. Zinc is also required for the transport of Vitamin A to be used by the cell. Low zinc can prevent the creation of stomach acid, which can lead down to gut dysbiosis and nutrient deficiencies. Take with caution and watch your levels, as zinc can compete with copper for absorption.

- Copper: this mineral works alongside iron to help form red blood cells that transport oxygen throughout your body. It also plays a major role in energy production, nerve cell function, collagen formation, and immune health. Copper can be found in nuts, seeds, cocoa, leafy greens, legumes, whole grains, and organ meats. Because copper is required to help transport iron in the body, a copper deficiency may worsen or be a leading cause of iron deficiency.

- Selenium: aids in T4 to T3 thyroid conversion and may help to reduce thyroid antibodies. Selenium may also help to prevent damage of excessive iodine and reduce oxidative damage from antibody attack. Natural sources of selenium can be easily found in brazil nuts. Just 68-91 mcg is in on brazil nut.

- Vitamin C: this vitamin is required for preventing free radical damage, supporting a healthy immune system, and helping aid in iron absorption. It also plays a crucial role in adrenal function and deficiency can lead to adrenal stress and impairment of the HPA axis. Vitamin C can be found in citrus fruits, berries, broccoli, leafy greens, and peppers. High levels of vitamin C compete with copper so make sure to assess levels for a balance.

- N-acetyl cysteine: helps to support glutathione levels which are involved in immune regulation and liver detoxification. NAC may also aid in female egg quality and serve as a biofilm disrupter for gut dysbiosis.
- Iron: required for the conversion of T4 to T3 as well as production the production of red blood cells. Without iron, red blood cells can not carry oxygen to the body's tissues. Iron is also required to make hormones in the body. Iron deficiency can lead to anemia, hypothyroidism, GI upset, weakness, and a depressed immune system. Focus on heme sources (animal sources) of iron such as eggs, chicken, red meats, and liver. Iron excess can heavily increase inflammation in the body (hemochromatosis), therefore make sure to do a full iron panel prior to supplementation. (Look for serum iron, % saturation, TIBC, ferritin, and hemoglobin levels)
- Iodine (depending on blood iodine levels): required for the synthesis of thyroid hormone. Too much or too little can cause hypo or hyperthyroidism. Iodine is required for almost every cell of the body. Iron competes with copper, so make sure to balance with this mineral.
- Digestive enzymes and probiotics, if warranted: can help in the digestive and absorption of food and participate in a healthy gut microbiome.

Supplements for Hyperthyroidism

- Ashwagandha- helps to increase T4 to T3 conversion
- Motherwort- may help reduce symptoms of hyperthyroidism yet doesn't act on the thyroid gland itself

- Guggal
- Bugleweed- may help to reduce thyroid synthesis, decreasing circulating thyroid levels; Also acts by preventing antibodies from binding to the thyroid gland
- Blue Flag
- Lemon Balm- may aid in blocking thyroid hormone receptors and preventing antibodies from attaching to the thyroid
- L-tyrosine- required for creation of thyroid hormones and most likely can be obtained through protein in the diet. Too much can worsen high cortisol levels through the production of norepinephrine and epinephrine.
- L-carnitine- may help reduce symptoms of hyperthyroidism as well as block the action of thyroid hormone in the cells
- CoQ10- aid in energy production and serves as antioxidant

To my fellow thyroid warriors- I have been in your shoes. I know the confusion & frustration that comes with being hypothyroid. Thyroid fatigue is real and combine that with not feeling like you are in control of your body- it can be crippling! From brain fog, hair loss, to digestive distress- I promise, you can and will get better and feel better. You must keep digging and refuse to let your disease rule your life. Keep searching for answers and stand firm in your right to have optimal health. Take your health back into your own hands by being your own health advocate. It's not normal to feel "off". Keep searching until you feel like your best self again.

9

THE CORTISOL CONNECTION

Cortisol imbalances can be crippling. Alterations in a healthy cortisol rhythm can lead to weight gain, trouble losing weight, poor immune function, blood sugar imbalances, brain fog, chronic fatigue, aches and pains, salt and sugar cravings, insomnia, hormonal imbalances, gastrointestinal distress... you name it! Many times when clients come to me, they have been put through the ringer with chronic, debilitating symptoms. After addressing diet, exercise, supplements, and digestive support, they still don't feel like themselves and can't balance their hormones. They are confused, frustrated, and want to give up. The culprit? Many times, it's cortisol.

Cortisol and adrenal imbalance are the biggest demons to your health, happiness, and well-being. In fact, my hypothyroidism was induced by cortisol imbalance. Chronic stress from attempting to do my Master's degree, dietetic internship, and remain a full-time online coach resulted in self-induced hypothyroidism. Not only did it cause my health to spin out of control, but it also impacted my mood, mental clarity, hormones, and metabolism. I wouldn't take back how I handled that time in my life, however it sparked a genetic susceptibility to hypothyroidism, and create my own issues by neglecting my cortisol and self care.

Do not be like me, ladies. You deserve better. Don't grind into the ground like I did. You will shoot yourself in the foot. Nobody wants that.

Do these questions sound like you?:

- Am I constantly tired, even when getting 8-10 hours of sleep?
- Do I feel energized, or worn out after exercise?
- Do I notice blood sugar swings throughout the day or random mood swings?
- Do I wake up in the morning not feeling refreshed?
- Do I need coffee and caffeine to get through the day?
- Do I wake up in the middle of the night?
- Am I "tired but wired" at night?
- Do I get sick often?
- Does my body feel inflamed and puffy?
- Do I feel stressed or have a lot on my mind?
- Do I notice aches/pains, especially in the morning?
- Do I have a craving for salty and/or sugary foods?
- Do I have a sensitivity to chemicals or fragrances?
- Do I have problems concentrating, remembering things, or deal with brain fog?

If you said "yes" to at least five of the questions above, you may have problems with cortisol or adrenal imbalance!

How do your adrenal glands and cortisol work? Your adrenal glands sit right on top of your kidneys and are a part of the intricate HPA axis (hypothalamic-pituitary-adrenal axis) that influences your thyroid and hormonal health. They are in charge of secreting hormones like cortisol, epinephrine, and norepinephrine (also known as adrenaline and noradrenaline, respectively). Together, they influence your flight-or-flight response- aka the stress response.

Your fight-or-flight response helps you react to emergencies and times of stress based on internal and external stimuli. Whether the stress is a tiger running at you, an upcoming exam, or your sister throwing a wrench in your party plans, your adrenal glands work to produce hormones to help your body in mitigating stress and preventing its repercussions.

What is stress? Stress is defined as "a subject to pressure or tension." Think about it, whether the tension is from your mother yelling at you about forgetting to defrost the chicken (we have all been there), an important deadline at work, or a grueling, heavy weight training workout, your body adapts to respond to the pressure or tension it's facing. This is stress.

The hard truth is that your body can't distinguish between types of stress, whether it is physical, mental, or environmental. To your body, stress is stress. Whether the stress is intentional (such as dieting, over-exercising, poor sleep, or poor diet quality), or unintentional (such as emotional or mental stress, inflammation, or disease/infection), stress will play out the same way physiologically. Long term, any chronic stress not addressed can lead to cortisol, adrenal, hormonal, and digestive imbalances.

Don't get me wrong- not all stress is bad, and neither is cortisol. Although chronic stress and high cortisol can be devils that wreak havoc on your health, we need cortisol in our bodies. Cortisol is essential for life and can:

- Regulate blood sugar and blood pressure
- Manage the sleep-wake cycle
- Maintain immune function
- Improve insulin sensitivity
- Impact digestion
- Respond to stress and danger
- Decrease inflammation
- Regulate digestion, growth, and reproduction

Cortisol is part of the glucocorticoid family in your body (aka- it raises your blood sugar). This is important because it helps to increase glucose levels and release them from the liver in times of stress and starvation when glucose is needed. Your body thrives on glucose. Ever have a terribly rough workout or go hours without eating? Your body pumps out cortisol to signal for more glucose to be released for energy! You need cortisol in your life. Just not too much, or too little.

Let's dive deeper into how your adrenal glands work. When your adrenal glands are stimulated, they activate either your parasympathetic or sympathetic nervous system. Both of these systems are a part of your autonomic nervous system (ANS), which is controlled by your central nervous system (CNS). Your nervous systems are a beautiful web of nerve cells (neurons) that transmit messages to each other through electrical impulses. Think of these impulses like text messages. Your neurons text each other to communicate. Neurons communicate with other neurons, but also with your muscles, tissues, and other bodily organs and glands. Through this communication, they control all of your body's functions, voluntary or not, and transmit signals back and forth between your body's cells and your brain.

The signals transmitted can result in voluntary or involuntary responses. The ANS works by helping your body regulate non-voluntary (autonomic = automatic) actions, such as controlling your heart rate, blood pressure, breathing, digestion, fluid balance (such as saliva and sweat), and sexual desire. On the other hand, your somatic nervous system (SNS) is responsible for voluntary actions of your body, including muscle movement and sense organs. When you lift your arm, walk, itch your leg, or smell a freshly baked cookie- that's your SNS. When your breathing quickens, you're digesting your food, sweating in the gym, or experiencing sexual desire- that's your ANS.

To make it even more confusing and complex, your ANS then divides into your parasympathetic or sympathetic nervous system, which together, work to control everyday life and activities. Your parasympathetic nervous system takes control of "rest and digest" mode, while your sympathetic nervous system takes action when meeting or facing a stress or challenge (aka your fight-or-flight response).

For example, when you eat a meal, your parasympathetic system sends signals to your body to increase blood flow to your digestive organs, allowing for the digestion of food and absorption of your food's nutrients. When you work out, your sympathetic nervous system accelerates your breathing and heart rate in order to increase the oxygen delivery to your cells, allowing for continued work.

Additional actions from your different nervous systems include:

- Sympathetic: pupil dilation, accelerated heart rate, constriction of blood vessels, inhibition of digestion and GI motility, stimulation of blood glucose from your liver, stimulation of epinephrine and norepinephrine from your adrenal glands, stimulation of orgasm, bladder release
- Parasympathetic: pupil contraction, slowed heart rate, stimulation of food digestion and digestive enzyme release, bladder constriction

Both of these systems need to work together. However, when your sympathetic nervous system becomes dominant, this is where cortisol and adrenal trouble starts to develop.

How does the stress response work? When a stressor is noticed, your hypothalamus releases a hormone called corticotropin-releasing hormone (CRH) and arginine vasopressin hormone (AVP). These hormones then trigger the release of adrenocorti-cotropic hormone (ACTH) from the pituitary, which then triggers the adrenal gland to release cortisol, epinephrine, norepinephrine, and aldosterone from your adrenal medulla and adrenal cortex. This increases the mobilization of fat, amino acids, and glycogen

306 | THE WOMEN'S GUIDE TO HORMONAL HARMONY

within your body, allowing for energy use. Think about when you are running from a tiger- you need that energy to get away! Your body responds to a stressor in this same way, regardless of the type. The stressor is noticed, the adrenal glands release their hormones, and in turn, a cascade of additional sympathetic activity, including increases in blood pressure, heart rate, and constriction of blood vessels, occurs.

Let's go step by step!:

1. When a stressor is noticed, your hypothalamus releases hormones called corticotropin-releasing hormone (CRH) and arginine vasopressin hormone (AVP).
2. These hormones then trigger the release of adrenocorticotropic hormone (ACTH) from the pituitary, which then triggers the adrenal gland to release cortisol, epinephrine, norepinephrine, and aldosterone from your adrenal medulla and adrenal cortex.
3. This increases the mobilization of fat, amino acids, and glycogen in your body, allowing for energy use (aka blood sugar release)! It also starts the cascade of additional sympathetic activity, including increases in blood pressure, heart rate, and constriction of blood vessels, along with inhibition of digestion and slowed motility.

Stress as you now know can be good or bad. Have you heard of the story of the three little bears? Where Goldilocks found the porridge that wasn't too hot, or too cold, and was "just right"? Same goes for where you want cortisol to be! When stress is short term and you can overcome it, you reach the Goldilocks effect. When your short-term stress turns into a long-term constant, this is where the porridge can be harmful.

Short-term stress, aka acute stress, helps the body in reacting to immediate stimuli and can be overcome by periods of relaxation and rest. This is where the parasympathetic nervous system (think rest and digest) takes over to help the body recoup from sympathetic stimulation (aka the fight-or-flight response). Acute stress occurs during times of illness, injury, or infection, sending white blood cells to the rescue to fight. It also occurs anytime something or someone stresses you out, you get scared, sense danger, go on a run, or lift weights. That acute stress and cortisol released by your adrenals are required for you to properly regulate your blood pressure, heart rate, energy levels, recover, and heal properly. To reiterate- not all cortisol is bad. If you don't have enough, this can lead to electrolyte imbalances (which can be life-threatening), chronic fatigue, bone loss, hypothyroidism, hormonal imbalances, dizziness, muscle loss and weakness, as well as anxiety and depression.

So we want acute stress. Gotcha. What we don't want is chronic stress and chronic high cortisol. This leads to chronic overstimulation of your sympathetic nervous system (fight-or-flight mode), which keeps cortisol and your adrenal hormones elevated for so long that it sends a surge of chaos throughout your body. This is where cortisol starts to compromise your health and can harm rather than help you.

CORTISOL IMBALANCES

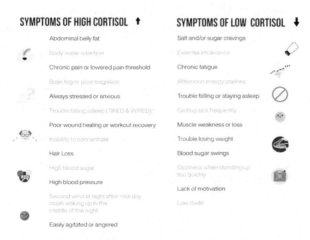

SYMPTOMS OF HIGH CORTISOL ↑	SYMPTOMS OF LOW CORTISOL ↓
Abdominal belly fat	Salt and/or sugar cravings
Body water retention	Exercise intolerance
Chronic pain or lowered pain threshold	Chronic fatigue
Brain fog or poor cognition	Afternoon energy crashes
Always stressed or anxious	Trouble falling or staying asleep
Trouble falling asleep (TIRED & WIRED)*	Getting sick frequently
Poor wound healing or workout recovery	Muscle weakness or loss
Inability to concentrate	Trouble losing weight
Hair Loss	Blood sugar swings
High blood sugar	Dizziness when standing up too quickly
High blood pressure	Lack of motivation
Second wind at night after mid-day crash waking up in the middle of the night	Low libido
Easily agitated or angered	

*You can have signs of both, as cortisol can be high or low at various points

High Cortisol & Your Health

High cortisol can then deplete your body of its immune reserves, leading to increased risk of infection, inflammation, and slowed recovery or healing.

Chronically high cortisol can:

Shift your hormone creation and conversion- such as inhibiting ovulation and reducing progesterone secretion, leading to PMS, infertility, or irregular menstrual cycles. The limit does not exist on how high cortisol can wreak havoc on your hormones.

- Upregulate your regulate androgen and DHEA levels, contributing to acne, weight gain, male pattern hair loss, or PCOS
- Impair your thyroid hormone conversion, reducing the amount that is able to be utilized by the cell. It also can inhibit the absorption of thyroid hormones into the cell.
- Slow digestion and prevent release of digestive enzymes from your stomach, pancreas, and gallbladder, contributing to constipation, food intolerances, gas/bloating, and risk of bacterial overgrowths
- Decrease insulin sensitivity and increase insulin output, contributing to blood sugar dysregulation, weight gain, and accelerated aging
- Accelerate the continued release of glucose from your liver contributing to insulin resistance and weight gain (also leading to acne and blood sugar dysregulation)
- Decrease your immunity and increase risk of illness and infection- causing you to get sick often or decrease your ability to fight illness
- Impair workout recovery and contribute to muscle and joint pains- making you feel like you got "hit by a truck" (at least that is what it felt like for me!)
- Impact mood and motivation – in turn increasing anxiety or depression

- Inhibit sleep and sleep quality- further contributing to your chronic fatigue
- Increase cravings for salty and sugary foods, further troubling issues with weight loss
- Increase total body inflammation and decreasing the capability fight and reduce inflammation, which can increase your risk of autoimmune flare-ups, development of chronic disease, and further hormonal imbalances

I hope you said "Dayum." Yes, girl- too much cortisol can wreak havoc. It produces a domino effect in your body that causes your health to take a slippery slope downward. Your hormones go down the hill with it.

High cortisol levels shift your reproductive hormones, causing disruptions in your hormonal symphony. Your hormones all start with the creation of pregnenolone. Pregnenolone then metabolizes into progesterone, cortisol, DHEA, testosterone, or estrogen. It's quite a complex process and each step can be hindered or accelerated through multiple mechanisms. In relation to cortisol, cortisol can prevent the conversion of progesterone and shift your hormones to produce cortisol instead!

Chronically high cortisol suppresses GnRH from pulsing to drive sufficient FSH and LH in your body. Remember, LH and FSH have to surge to trigger ovulation. Without ovulation, you can't produce progesterone, and without progesterone, you can't have a period! High cortisol can both suppress ovulation and lower progesterone levels created during your luteal phase. This can lead to amenorrhea, a luteal phase defect, or luteal insufficiency, or PCOS. Cue PMS problems, anxiety, infertility, long luteal phase (late menstrual cycle), or mid-cycle spotting.

With chronic stress, the body has no clue what type of stressor is coming its way. For all it knows, there could be a tiger running at it. The body reacts to conserve energy and puts its efforts into maximizing your alertness. It goes into "survival mode." Would it be safe to reproduce or put effort into digesting when a tiger is coming? Heck no. Your body adjusts to help you survive. It diverts its efforts from digestion and reproduction as a safety mechanism.

Chronic high cortisol levels and chronic stress lead to multiple stages of adrenal dysfunction. Each stage requires different treatment protocols based on what is, or is not, imbalanced. Don't get it twisted. There is no such thing as "adrenal fatigue." Let me repeat- adrenal fatigue does not exist. However, adrenal dysfunction and imbalance does, and its symptoms and effects on health can be crippling.

The ability to manage acute stressors and prevent them from causing cortisol chaos depends on each person's stress bucket size. The ability to handle stress is person by person dependent. It also depends on the type of stressor. One person's stressor may be another's relaxation. It truly varies between women. Your ability to mitigate stress is influenced by your genes, hormones, inflammation, diet quality, sleep quality, environment, and relationships. These factors influence how small, or large, your stress bucket is. For me, I think of my stress bucket as a teaspoon. For other women, their bucket is more like a swimming pool. Those lucky women can bounce back easily from stress. Whether that's due to increased stress resilience, a foundation of healthy stress coping strategies, or the luck of the draw in genetics, I am quite jealous of them.

Remember the COMT gene I mentioned in a previous chapter? Having the homozygous ++ COMT gene results in decreased enzyme clearance of your estrogen, epinephrine, and norepinephrine, resulting in increased levels in the blood for longer periods of time. This can leave someone with increased cortisol levels for longer, increasing their risk for chronic stress and burnout! On the other hand, the lucky women with the homozygous - - COMT gene have increased clearance of these hormones, which results in faster clearance of cortisol. This means they are more likely to get over a stressor and are less susceptible to burnout.

· · ·

Low Cortisol and Your Health:

Though you won't hear about it in conventional medicine, and some conventional doctors may deny its existence, subclinically low cortisol levels can be a devastating cause of chronic aches and pains, fatigue, low thyroid, and hormone imbalances. Conventional doctors may not recognize this without the diagnosis of Addison's disease or an adrenal crisis, however what I call "subclinical hypercortisolism" is real, and can be crippling.

Low cortisol levels can:

- Downregulate sex hormone production, leading to total low sex hormones and infertility
- Contribute to low blood sugar and low blood pressure (including orthostatic hypotension or dizziness upon standing quickly), creating energy crashes throughout the day and possible caffeine sensitivity
- Create electrolyte imbalances, leading to alterations in blood pressure, salt and sugar cravings, water retention, increased urination, and heart palpitations
- Decrease immunity and wound healing capabilities
- Worsen chronic fatigue and fibromyalgia- leading to a vicious cycle of low energy, motivation, impaired memory, and chronic pain
- Increase risk for bone loss- leading to increased fracture risk and osteoporosis
- Disrupt sleep – causing insomnia, abnormal cortisol rhythms, and muscle loss
- Cause weight gain (especially around the abdominal region) or trouble losing weight
- Create exercise intolerance- in which any form of exercise makes you feel worse and worse
- Heighten stress, anxiety, and depression

I know what you're thinking. Good lord. Cortisol too high or too low can be a demon. It sure can!

In the case of low cortisol, the top causes in the conventional medicine world include:

- Addison's Disease (primary adrenal insufficiency): This is where the adrenal glands are unable to produce enough cortisol, either from gland destruction or malfunction. Autoimmune disease is the most common culprit for the development of Addison's. Other causes include long-term use of glucocorticoids (such as prednisone), infections, head trauma, radiation, or cancer.
- Congenital adrenal hyperplasia (CAH): In this rare condition, you inherit a gene that can't code for the enzyme adrenal steroid 21-hydroxylase. Without this enzyme, your adrenal glands may be unable to produce enough cortisol or aldosterone. They may even make too many androgens.
- Hypopituitarism: When this occurs, the pituitary does not create enough hormones (including sex, thyroid, and adrenal), which causes hormonal imbalances and low cortisol levels. Also seen is lack of antidiuretic hormone (ADH) creation, which leads to increased thirst and urination. Common causes of hypopituitarism include head trauma, infection, genetics, hypophysitis, cancer, or radiation.
- Secondary adrenal insufficiency: This insufficiency involves the pituitary's inability to produce adrenocorticotropic hormone (ACTH). Without ACTH, adrenal hormones are not created, including cortisol. Causes of secondary adrenal insufficiency include head trauma, genetics, cancer, medications, or autoimmune disease. It can also be caused by overuse or chronic use of hydrocortisone or medications such as prednisone.

The causes above can be diagnosed through a blood test, MRIs, and ultrasounds. What I see in my patients is quite different, and does not involve zero cortisol or adrenal production, but does include suboptimal production. This can be tested through a four point salivary cortisol test (such as ZRT) or a DUTCH Plus or DUTCH adrenal test. With these tests, you can assess for not only total cortisol production but also for your cortisol pattern and rhythm.

Again, conventional doctors may not believe in subclinical cortisol levels. Some may not believe in testing salivary cortisol. However, I find it is the gold standard for assessing cortisol, especially in the case of subclinical levels.

The top causes of sub-clinically low cortisol I see in my clients include:

- Hypothyroidism
- End stages of the stress response (more on that in a bit)
- Medications
- Nutrient deficiencies

In working to find the root causes of my client's struggles, assessing cortisol levels to rule out both high and low levels is critical. I also love assessing their cortisol rhythm, as most need a little love in rebalancing a wonky rhythm.

Your Cortisol Rhythm:

Your body has a natural diurnal rhythm of cortisol production that helps give you the right amount just when you need it most. A healthy cortisol rhythm starts with your cortisol awakening response (CAR) in the morning, where cortisol levels should be the highest, and then slowly drops throughout the day, until cortisol reaches its lowest levels in the evening. Your CAR is what kick starts your cortisol production in the morning. It also participates to help scavenge free radicals through a process called apoptosis (aka killing of "failed cells") and combat inflammation. Ever notice increased aches and pains in the morning that go away in the evenings? This can be tied to a disruption in your CAR, or the lack of one.

Your cortisol levels should follow a downward slope from the time you awaken to the time you go to bed. When light hits your eyes in the morning, this triggers your hypothalamus and adrenal glands to release the burst of cortisol you need in the morning to conquer your day. Your cortisol then steadily drops throughout the day until it reaches its evening low. This low allows for the production of melatonin, which helps you to fall and stay asleep, as well as triggering the secretion of growth hormone. Melatonin is produced by your pineal gland in response to darkness. This production of melatonin can be interrupted by artificial and blue light, which prevents your body from releasing melatonin as well as alter your natural cortisol patterns.

Are you a nighttime Netflix binger or social media scroller? Are you guilty of checking emails late at night? By doing so, and increasing your nighttime artificial and blue light exposure, you are preventing your body from creating adequate melatonin. Over time, this throws off your hormones, cortisol, and sleep patterns! Hello insomnia, chronic stress, and hormonal chaos. It can even turn your cortisol pattern upside down, creating an inverse slope. This is far from optimal for your body. If you're guilty of the nighttime blue light, the first step is to minimize or eliminate it through reducing electronic use in the evenings, using a blue light filter, or wearing blue light blocking glasses in the evenings. I suggest wearing blue light blocking glasses for at least two hours before bedtime and then cutting off any and all electronics at least thirty minutes prior.

Adequate melatonin levels are critical to more than just your hormonal health and cortisol rhythms. Melatonin impacts your insulin sensitivity, immunity, energy levels, ability to heal and repair, and also influences inflammation. This is why those with jet lag or work night shifts can have trouble with weight gain, as they not only lose insulin sensitivity, but can have increased cravings and appetite. Symptoms of low melatonin include insomnia, chronic fatigue, poor immunity, constipation, increased appetite, weight gain, and mood instability.

The Stages of Adrenal Imbalance:

In the functional medicine world, there are four main stages of adrenal imbalance. As someone moves through these different phases, not only are their adrenals affected, but so are their sex hormones, thyroid, and digestion. The start of high cortisol results in the body burning through key nutrients required to make adrenal hormones, such as B-vitamins, glutamine, magnesium, and amino acids (specifically l-tyrosine), which further leads to nutrient deficiencies and worsens health, happiness, and hormonal harmony. Happy neurotransmitters become depleted, increased pain and aches set in, and the body's original beneficial stress response becomes harmful instead of helpful.

These stages are quite different from the two types of diseases recognized in general medicine that are affected by either increased cortisol production (Cushing's Disease), or low to no production (Addison's Disease). Cushing's disease can be caused by glucocorticoid therapy or pituitary tumors, while Addison's disease can be caused by autoimmune disease that damages the adrenal gland. Both of these diseases are endocrine disorders that are recognized within conventional medicine and are not caused by chronic stress.

Cortisol Phases 101

- Stage 1- You are a Boss B*tch. Getting the job done and high on life! Adrenaline kicks in and some feel the energy bunny effect (I sure do!)
- Stage 2- You are wired and tired. You start to develop energy crashes midday or blood sugar swings, low motivation, trouble falling asleep or waking up in the

middle of the night, poor recovery, and getting sick easily. You may be relying on caffeine.

- Stage 3- You are anxious and tired, but pushing through. You may notice extreme morning fatigue, irritability, aches and pains, salt and sugar cravings, exercise intolerance, and brain fog. Caffeine may not do the job anymore or make you feel worse!

- Stage 4- You are just plain exhausted. Nothing can get you through the day. Everything hurts and you may be depressed and anxious all the time. You are constantly craving food and salt and gaining weight, especially in your abdominal region.

THE **4 STAGES**
OF THE STRESS RESPONSE

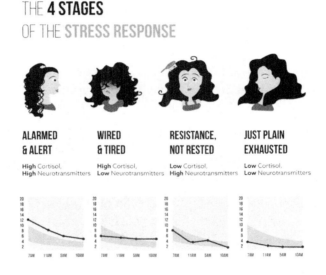

ALARMED & ALERT	WIRED & TIRED	RESISTANCE, NOT RESTED	JUST PLAIN EXHAUSTED
High Cortisol, **High** Neurotransmitters	**High** Cortisol, **Low** Neurotransmitters	**Low** Cortisol, **High** Neurotransmitters	**Low** Cortisol, **Low** Neurotransmitters

Stage one tends to be skipped or not noticed. During this "alarmed and alert" phase, all hands are on deck to get a job done or push through a stressful day or week. You may feel stressed and anxious, but don't notice any changes to your overall energy levels or sleep. Digestion may take a hit, however this phase is mostly short-lived and doesn't lead to long-term repercussions.

The second stage of adrenal dysfunction (what some may call "adrenal fatigue") is the "wired and tired" stage. During this phase, you may notice trouble sleeping (or waking up in the middle of the night), wake up exhausted, crave salty or sugary foods, and have more bouts of anger, irritation, and mood swings. The body attempts to adapt to the stressors thrown at it and is able to handle them by upregulating adrenal hormones. During this phase, it's common for people to run to caffeine for energy, or not even need it, running on an adrenaline high, and be able to still focus and complete necessary day-to-day tasks without much hindrance. Regarding testing, DHEA levels tend to remain normal or be elevated, not yet affecting other hormones, and if tested, epinephrine and norepinephrine may be elevated. Cortisol may be elevated at one or more points in a four point salivary cortisol, may only be elevated at night, or there may be an exaggerated cortisol awakening response (CAR).

The third phase involves "cortisol adaptation" in which your body attempts to overcome the stressors and starts to signal alarms for help to overcome them. During this phase, one might notice blood sugar and blood pressure swings, insomnia, digestive distress, low sex drive, shortness of breath with minimal exertion, low motivation, trouble concentrating, joint and muscle pain, and have caffeine dependence. During this phase, thyroid and hormonal problems can start to arise. DHEA and sex hormones may drop, including progesterone, which can inhibit ovulation (causing an irregular cycle, mid-cycle spotting, or the loss of the menstrual cycle). Women may also have extreme PMS and heightened anxiety or depression. Low progesterone can also further influence GABA levels, which is a relaxing neurotransmitter. Lack of GABA decreases stress resilience and worsens sleep. Cortisol levels during the adaptation phase may be up or down throughout the day, with one low or high cortisol point and imbalanced cortisol curve.

During the last phase, you reach chronic exhaustion, aka "too tired to be tired." This is the burnout phase that leads to crippling and debilitating fatigue and pain for many. People tend to reach this phase when they go so long under chronic stress and don't (or can't) mitigate it, that their body is no longer able to adequately maintain sufficient cortisol levels to deal with the stressor. The body starts to divert from sex hormone creation to stress hormone creation, going into preservation and conservation mode. DHEA levels drop, causing or contributing to low testosterone and estrogen levels. Symptoms during this phase include chronic fatigue and exhaustion, low blood pressure and orthostatic hypotension (blood pressure drops when standing quickly), constipation, brain fog, low resting heart rate, trouble losing weight or weight gain, and hypoglycemia. Cortisol levels during this phase may all be low with no curve at all, or present as a flat cortisol awakening response.

Having healthy adrenals involves learning to listen to your body and what it can handle! Optimizing your nutrition via a healthy diet, ensuring adequate sleep, exercising in a way that makes you feel good, focusing on stress reduction, talking with friends or a loved one, and learning when to say "no" are all crucial components of adrenal management.

Lifestyle strategies such as sleep hygiene, ensuring adequate food intake and diet quality, stress management, and not overr-training are essential steps for you to keep in practice in order to have healthy adrenals. However, there are also some incredible supplements and herbs that can be powerful to help your adrenals adapt to the stressors in your life. Notice the keyword in the name: "adapt"ogens. Adaptogens can serve as a "stress shield" to help the body cope with stress and in turn, deal with high cortisol! They also play a role in nourishing the adrenals, promoting healthy hormones, and can help to even enhance your mood and energy levels! I have found them extremely helpful in practice and in helping aid in sleep, combat stress, balance hormones, and ward off PMS. Not all adaptogens are the same, however. Some adaptogenic herbs stimulate, while others relax and nourish. Taking what you need based on your own cortisol curves and dysregulation is important in order to help you achieve an improved cortisol rhythm, versus making it worse. Adaptogens aren't magic. They won't do the sole work and cure all your problems, but they can be powerful to help your body adapt to the highs and lows of a rollercoaster life by making the highs and lows more manageable!

Adaptogens:

Adaptogen	Benefit	Effect & dose
Ashwagandha	Anti-inflammatory; reduces stress, anxiety, & cortisol; reduces oxidative damage; boosts libido; increasing T4 to T3 conversion	SOOTHING (an be stimulating for some); 100-300 mg Sensoril brand, 500-1200 mg KSM 66 brand or 1-2 g leaf & root
Holy Basil	Anti-inflammatory, fights fatigue, combats stress, enhances energy, lowers blood glucose	ENERGIZING; 300-400 mg not safe for women trying to get pregnant
Rhodiola Rosea	Anti-inflammatory, fights anxiety & stress, boosts immune system, enhances mood & libido, may improve mental and exercise performance	STIMULATING & NOURISHING; 300-600 mg
Maca	Improves energy and memory; reduces anxiety; enhances concentration; may help boost low testosterone & estrogen levels (can help with night sweats, hot flashes & low libido)	STIMULATING & NOURISHING; 1500-3000 mg
Cordyceps Mushroom	Anti-inflammatory, fights fatigue, regulates blood sugar	ENERGIZING
Reishi Mushroom	Improves immunity, aids in sleep, helps natural liver detoxification, stabilizes blood sugar	CALMING
Ginseng	Enhances concentration, fights fatigue, supports the immune system	STIMULATING
Licorice Root	Anti-microbial, helps increase energy & fight fatigue, helpful with high androgens	STIMULATING (not good for people high blood pressure)
Reishi Mushroom	Fights fatigue, helps boost immune system	NOURISHING
Lemon Balm	May help improve sleep, aid in stress relief & anxiety, supports the nervous system, improves cognition	CALMING
Valerian	Relaxes and aids in sleep, reduces anxiety, may help in restless leg syndrome	SEDATING

Heart Rate Variability

Another method to help in assessment of your adrenal health is checking your HRV (heart rate variability). You can track this through an app like Elite HRV on your smartphone, which tests your finger pulse to look at variability in your heart's pulse rate, which is essentially the time between each beat of your heart. You can also use HeartMath, an Oura ring, or Whoop strap. Do keep in mind, HRV decreases naturally with age, and HRV is very individualized. For example, athletes tend to have a higher HRV than non-athletes, and men have a higher HRV than women. Always compare your data to yourself! It's the trends that matter.

What can HRV tell you? Well, it can help you in assessing the balance of your parasympathetic (rest and digest), and sympathetic (flight or flight) nervous system. Using HRV, you can potentially make crucial decisions in your lifestyle and training to help you better manage your adrenals and ANS response! For example, having a low HRV may indicate that your body needs a little more rest and love, and doing a hard high intensity workout may not be the best for you then. You may want to focus on more relaxing activities and ensure proper sleep, nutrition, hydration. Your low HRV may put you further at risk for getting sick and be a sign you need extra recovery time. Having a "normal" higher HRV may indicate that you are well rested, hydrated, and ready to crush a workout! That higher HRV means that your body's parasympathetic system is dominating, while low HRV means that sympathetic is most likely dominating. Would you want to add more stress on an already stressed system? No! Then tracking HRV can help you potentially prevent from doing so.

HRV can decrease due to factors such as poor sleep, sickness, high stress, poor diet, poor recovery of workouts. Try using HRV to help you make intelligent decisions on training, staying on top of self care and relaxation techniques, and helping to motivate you to ensure proper hydration, food quality, and sleep hours!

Cortisol Review:

- Stress is stress. Any stressor- physical (such as training), emotional (such as a break up or trauma), mental (such as long periods of studying), or physiological (such as low blood sugar) - can spark cortisol production. We WANT this short-term, but elevated cortisol for too long is where you start to cause shifts in your hormones, thyroid, digestion, and both physical and mental health.

- Your cortisol response is controlled through your hypothalamus, pituitary, and adrenal glands, however cortisol impacts almost every tissue and cell of your body! Any disease or dysfunction in your HPA axis can influence your cortisol levels.

- Chronically high cortisol ultimately leads to the exhaustion phases of the stress response. No- not adrenal fatigue. That doesn't exist. INSTEAD- your body notices that cortisol isn't doing the job, up-regulates epinephrine and norepinephrine (flight-or-flight hormones), and DHEA levels (though these later drop) to try to serve as an alternative. High cortisol leads to low cortisol over time. Each phase of the adrenal response needs its own strategic healing protocol. Always test, don't just guess. Not all symptoms are cortisol related and may indicate another health issue that needs attention. Always work with a clinician or practitioner.

- You can't fix your cortisol issues if you aren't fixing what is causing them to be high or low in the first place. If you can't remove the stressors, infections, overgrowths, mold, or prioritize self care, sleep, and slothing- you won't get truly better!

My Top Tips for Adrenal Health:

- Learn to say "No"- if it doesn't serve you or depletes your life of happiness or impacts your health, cut it out. Including toxic relationships with friends or significant others, and toxic relationships with yourself.

- Ensure you are eating a nutrient-dense diet full of the vitamins and minerals involved in your stress response. These include vitamin C, vitamin D, GABA, zinc, folate, B-12, iron, magnesium, and trace minerals. Incorporate healthy fats, various colors from fruits and vegetables, healthy fibers, and lean proteins. Avoid too many added sugars, refined grains, and processed vegetables oils, and if you suspect a food intolerance or sensitivity, work with a healthcare professional to help eliminate it. Remember, high stress causes your body to burn through these nutrients, so you may need more than normal, especially if you have already gotten your body to a place of deficiency.

- Don't be afraid to go to therapy or counseling. Talking with someone can help you to acknowledge your feelings and emotions, and channel them into energy to help you accomplish your life goals instead of holding you back.

- Focus on sleep and your cortisol rhythms. Start each day with getting into the sunlight as soon as possible, even try taking a walk or using a happy light if you don't have light upon waking! -Don't skip meals (unless strategically practicing intermittent fasting), and avoid the use of blue light at least two hours before bed that can block your body's ability to produce the melatonin you need to go to sleep! Blue light blockers can be excellent to help with this, whether they are glasses or a setting on your phone or laptop (or blue light blocking screen for your TV!)

- If you suspect adrenal imbalance- test, don't guess! (I am a huge fan of the DUTCH Salivary cortisol test or ZRT salivary four point cortisol test). Don't try to self-medicate with adaptogens or CBD oil alone. Be smart and invest in your health and yourself by doing proper testing. You want to make sure your testing involves four points to assess cortisol fluctuations throughout the day, and not just use a single cortisol level via blood test (like many conventional doctors will use to assess). These single blood markers can be helpful in assessing adrenal diseases of Cushing's and Addison's, but they will most likely not catch adaptive cortisol or cortisol dysregulation.

- Use adaptogens in a smart way. Again, you need to be

using what will help you! See the adaptogen table for details on some of my favorites!

- Practice gratitude! Starting your day with a grateful mindset can set the tone for a positive outlook on the day. Not only that, but your thoughts can either help or hinder your healing. Negative thinking can increase inflammation in your body, preventing you from healing both emotionally and physically! Start your day by journaling, praying, practicing yoga, or going for a walk. Drink a cup of tea (or coffee if your adrenals are able to handle it), and cuddle with your pet (which I hope is a cat- just saying).

- Journal down your thoughts so that you can recognize, release, and respond to them and your emotions. I like writing down one thing each day that I love about my life, one thing that I love about myself, and one thing I am grateful for.

- Have an orgasm. Yes, girl- do it. Orgasms can lower your cortisol levels and flood your brain with the happy neurotransmitter oxytocin. Help your brain choose pleasure over stress.

- Learn how to "sloth mode." This is a grand skill and one I can now claim on my resume after being in burnout several times. Slothing means doing nothing. Being a pure sloth. Slow, relaxed, and recharging. Slothing isn't just physical- it is also mental and emotional! Silence your phone, sit or lay on your couch, and watch a funny or happy movie. Learn to sloth when you need it and it will become a superpower. #SlothingSavesLives

- Detox your social media. If following someone increases stress, self-hatred, or causes comparison to yourself or your body, kindly unfollow or mute the person. You need to do what is best for YOU. If that means deleting social media, do it. Sometimes a social media detox for a week is enough, other times it may be time to cut it out for good.

- Laugh, cuddle, hug people, and have sex (get that orgasm girlfriend!). Then do it again. Seriously though, this boosts levels of oxytocin in your brain, which leads to feelings of happiness, as well as relaxation. Plus, who needs an excuse to have an orgasm?

- Limit consumption of refined sugars and carbohydrates to help balance your blood sugar. Focus on smart snacks- always pairing two macronutrient components together!

- Track your heart rate variability (HRV). As previously discussed, this can help you when you may need more rest, relaxation, and recovery.

- Limit your caffeine intake, especially if you are a slow caffeine metabolizer (CYP1A2-1F are slow, while CYPA2-1A are fast). Having caffeine too late in the day can keep you wired at night, affecting your sleep. It can also increase cortisol in your body, which you don't want when your cortisol levels and adrenals need some love. You don't need to cut out caffeine cold turkey, but think of weaning yourself down bit by bit. A great goal is keeping your caffeine under 400 mg per day, if possible. If caffeine makes you jittery or causes low blood sugar, it's a great sign caffeine is not for you.

Supplementation for Cortisol Imbalances

Please do not do this blindly. Test your cortisol levels and work with a healthcare professional prior to starting or stopping a cortisol-supporting herb or supplement. You don't want to increase what may need to decrease, or decrease what may need to increase! I truly believe that everyone responds differently to adaptogens and herbs, and what may work for you may not work for someone else. Be willing to experiment (under guidance) to find what may make you feel best! That being said, also be willing to give a supplement, herb, or adaptogen time to work. Most adaptogens and herbs work best when taken consistently for at least two months.

Supplements for overall adrenal health include:

- B-vitamin Complex (don't add to a multivitamin)
- Magnesium biglycinate: 400 mg/day
- Vitamin C: 1-2 g/day
- Omega-3s: 1-2 g/day
- Vitamin D: 1000-5,000 IU/day, depending on labs (deficiency may need up to 10,000 IU)
- Zinc: 10-50 mg based on needs, deficiencies, and copper levels
- Reishi mushroom: 300-2000 mg/day

Supplements for High Cortisol	Supplements for Low Cortisol
Ashwagandha: 1-4 g/day	Ashwagandha: 1-4 g/day
5-HTP (do not use if on an SSRI): 50-200 mg/day	Cordyceps: 1-2 g/day
L-theanine- 100-600 mg/day	DHEA: 10-50 mg/day
Phosphatidyl serine 100-1000 mg/day	L-tyrosine: 500-1000 mg/day
Passion flower: 1-2 g/day	Panax Ginseng: 100-400 mg/day
Holy Basil: 100-500 mg/day	Licorice: 100-400 mg/day (monitor blood pressure- don't use with hypertension)
Valerian root: 100-400 mg/day	Magnolia flower: 100-400 mg/day
Schisandra: 100-200 mg/day	Pregnenolone: 10-100 mg/day
Magnolia flower: 100-400 mg/day	Hydrocortisone: *based on MD recommendations*
Cordyceps: 1-2 g/day	Schisandra: 100-500 mg/day
Rhodiola standardized to 3% rosavins and 1% salidroside: 200-1200 mg/day	Maca: 500-2000 mg/day
Maca: 500-2000 mg/day	

Sleep: Your Body's House Cleaning Service

About 30% of your life is spent sleeping. To all you "grinders" that think that's a waste of time, I want you to think again. Sleep is what helps you prepare and recharge for the daily grind! It's what helps you not only maximize your cognition but also gives you the dedication, drive, and energy to get through your day-to-day life! Think of sleep as your superpower against grinding into the ground. Sleep is your best friend to ensure you have a healthy mind and body. Optimal sleep is crucial for energy, but it's also when your body's "clean up crew" comes in. Sleep is actually your body's free house cleaning service. During sleep, damaged and destructed cells and toxins are removed from your body, which plays a crucial role in combating and reducing inflammation. Ever woken up with more pain and inflammation that dissipates later during the day? This can be due to lack of deep or REM sleep, due to your "clean up crew" not getting to complete their jobs!

Lack of sleep can negatively affect your hunger levels by increasing ghrelin hormone levels and increasing fatigue. This can lead to increased cravings, lack of control with food, as well as decreased satiety with meals. It can also increase your risk of developing chronic diseases such as high blood pressure, cardio-vascular disease, diabetes, and obesity. Lack of sleep or poor quality of sleep can also increase inflammation, decrease recovery, inhibit optimal thyroid and hormone production, and decrease your immunity. This is extremely important, because it essentially means that sleep quality and quantity can affect your whole body, along with your current and future health!

How does sleep work? There are essentially four stages of sleep. In stage 1, which lasts just a few minutes, your heart rate and breathing slow, and muscles relax. This is your lightest and shortest sleep stage. You can be easily woken up during this phase. Stage 2 sleep remains a light sleep as you transition into Stage 3. Stage 2 involves the further lowering of your heart rate and breathing, and it's here that your eye movements stop. About 50-60% of your sleep is light sleep (4-7 hours a night, depending on your total sleep amount).

Stage 3 is classified as deep sleep, in which your body's heart rate and breathing are at their lowest points. It's here that your body performs rebuilding and repairing, as well as secretes growth hormone and rebuilds the immune system. This stage is all about helping heal and repair your body by eliminating the damaged cells from oxidative stress and inflammation. About 10-25% of your total sleep can be Stage 3 sleep. Lack of deep sleep results in unrefreshing sleep (cue morning fatigue and grogginess). Stage 3 sleep is where sleep talking or walking, night terrors, or bedwetting can occur.

Stage 4 sleep, or REM (rapid eye movement) sleep, is where your magical dreams happen! Stage 4 is all about the brain, and though your body actually becomes temporarily paralyzed, your brain is working at its highest capacity. This stage is extremely important for helping with the "filing" of your long term memory! Memory filing also occurs during Stage 3 sleep. This filing is actually rippling waves of brain oscillations from your hippocampus that activate selective memories, strengthening long term memory within your brain's cortex. Your eyes may move back and forth and your breathing may be irregular during this stage. REM sleep is completely during the second half of the night, and any early rising or cutting your sleep short can drop the amount of REM sleep that you get.

What does sufficient sleep look like? Just like with nutrition and exercise, everyone's body is different and has unique needs. In general, most people function best with seven to nine hours of sleep per night. However, just because your eyes are closed and you are lying horizontally does not mean that you are getting proper rest. According to the National Sleep Foundation, the key determinants of quality sleep include (1) sleeping at least 85 percent of the total time while in bed; (2) falling asleep in 30 minutes or fewer; (3) waking up no more than once per night; and (4) being awake for 20 minutes or less after initially falling asleep.

I don't know about you, but I have had my periods of poor sleep. Lying wide awake, wired, staring up at the ceiling. When my cortisol issues were at their worst, I would have 2 am waking periods of tossing and turning, and would wake up forever feeling unrested.

. . .

What Can Go Wrong to Screw With Your Sleep?

- Hormone imbalances
- Thyroid disorders
- Gut infections
- Nutrient deficiencies
- Adrenal imbalances
- Poor nutrition
- Blood sugar imbalances
- Mold toxicity
- Under-eating
- Poor liver health

To fix your sleep, focus on fixing the basics that involve nutrition, environment, mindset, and supplementation changes. Truth is- sleep is one of the most underrated aspects of health. Lack of sleep will disrupt your hormones, increase your hunger, and steal away your energy, and happiness.

My Secret Sleep Tips:

- Cut off blue light from electronics at least two hours before bed. You can use a blue light filter on your phone or laptop, blue light blocking glasses, or a blue light blocking screen. Blue light exposure can disrupt your circadian rhythm at night and prevent the release of melatonin that helps to relax you prior to sleep. Blue light can also keep cortisol elevated during the night, keeping you tired and wired. Put blue light blockers on around 8 pm when melatonin naturally starts to rise.
- Stop the use of electronics 30 minutes prior to bed. Electronics, even without blue light, may keep your brain wired and prevent you from relaxing and being able to fall asleep. I know you know this feeling- especially if you were watching an intense Netflix show!

- Have a consistent sleep time AND sleep routine. A consistent wake time is also suggested, as doing this will help train your circadian rhythms to follow a natural cycle.
- Optimize your bed room environment. Keep your bedroom cool: 65 to 70 degrees F is optimal for most people. If you struggle with sleeping hot, think of using breathable sheets such as bamboo or silk. Invest in comfort as well- if your mattress or pillow are uncomfortable, hot, or causing you pain, that can be a huge underlying cause of sleep issues! I suggest investing in a non-toxic mattress without fire retardants, plastics, synthetic latex, or petrochemicals that can release VOCs (volatile organic chemicals) linked to a host of health problems from hormone imbalances, respiratory issues, allergies, to cancer. I own a Brentwood Homes Oceano- but other good brands include Avocado Green, Happsy, Tuft & Needle, Saatva, PlushBeds, Bear, DreamCloud, Loom & Leaf, and Zen Haven. You spend almost half of your day in your bed- so make sure you aren't breathing in detrimental chemicals while you're lying there!
- Use blackout curtains, which may help from early awakening, as well as a white noise device such as a box fan to help minimize external noise exposure. Nothing fancy is needed- a box fan will do!
- Avoid caffeine after 5 pm, or even earlier if you are a slow caffeine metabolizer or sensitive to caffeine. Caffeine can remain elevated in your blood for up to 8 hours, so reducing prior to bed is essential.
- Watch your liquids and aim to drink more water during the day vs night. If you find yourself waking to pee a lot, it may be that you are drinking too many liquids in the evenings. Try getting at least ¾ gallon in by 4 pm. If you then still struggle with peeing a lot during the night, it may be a sign that something else is wrong, such as adrenal imbalance or mold toxicity.

- Monitor your medication timing. Some medications may keep you wired or increase the amounts of adrenaline produced in your body. Others may make you sleepy! Medications that inhibit sleep include T3 or a desiccated thyroid hormone, SSRIs, corticosteroids, diuretics, Excedrin, Sudafed, and beta blockers. Make sure to speak with your clinician about how and when to take your medications.
- Try stress reduction activities such as stretching, yoga, journaling, prayer, deep breathing, or meditation before bed. You want to stimulate your parasympathetic nervous system. If you like apps, try the Calm app or Headspace app- but be careful of the blue light and use your blue light blockers. You could also try listening to a lullaby or soothing binaural beats.
- Make sure you aren't under-eating, which can cause difficulty sleeping and insomnia. This is why many people may struggle with sleep when dieting!
- Fix your mindset! If you are stressed and have to do's or things on your mind, it's highly likely your sleep will take a hit. Do a brain dump. Write all your anxious thoughts down on paper. Let them go. Spill your secrets on paper and soothe your soul.
- Try to eat a complex carb-based snack with adequate protein (15-30 g) and/or a high quality fat source (8-10 g) to help with boosting serotonin levels in your brain and balancing your blood sugar prior to bed. Blood sugar crashes during sleep can cause early cortisol spikes causing mid-sleep awakening or early rising. My favorite pre-bed snack is oatmeal with a scoop of protein powder and 1 tbsp of almond butter or some protein pancakes.
- If you still struggle with sleep after making the above changes or recommendations, think about doing a sleep study to assess for sleep apnea, which is caused by inconsistent breathing that can cause insomnia. This condition is more common in men, but women may still

struggle. Sleep apnea can be aided by the use of a CPAP (continuous positive airway pressure) machine.

Sleep Aid Supplements: Supplements can help you either fall or stay asleep by relaxing you or promoting a health REM cycle. Always strive to start with diet and lifestyle changes first- then grab you a natural sleep aid! I suggest starting with one to two supplements at a time, giving yourself at least one week to notice an effect. Remember, supplements only work if health, nutrition, environment, lifestyle, and mental health are addressed.

- Melatonin: Melatonin is a hormone naturally produced by your body that helps in increased relaxation. Start low around 0.3 mg and increase up to 10 g. Keep in mind that melatonin needs are person-by-person specific. If you wake up feeling groggy and worse (I call it the "hit by a train" effect), you took too much. My sweet spot is 3-5 g, however someone else's may be much lower or even higher! Melatonin also has potential roles in helping to increase insulin sensitivity, and can be extremely helpful to negate circadian rhythm dysregulation from night shift work or overseas jet lag from time zone differences. Want some natural melatonin? Consume some dark cherries or sip on some tart cherry juice!
- Ashwagandha: a popular (and my favorite) adaptogen, this herb helps your body "adapt" to stressors. Look for a full-spectrum, standardized root and leaf extract and go for organic. Take 600-1200mg every night. Good news – it also helps nourish your thyroid metabolism and reduces stress!
- Valerian: this ancient herb is referred to as "nature's vallium", and can both promote sleep and reduce anxiety. It acts by helping to regulate gamma-aminobutyric acid (GABA) levels, resulting in feelings of tranquility and

reduced anxiety. Take 300-600mg up to 2 hours before bed. Valerian is sedating, so I don't suggest taking during the day.

- Magnesium: this mineral can improve sleep quality and duration by activating the parasympathetic nervous system. It also can help to fight inflammation, aid symptoms of PMS, relieve constipation, and lower blood pressure. There are many forms of magnesium that each have their own therapeutic roles. Magnesium glycinate is my favorite. Be cautious with magnesium citrate and oxide, which both can be used as laxatives. Try 300-400mg about an hour before bed.

- CBD: cannabinoids are natural compounds found in marijuana and hemp plants that attach and bind to receptors within your central nervous system. They have powerful anti-inflammatory effects and are used by many to promote relaxation, aid in sleep, decrease pain levels, as well as fight inflammation. They are a variety of cannabinoids that have varied effects within the body. The two main cannabinoids are CBD and THC. THC is the cannabinoid most known for causing the "buzz" or "high". Some states do not allow for the sale of THC containing products.

Many companies sell CBD oils, edibles, or vapes with low concentrations (legally must be less than 0.3%) of THC. Companies also sell THC free products. CBD can be extracted from either the cannabis or hemp plant, which will vary its total cannabinoids and THC content based on species and plant extraction methods. Therefore, it's best to do your research to find the product that you want based on the benefits you are searching for. Companies have developed extracted CBD oils that contain specific CBD isolates, CBD compounds, and may or may not contain THC. While taking CBD oil alone won't get you high, it may promote relaxation, fight inflammation, reduce cortisol, and aid in digestion support. Make sure that you're buying a full-spectrum extract from a third-party tested brand. I suggest taking 50-80mg about an hour before bed for best sleep support.

- Chamomile: this flower extract has been used since the time of Hippocrates for helping with insomnia, anxiety, fevers, and digestive upset. It's packed with phenolic compounds, including apigenin, which give its many therapeutic qualities. Sip a mug of chamomile tea before bed or take 200-270mg of extract before bed to get some relaxation.
- L-theanine: this amino acid is found naturally in tea leaves and promotes relaxation without causing drowsiness. Though it may sedate you, it can aid in relaxation and stress reduction, helping you to unwind and fall asleep more easily. L-theanine helps by elevating relaxing neurotransmitters in the brain, including GABA and serotonin levels. It can also serve as a focus and memory aid, and pairs quite well with a cup of coffee for studying and cognitive enhancement. L-theanine gives you the beauty of both worlds with its ability to aid in daytime focus and nighttime relaxation. For best sleep, try taking 100-200mg 1 hour before bed.
- GABA: this naturally occurring amino acid and inhibitory neurotransmitter (gamma aminobutyric acid) functions as a chemical messenger in your brain to help produce a feeling of calmness. It's commonly used for stress reduction, sleep, and anxiety. A combination of GABA and l-theanine can help to reduce the time it takes to fall asleep, while increasing sleep duration. Some argue that GABA in supplemental form can not cross the blood-brain barrier to be used, however studies show that supplementation may still help by promoting relaxation and reducing anxiety. I suggest starting at a low dose of

100mg before bed in a combination formula with l-theanine and/or melatonin.

- 5-HTP: 5-hydroxytryptophan is another amino acid naturally occurring in your body that serve as a precursor to serotonin. Low levels of serotonin are associated with anxiety and depression, and therefore serotonin has been coined the "happy" neurotransmitter. Supplementation may help restore serotonin levels, reducing feelings of depression, anxiety, and normalizing sleep patterns. Try taking 100-300mg before bedtime, however if prescribed an SSRI or medication, you must be cleared by a doctor to supplement. Too much serotonin can be lethal, leading to serotonin syndrome.
- Glycine: this non-essential amino acid can help improve sleep quality and reduce the time it takes to fall asleep. It also has been shown to reduce feelings of fatigue and sleepiness after a night of sleep restriction. Try taking 3g one hour before bedtime on nights you know you may get less sleep than normal.
- Lemon balm: this herb (known also as Melissa officinalis) can help to relieve stress, aid in relaxation, and reduce restless sleep. Lemon balm can be taken in tea form, or a concentrated extract. It also has free radical scavenging effects due to its concentration of antioxidants! Take caution if you have hypothyroidism. This herb may helpful in reducing symptoms associated with hyperthyroidism and may mildly reduce thyroid levels by blocking hormone receptors and preventing antibody attachment to the thyroid. Take caution or avoid if you have hypothyroidism.
- Reishi: this medicinal mushroom and adaptogen can help to boost your immune system, reduce stress, and enhance sleep quality. It can be taken in liquid, capsule, or powder form. With taking reishi or any adaptogenic mushroom, ensure to look for a high quality extract or powder that contains both the mycelium (roots) and fruiting body

(mushroom itself). The mycelium and mushroom are not the same and have different concentrations of healthful compounds. Low quality mushroom products can contain high amounts of carbohydrate fillers, as their growth and cultivation is done often on grain, and will be labeled as "mycelium on grain". Be cautious of "full spectrum" products as well, which just indicate presence of the entire plant. To get your bang for your buck and benefits, look for an organic mushroom extract with guaranteed concentration of beta-glucans. Shoot for 750-1500mg before bed.

My last and final tip: don't stress about it. Do what you can to promote better sleep, but don't fixate on logging a set amount of hours for the rest of your life. Allow yourself to enjoy late nights on special occasions, and just go to sleep a little earlier the next night. Sleep enough to optimize your health and happiness.

10

THE GUT GUIDE

Have you ever heard the saying "you are what you eat"? Well actually, you are only what your body is able to digest and absorb. Poor digestion can be an issue for many people, especially those with irritable bowel syndrome (IBS), inflammatory bowel disease (IBD), gastroesophageal reflux disease (GERD), gallbladder problems, and intestinal overgrowths or infections. However, they can also be symptoms and underlying causes of autoimmune diseases, skin disorders, migraines, hormonal imbalances, hypothyroidism, and nutrient deficiencies.

Your gut controls key functions of your health, including the production and conversion of hormones, neurotransmitters, and micronutrients (yes, you produce micronutrients in your gut too!). Your gut is also your most important immune system barrier, as 80% of your immune system resides in your gut.

When you optimize your digestion, your body is able to take the foods that you eat and utilize them to keep your body thriving. If there is any disorder, nutrient or digestive enzyme deficiency, overgrowth, infection, parasite, malabsorption, intestinal permeability, or intestinal adhesion, then your body can't thrive. Instead, it's thrown into a downward spiral that can lead to full-blown health problems.

Here are some signs that your gut is out of whack:

- Abdominal pain
- Bloating
- Reflux
- Diarrhea/loose stool
- Steatorrhea (fat in stool)
- Constipation
- Weight loss
- Muscle wasting
- Micronutrient deficiencies
- Hair loss
- Dry, brittle hair
- Dry, flaky skin
- Brittle nails
- Fluid retention
- Anemia
- Acne

We're going to take a deep dive into digestion by first talking about the entire digestive process, and then we will go over what can go wrong!

Your digestive system is pretty amazing and complex. Did you know that digestion begins before food even enters your mouth? Just thinking about food, smelling food, or seeing food can activate your digestive system. In the mouth, your food is chewed and mixed with saliva. It then passes into your stomach via the esophagus, where your protein digestion (and only protein digestion) takes place.

After food has been broken down in your stomach, it moves into your small intestine. This is where most of the digestive magic happens. Your small intestine is lined with a highly absorptive surface area covered in microvilli. These microvilli help to increase absorption by increasing the surface area of your gut lining. Think of them like a super absorbent paper towel. They soak up the good stuff! (And the bad stuff if you have intestinal permeability, but more on that later).

Completed digestion and absorption of your carbohydrates, proteins, and fats occur here in the three main parts of your small intestine: the duodenum, the jejunum, and the ileum. After digestion in the small intestine, undigested food, waste, and water pass through your large intestine before being excreted. Your large intestine then reabsorbs water, electrolytes, and produces nutrients such as Vitamin K and short-chain fatty acids, which are absorbed by your body prior to the last step of your digestion defecation (aka pooping)!

See the diagram below to see where each macro and micronutrient is absorbed.

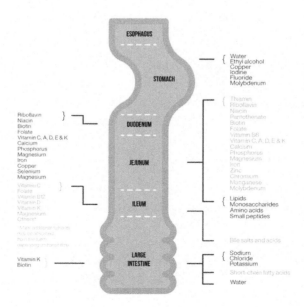

Digestion Mechanics

There are three types of digestion: mechanical, chemical, and bacterial. Each of these processes occurs in different places and phases within the process of digestion. They intertwine together to maximize the digestion and absorption of the foods that you eat. Any issue with one type can leave you with gut-related disturbances, which can feed into health disturbances down the line!

Mechanical Digestion

Mechanical digestion begins in your mouth when your teeth help to break down the foods that you eat. This is such an underrated and forgotten part of the digestion process, and many people (me included) sometimes forget to optimize the first and one of the most helpful parts of digestion! Chewing your food sets the stage for what is to follow. The process of chewing sends signals to your stomach to start producing gastric juices. Basically, it says, "Get ready! Food's coming!"

If you are "inhaling" your food and not taking time to properly chew it, your stomach isn't getting that time to prepare. Your salivary amylase is also not produced to the same extent, which can impact the beginning of your carbohydrate digestion. By chewing your food thoroughly (about 20-30 times per bite), you are helping all later digestion phases to work more efficiently.

There are many additional benefits to eating more slowly and mindfully! Eating too quickly can lead to the swallowing of air (known as aerophagia), which can cause unnecessary bloating and gas. In addition, eating slowly allows you to better recognize your satiety and hunger cues. This allows you to better sense your hunger levels both during and after your meal, as well as allows you to be present, fully enjoying and tasting the foods that you eat! I am going to age myself here and remind you of the Spongebob episode where Patrick eats his (and Spongebob's) chocolate bars so quickly that he forgets he even ate them. Can't relate to that?

What about when you are consuming popcorn or chips watching a movie and you go for another one and hit the sad bottom of the container or bag? Yeah- the worst. Eating slowly, chewing properly, and paying attention to your food while you eat helps you to properly digest and enjoy it!

Mechanical digestion also occurs with muscular contractions, which include peristalsis, segmentation movements, and tonic contractions that help to move food throughout your digestive tract.

Your gut motility can be affected by your migrating motor complex, or MMC for short. Your MMC occurs during fasting or periods between meals and serves as the "housekeeper" within your gut. It helps to "sweep" undigested food particles through your intestines, specifically the stomach and small intestine. Your MMC is halted with the ingestion of food as well as reduced by high stress.

Why is the MMC important? Without your housekeeper, the undigested food particles in your gut can leave you feeling heavy, sluggish, and too full after eating. Your slowed MMC also increases the time that undigested particles and any bacteria, toxin, or yeast stay in your gut. If they stay for too long, this can cause over-fermentation (cue gas and bloating), and down the line lead to bacterial or fungal overgrowths. Your MMC can also cause alterations with the reabsorption of estrogen in your gut, contributing to hormonal imbalances.

There are many things that can affect your motility and MMC, including caffeine, alcohol, stress, food intolerances, meal frequency, and thyroid hormones. Your parasympathetic nervous system also plays the role of the most important roles in gut motility. There is a reason why it's called "rest and digest." Being in a parasympathetic state allows for the release of your digestive enzymes and sweeps of your MMC. When you are in a sympathetic state (aka fight-or-flight mode), your body turns to focus energy away from digestion and instead focuses on the stressor it's thrown. Remember- any stressor is stress to your body. For all it knows, there is a tiger coming its way!

What can help increase parasympathetic activity?

- Yoga, meditation, or mindful breathing
- Singing/chatting loudly (I call it "Beyonce-ing")
- Humming
- Listening to relaxing music
- Gargling vigorously
- Acupuncture

Chemical Digestion

There are many hormones, chemicals, and enzymes secreted in your body that help you to properly break down your food. In your mouth, saliva contains lingual lipase and salivary amylase, which begin the breakdown of some carbohydrates and fats. In your stomach, HCl (stomach acid or hydrochloric acid) stimulates protein digestion. With the low pH of your HCl and the use of chyme, chemical digestion in your stomach helps to kill pathogens, bacteria, and break down your proteins.

In your small intestine, both bile and pancreatic enzymes are released to digest your carbohydrates, fats, and the rest of your proteins. It's here that most of your food is both digested and absorbed. Here, pancreatic enzymes further break down your proteins into amino acids, and complete the breakdown of carbo-hydrates and fats in your diet through pancreatic proteases, amylases, and lipases.

Bile, one of your BFFs for digestion and hormonal health, is made by the liver and stored in your gallbladder. There are three impor-tant functions of bile:

1. Bile acids are critical for the digestion of fats and fat-

soluble vitamins (vitamins A, D, E, K) in the small
   intestine.
2. It is a critical part of detoxification. Waste products are
   bound and excreted from the body via bile.
3. Bile acids contribute to the majority of cholesterol
   breakdown in the body and help control cholesterol
   homeostasis.

Bacterial Digestion

The trillions of microbes that reside in your gut play a huge role
in your immunity, hormonal health, and digestion. Your large
intestine hosts a beautiful ecosystem or "microbiome" that help to
ward off pathogens and synthesize micronutrients such as vitamin
K and B-vitamins. These microbes also help to convert consumed
fiber into short-chain fatty acids, which are then used for the regulation of your metabolism and the maintenance of your gut lining.
The relationship between your digestive system and "gut ecosystem" is mostly symbiotic, meaning that both you and the bacteria
benefit from each other. However, if there is an overgrowth of a
certain species, pathogen, or poor gut immunity (as in the case of
heightened intestinal permeability), this is when a gut rebellion
can occur.

A Healthy Microbiome = A Healthy Gut

Your gut microbiome is as unique as your fingerprint! The truth is
- we don't even know what a "healthy microbiome" truly looks like
yet. We also don't fully know how each bacteria strain can affect
our body's metabolism, mood, disease risk, nervous system,
immune system, etc. We don't even know all the microbes that
reside in our gut! Trying to understand our gut microbiome is like
trying to understand all the stars and planets in our galaxy. New
studies are being conducted every day, so stay tuned.

Have we learned a lot? Yes, we have established many correlations, some causations. But- there is so much that we don't know yet. I am not a gut health expert and won't claim to be. However, I will do my best in this chapter to explain what can influence your gut, how to support a healthy gut, and what to do when things go wrong.

What Influences a "Healthy Microbiome"?

Many factors influence the health of your microbiome, including:

- Exercise and sleep habits
- Diversity of plants in the diet- including fiber and prebiotics
- Amount of digestive enzyme secretion (including stomach acid, pancreatic juices, and bile)
- Environmental toxins and pollutants (including mold, endocrine disruptors, and heavy metals)
- Geographic location
- Stress levels (which can damage the gut lining and heighten your risk of infection and intestinal permeability)
- Antibiotic usage
- Artificial sweeteners and food additives
- Intake of fermented foods and probiotics
- Diet quality- mostly plant based vs animal based and highly processed vs whole food based
- Birth and infancy- the way you were born (natural vs C-section), bottle-fed vs breastfed, how your mom ate during pregnancy and her environmental exposures

As you can see, your gut can get help or take a hit without any specific intentional change made by you! You aren't fully in control of what happens to your microbiome. Especially if you get hit with food poisoning or develop poor digestion from a thyroid or hormonal disorder.

. . .

The Common Culprit- IBS

IBS, or "irritable bowel syndrome" is one of the most common diagnosed gut disorders in both men and women. Sadly, IBS has become an umbrella diagnosis for "Hmm... we aren't sure."

What can cause IBS?

- Gut infections, overgrowths, or dysbiosis
- Food intolerances
- Stress
- Liver dysfunction
- Inflammation
- Low digestion enzymes or stomach acid
- Hypothyroidism
- Heavy Metals
- Intestinal permeability (or "leaky gut")

Conquering irritable bowel syndrome is all about figuring out and uprooting the root cause. IBS symptoms vary from person to person, however diagnosis is made based on the Rome III Criteria – which includes having two of the following symptoms for at least three months:

- Improvement with defecation (pooping)
- Onset associated with change in frequency of stool
- Onset associated with change in form/appearance of stool

Pretty generic, right? That's why IBS is one of the most commonly diagnosed digestive disorders. Many doctors will slap "IBS" on you if you have these symptoms and then proceed to give you a laxative or Metamucil. No bueno! IBS affects your digestive system causing irregular bowel contractions, risk of nutrient deficiencies, and chronic pain to the point where some people can't even live their daily lives. Have you been diagnosed with "IBS"? It's time to figure out what the root cause is.

Gut Rebellion- How to Fix Your Gut

Is your gut crying for help? Do not just slap a band-aid on it! Your gut can be complicated. Healing your gut can be complicated too. The 4R approach may address and correct the underlying causes to your digestion issues! Keep in mind, thyroid and hormonal imbalances can actually stem from the gut, without gut-specific symptoms being present. Just because you think you have a healthy gut doesn't mean that you do. You don't know what you don't know.

My "Heal Your Gut Starter Pack"- 4R Approach:

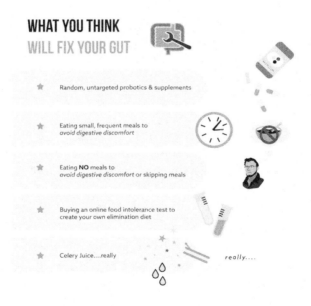

Please work with a professional to do this. Don't blindly drive your "car." You could crash it.

Step 1- Remove:

Identify and eliminate factors that may be contributing to your symptoms, including allergens, intolerances, infections, over-growths, and parasites. The removal agents that you use will depend on your situation and needs. For example:

- Anti-fungals (such as caprylic acid) may help eradicate yeast overgrowths such as Candida
- Anti-parasitics (such as black walnut, goldenseal, wormwood, and oil of oregano) may help to clear out parasites
- Anti-microbials (such as allium from garlic, berberine-containing herbs, neem, and oil of oregano) may help to diminish SIBO and aid in dysbiosis – may be used in single products or combination products
- Products such as activated charcoal and modified citrus pectin may be helpful in removed mold or heavy metals

Step 2- Replace

Replacement includes HCl, pancreatic enzymes, and bile acids based on your specific needs. Be careful, more is not better. Too much HCl can cause stomach burning and lead to ulcerations if H pylori is present. The replace phase also includes replacing and ensuring adequate sleep, stress reduction, and switching from a low quality, processed food diet to a whole food based diet.

Step 3- Reinoculate

Repopulate your microbiome with good bacteria by taking a targeted probiotic supplement and eating fermented foods. You can also repopulate your gut by consuming prebiotics that will serve as additional fertilizer for your gut bugs.

My favorite reinoculation products include:

- PHGG (partially hydrolyzed guar gum) or "Sun Fiber"- acts as a prebiotic to stimulate the growth of healthy gut bacteria. It is slow to ferment, reducing the risk of gas and bloating that other prebiotic fibers can cause, and may help to reduce symptoms of both diarrhea and constipation dominant IBS
- S. Boulardii probiotic- this is a yeast-based probiotic that can help to reduce inflammation, eradicate infections, and aid in healing a weak intestinal lining
- Megaspore- this product is spore-based, broad spectrum probiotic, meaning that it was formulated to survive through the digestion tract to ensure short-term colonization within the GI tract. Megaspore may help to increase microbial diversity, reduce metabolic endotoxemia (aka "leaky gut"), strengthen the immune system, and reduce symptoms associated with "IBS"

Step 4- Repair

Help seal the gut lining through diet, lifestyle, and supplementation. You should always be repairing in every one of these steps. A quick note- repairing can't truly happen if an infection is present, or if mold and heavy metals continue to circulate their toxicities throughout your body. You have to find the root source to prevent your health issue from coming back and flourishing.

My favorite products for repairing the gut include:

- Glutamine: serves as a fuel source for your intestinal cells, helps in the maintenance of your intestinal lining, and stimulates gut mucosal cell proliferation
- Zinc carnosine: may help aid in the repair of the gut lining and reducing inflammation

- Bovine colostrum/immunoglobulins: colostrum comes from the first milk produced after an animal gives birth- reduces inflammation and stimulates the immune system
- Deglycyrrhized licorice: helps to soothe the gut lining, lower inflammation, and promote healing of the mucosal lining
- Saccharomyces boulardii: a beneficial yeast probiotic that can help to preserve and restore gut barrier infection, increase secretory IGA levels, and combat conditions such as H pylori, SIBO, and food poisoning
- Full spectrum CBD oil: lowers inflammation and pain levels- may enhance the healing of the gut lining

During these four phases, remember that diversity of plants in your diet is one of the biggest contributors to a healthy gut. Fiber is your friend! Prebiotics and fiber ferment to produce SCFAs (short-chain fatty acids) that serve as fuel sources to help maintain your gut lining health, reduce inflammation, combat pathogens, lower cholesterol levels, as well as influence your immune, cardio-vascular, and nervous system. They also help to enhance the diversity of your gut microbiome, which is what you want in order to have a healthy, not rebellious, gut.

The quality of your diet also plays a significant role in the diversity and balance of your gut microbiome. Western diets high in refined grains, saturated fats, and processed vegetable oils not only lower bacterial diversity in the gut, but increase gut inflammation. On the other hand, plant-based diets appear to increase diversity and richness of your gut microbiota, with an anti-inflammatory and gut-protective effect.

What does this mean for you? Plant-based eating doesn't mean eat only plants and go vegan or vegetarian. It just means eat more plants! Try to consume at least three cups of plant-based foods per day, hit your fiber goals, and focus on the quality of your overall diet.

. . .

What Is a Probiotic?

Probiotics can be defined as "live microorganisms which, when administered in adequate amounts, confer a health benefit to the host." Probiotics can be incorporated into supplements through capsules, powders, and tablets, as well as added into food, such as yogurts, milks, and even breakfast cereals.

Though normally thought of as a naturally occurring probiotic, fermented foods including kefir, sauerkraut, and yogurt are actually not considered probiotics themselves. Instead, they are considered to contain "live and active cultures." This is because foods contain an undefined bacterial strain content, strain composition, and quantity, and in turn, therapeutic effects cannot be well controlled.

How Can Probiotics Benefit You and Your Microbiome?

Within a species of bacteria there are numerous amounts of strains. Each strain has its own mechanism of action, as well as condition-specific benefits. Though there may be similarity between strains of the same species, that does not mean that they will produce the same benefits to a host. Some strains help to fight off pathogenic bacteria and interact with the immune system, while others are unable to even survive as they travel through your digestive tract. This is imperative to understand. If you choose to use or consume a probiotic, you do not want to be wasting your money on a strain that won't even get to work in your gut!

To give you an example, when looking at a probiotic label- you may see names such as Lactobacillus rhamnosus. That tells you the probiotic species, but what is the strain? As the strain Lactobacillus rhamnosus GG (found within Culturelle), has been studied and clinically proven to help prevent antibiotic-associated diarrhea and aid in the eradication of H. pylori. However, all L. rhamnosus strains won't do this. This is confusing to even medical providers, as companies are very good with their tricky wordy and marketing! I suggest using the "US Probiotic Guide" found at www.usprobioticguide.com as a tool for yourself when assessing probiotic needs, or entrusting your healthcare provider to make the best informed decision based on your needs.

Though many people will say that probiotics help to "colonize" the gut (and they do!), however, this is a short-term modification. Probiotics do not, as of now in the literature, cause permanent colonization and changes to your gut microbiome. They are place-holders with short-term effects. Think of them like a fertilizer. They can sprinkle in benefits, but those benefits don't stay there long term. As of now, only diet changes or fecal stool transplants have been found to permanently change your gut microbiome.

Just because the effect is short term does not mean it's not benefi-cial! There are many benefits to using probiotics (and specific strains) to help in certain diseases and conditions. Make sure to not slap a probiotic on yourself without knowing what it is and how it can help. Probiotics aren't always beneficial. Sometimes in a state of dysbiosis or overgrowth, using one can be like throwing fire fluid on a fire (especially in the case of SIBO!).

Common Clinically Proven Probiotic Benefits of Single and Multi-Strain Products:

- A- Saccharomyces boulardii CNCM I-745 (found within Florastor) can help prevent antibiotic associated diarrhea, help to eradicate H. pylori, fight off Clostridium difficile-associated diarrhea, prevent traveler's diarrhea, and even aid in the management of ulcerative colitis (a form of IBD).
- B- Lactobacillus rhamnosus GG can help prevent antibiotic associated diarrhea and aid in the eradication of H. pylori.
- C-Visbiome (a combination of Lactobacillus, Bifidobacterium, and Streptococcus strains) has been

used in the treatment and maintenance of ulcerative colitis, IBS, and antibiotic-associated diarrhea.

- D- Fem-dophilus (a combination of two Lactobacillus strains- L. reuteri RC-14 and L. rhamnosus GR-1) – may help to prevent recurrent UTIs and support a healthy vaginal flora.

Dysbiosis and Overgrowths

The presence of dysbiosis or an overgrowth of bacteria in your gut can spell a recipe for disaster to your thyroid, hormones, metabolism, and your overall health. Not only can digestive symptoms occur, but so can nutrient deficiencies, autoimmune attack, low immunity, hormonal imbalances, and poor thyroid conversion.

What does "dysbiosis" mean? How does it develop to cause harm?

You actually have billions of bacteria in your body. These bacteria, when in balance, make up what is called your microbiome. They live together in a state of symbiosis, aka they are close neighbors that help each other out and help to protect you against infections, influence the production of your neurotransmitters, make vitamins, and influence your hormones and metabolism.

When food particles such as undigested carbohydrates or protein can't be absorbed into your bloodstream, this causes them to be over-fermented by the bacteria in your intestines, leading to symptoms of gas, bloating, and for some, constipation or diarrhea. In the short term, undigested food particles won't cause an issue. However, with chronic undigested food, plus slowed gut motility and heightened intestinal permeability, this is where gut damage and health chaos occur.

Contributors to Dysbiosis include:

Dietary factors (low fiber, high processed foods, high intake of artificial sweeteners, added sugars/sugary foods, food additives or preservatives)

- Environmental toxins (mold, heavy metals, etc)
- Impaired digestion
- Nutrient deficiencies
- Medications such as birth control, proton pump inhibitors (PPIs), antibiotics, NSAIDs
- Diabetes
- Viral, bacterial, or parasitic infections
- Poor oral health
- Low stomach acid, pancreatic enzymes, or bile acids
- Intestinal adhesions
- Chronic stress (physical or emotional)
- Undereating
- Food poisoning
- Ileocecal valve malfunction (lies between your colon and small intestine)

Without proper digestion and absorption, you can start to develop nutrition deficiencies that then further the vicious cycle of health issues. For example, you need B12 and zinc to make stomach acid. If you have low digestive enzyme output from hypothyroidism or an overgrowth like H. Pylori, this can decrease the digestion of protein and nutrients in the stomach. Not only will the protein then over-ferment in your gut, but you then don't absorb the B12 and zinc you need to make stomach acid, and can't use them to help optimize your thyroid and hormonal health either. See how it goes in circles?

There are 3 main patterns of dysbiosis:

1. Low Beneficial Bacteria: causes include chronic stress &

inflammation, chronic antibiotic use, undereating, low-fiber diet, poor digestion, chronic antimicrobials, environmental exposures

2. High Pathogenic Bacteria: causes include poor digestion, lack of enzymes, low stomach acid, chronic stress, heightened intestinal permeability, parasites, yeast overgrowth, slow motility, chronic inflammation, food poisoning , poor oral health

3. Loss of Overall Microbial Diversity: causes include chronic stress & inflammation, chronic antibiotic use, undereating, low-fiber diet, poor digestion, chronic antimicrobials, medications, environmental exposures

The Main Overgrowths that I see in my clients are:

SIBO

SIBO- aka Small Intestinal Bacterial Overgrowth, is a condition caused by the overgrowth of bacteria in your intestines. Though labeled with "Small Intestinal," SIBO can also occur in your large intestine! Methane Dominant SIBO actually was renamed to be "Intestinal Methanogen Overgrowth" or IMO to account for this. The three main types of SIBO include on overgrowth of either (or a combination) of hydrogen, methane, and sulfur producing bacteria. It is estimated that approximately 60% of IBS sufferers have SIBO.

Symptoms of a small and/or large intestine overgrowth include: chronic bloating (especially present upon waking without having eaten food), belching, reflux, brain fog, chronic fatigue, chronic diarrhea and/or constipation, acne, eczema, hair loss, depression, joint pain, weight loss (or weight gain), hormonal imbalances, iron or B12 deficiency, heartburn/reflux, and hypothyroidism.

. . .

Common comments I hear from clients with SIBO include:

- "I feel pregnant all day long!"
- "Sugar and carbohydrates seem to make things worse"
- "I just can't eat anything without symptoms"
- "I've tried probiotics- they make me feel worse"
- "I just can't seem to get rid of my acne"
- "I am tired, irritable, and anxious. Nothing seems to help"
- "I can't poop no matter what" or "I have diarrhea despite any change in my diet"

In order to get rid of SIBO, you have to get rid of, or address, the cause of it. SIBO, though an accurate diagnosis, is really just a symptom and manifestation of a larger problem in your body causing the overgrowth to happen. There is a reason that the bacteria become overgrown, and in order to cure SIBO, you have to find and address the root cause.

Causes of SIBO include:

- Medications (ex. birth control, proton pump inhibitors, antibiotics)
- Low stomach acid
- Pancreatic enzyme deficiencies or bile acid deficiencies
- Mold toxicity
- Ileocecal valve malfunction
- Immunosuppression
- Traumatic brain injury
- Poor MMC- Migrating Motor Complex
- Chronic stress
- Chronic undereating or eating disorders
- Abdominal surgery
- Intestinal adhesions
- Slowed motility (ex. Gastroparesis)
- Nerve dysfunction

- Food poisoning
- Co-infections (H pylori, Candida)

There are three Main Types of SIBO that each have their own symptoms and treatments. More than one can be present at a time, and commonly, treating one can reveal another:

- Hydrogen-dominant: mostly produces chronic diarrhea
- Hydrogen Sulfide-dominant: mostly produces a mix of diarrhea and constipation with a "rotten egg" smelly gas
- Methane-dominant: mostly produces chronic constipation (though commonly causes both constipation and diarrhea)

SIBO could be the cause of your digestive distress, thyroid/hormonal imbalances, and IBS. Bacteria are an essential part of a healthy gut, but if you have too many of the "bad guys," this can contribute to overgrowths like SIBO and ultimately to "leaky gut" (aka intestinal permeability). Intestinal permeability can then reduce your ability to heal your SIBO, which becomes a vicious, demonic cycle.

How to test for SIBO? This is where it gets tough. Current gold standards for testing SIBO include a hydrogen and/or methane breath test using lactulose and/or and glucose as a substrate. This testing is based on the principle that the substrate produces hydrogen and methane gas from bacterial fermentation in the gut, that is then carried to your lungs and expired out through your mouth. The measurement of the gas produced after substrate ingestion is then compared to healthy controls to look for overfermentation and too much gas production. You can also see potential signs of SIBO on a stool test, such as a GI Map Test (though not yet clinically validated). The catch is that there is no perfect test, which makes it tricky. They all have their flaws and false negatives.

For example, you can get tested with a methane/hydrogen breath test and have a "negative" result—but that doesn't mean you don't have SIBO. It just means you may not have hydrogen or methane-dominant SIBO. It could be hydrogen sulfide SIBO, which currently has no validated test for diagnosis, or to make it even more confusing- the methane-dominant bacteria in your gut could actually be suppressed by the overgrowth of hydrogen-producing bacteria (as methane bacteria can feed off the hydrogen). Meaning, you could have an overgrowth of both! Complex, I know. SIBO testing also can be impacted by oral microbiome health (which can elevated starting gas production numbers) and is greatly impacted by the SIBO test prep diet. Testing should be performed & evaluated with caution to account for these issues. In working with my clients, I use testing as one tool in my toolbox for treatment, not as the sole bible for it.

Treatment in general for SIBO consists of either antibiotics or antimicrobial herbs, gut immune support, and diet modification. You need to get rid of the overgrowth, but also address why it occurred in the first place. A common mistake I see in treatment is people attempting to "starve" their SIBO. This isn't helpful. You need your gut bugs active to kill them off! Your SIBO will lie dormant if you don't feed them. Another mistake I see is using killing agents without addressing the root cause. Did the SIBO develop from low enzyme output, intestinal adhesions, poor gut motility, medications, traumatic brain injury, abdominal surgery, chronic stress, undereating or over-exercising, intestinal permeability, poor MMC activity, chronic antibiotic use, food poisoning, mold toxicity, or a heavy metal toxicity?

You have to address the why to address the what. Make sure to work with a professional to get rid of any overgrowth! My favorite antimicrobials for SIBO include compound formulas such as Metagenics Candibactin AR and BR, Biocidin with Olivirex, Biotics FC cidal with Dysbiocide, or a use of 2-3 herbs high dose of berberine containing herbs, oil of oregano, allicin (an extract of garlic), or neem. Herbals or antibiotics, diet, digestive support, and lifestyle therapies should all be used when healing SIBO.

The Top 8 Mistakes I see when people attempt to treat SIBO include:

- Not testing correctly or relying on testing as the sole treatment guide. A specific diet must be followed to properly test for SIBO. Not following test protocols beforehand can skew results.
- Only attempting to remove the SIBO without also focusing on repairing the gut lining and intestinal permeability. You can't eradicate an infection if your immune system in your gut is not optimal.
- Trying to "starve the SIBO" and in turn starving themselves and inhibiting its removal.
- Making SIBO your identity and letting it become a stressor and trauma that then prevents you from healing.
- Ignoring lifestyle factors that contribute to healing such as sleep, stress levels, exercise, and your environment. Yoga, meditation, hypnotherapy, acupuncture, abdominal massage, and cognitive-behavioral therapy can be extremely helpful for many cases.
- Not ensuring proper MMC activity and forgetting a prokinetic (if necessary)- may favorites include Motility Activator or Motil Pro.
- Not testing for additional disorders or causes to SIBO- including mold toxicity, heavy metals, or hypothyroidism
- Trying to treat SIBO alone without professional guidance.

Candida

Candida, aka Candida albicans, is an opportunist yeast that is naturally present in your intestines. However, when it becomes overgrown, it can compromise your immune system, deplete your good bacteria, and increase your risk of nutrient deficiencies.

Symptoms of Candida include:

- Skin, hair, or nail fungal infection
- Brain fog or poor mental clarity
- White tongue
- "Drunk" or tipsy feeling without drinking alcohol
- Digestive distress such as gas, bloating, or constipation/diarrhea
- Recurring UTIs or yeast infections
- Skin issues such as acne, rosacea, hives, or psoriasis
- Mood swings
- Worsening anxiety or depression
- Sugar or refined carbohydrate cravings
- Vaginal or rectal itching
- Chronic fatigue
- Sinus infections of worsening allergies

Candida can be caused ultimately by the same factors as intestinal permeability and SIBO, however I see it develop mostly in those that have been exposed to mold in their environment and/or have a diet high in refined, simple carbohydrates. It is also commonly see with its best friend, H pylori, as a co-infection.

The best tests for Candida include stool testing (such as the GI map by Diagnostic Solutions) and Candida blood antibodies via blood. To get rid of Candida, I suggest following the 4R Gut Repair approach using anti-fungals such as caprylic acid, garlic, grapefruit seed extract, undecylenic acid, or monolaurin. If you have or suspect Candida, a yeast-free diet low in added sugars is a must to eradicate it. "Candida diets" exist, but are not always necessary. Treatment also requires supporting the immune system and addressing the potential cause of infection.

. . .

General Supplement Recommendations for Clearing Candida:

- Anti fungal herbs: caprylic acid, garlic, grapefruit seed extract, undecylenic acid, or monolaurin
- Broad-spectrum antimicrobials: Biocidin, GI Microb-X, Candibactin AR and/or BR, oil of oregano, berberine containing herbs, olive leaf
- Digestive enzyme support: HCl, pancreatic enzymes, pancreatins, bile acids
- Saccharomyces boulardii probiotic
- Gut lining support- including bovine immunoglobulins, glycyrrhizinated licorice (DGL), marshmallow root, zinc carnosine, glutamine, bone broth, aloe vera, slippery elm, methylsulfonylmethane (MSM), citrus pectin
- Biofilm disrupters such as Interphase plus or n-acetyl-cysteine
- Binders for die off: activated charcoal, modified citrus pectin, humic or fulvic acids

What to avoid with Candida: fermented foods, cultured dairy, lactic acid, B-vitamins made from yeast, buttermilk, soy sauce or miso, MSG (made from fermentation), vinegar (unless apple cider), yeast extracts, preserved or aged meats, and alcohol. Coffee may also need to be avoided unless low mold.

H Pylori

H pylori is another the normal bacterial inhabitant that when overgrown, causes total health chaos!

Symptoms include:

- Burping/belching
- Difficulty digesting protein
- Bad breathe

- Heartburn or reflux
- Upper abdominal pain (esp right after meals)
- Acne
- Bloating & gas
- Constipation
- Headaches
- Nausea
- Undigested food in the stool

H pylori overgrowth can lead to:

- SIBO
- Candida
- Anemia
- Nutrient deficiencies
- Hormonal imbalances
- Hypothyroidism
- Stomach ulcers, gastritis, or gastric cancer
- Intestinal permeability

Why does a normal inhabitant overgrow? Typically, this occurs due to low stomach acid (hypochlorhydria). Stomach acid is your first line of defense against pathogens, bacteria, & parasites. Your immune system needs an acidic environment to kill them off. Low stomach acid allows H. pylori to survive in the stomach, & with a depressed immune system, this can lead to an overgrowth of H pylori. H pylori then can prevent you from breaking down the foods that you eat and absorbing your nutrients, leading to potential additional overgrowths such as Candida and SIBO. I quite often see Candida and H pylori together when testing.

The best way to test for H pylori is through stool antigens (such as the GI map), a breathe test (which tends to have higher false negatives), and an endoscopy or biopsy.

Treatment for H pylori involves eradicating the infection with antibiotics or antimicrobials such as mastic gum., berberine, and oil of oregano. Saccharomyces boulardii is also a beneficial yeast probiotic that can help in eradication. If an H pylori infection is present, you will want to follow the recommendations in the Low Stomach Acid section, excluding the using of Betaine HCl, which can cause potential mucosal damage with an H pylori Overgrowth.

Intestinal Permeability or "Leaky Gut"

Intestinal Permeability, or "leaky gut" as it is commonly called, is not a specific disease, but an explanation of how well your gut barrier is intact. When you have increased intestinal permeability, the lining of your intestinal tract and intestinal wall tight junctions become loose, allowing for undigested food particles, toxins, and microbes to escape your gut and enter your bloodstream. Having increased intestinal permeability simply indicates that your gut lining and gut barrier are not fully intact.

Within your intestines lie cells called enterocytes. These enterocytes are held together by tight junctions, which serve as a border between food in your intestines and your bloodstream. Think of your gut lining like your front door. You want the good guys to come in and the bad guys to stay out! This is the same with your intestinal tract. Your enterocytes and tight junctions work to keep your door closed when needed.

Fact- 90% of your immune system resides in your gut. If those tight junctions are loose, your immune system becomes weaker and you become at an increased risk for contracting infections, overgrowths, parasites, and viruses. Your intestinal door is open to molecules, both good and bad, passing into your bloodstream. This "leaky gut" creates a heightened immune response, as undigested food, bacteria, fungi, and toxins have a free pass to your bloodstream. This can increase the creation of cytokines and antibodies, triggering both a local and systemic (full body) inflammatory response.

If there is SIBO or an infection present, bacteria can produce lipopolysaccharides (LPS), that can further increase intestinal permeability. This can further increase inflammation, and cause the development of food intolerances (or "pseudo food intolerances,"), food allergies, malabsorption, as well as trigger chronic conditions or autoimmune disease.

Symptoms and Diagnoses associated with heightened intestinal permeability include:

- Anxiety
- Depression
- Asthma
- Allergies
- Brain fog
- Chronic fatigue or pain
- Indigestion
- Diarrhea or constipation
- Bloating
- Reoccurring illness or infections
- Multiple chemical sensitivities
- Exercise intolerance
- Acne or skin rashes/eczema
- Arthritis
- Autoimmune disease (ex. Crohn's disease, Type 1 Diabetes, Hashimoto's, Lupus, multiple sclerosis, Sjogren's syndrome)
- Celiac disease
- Ulcerative colitis
- Gluten intolerance
- Irritable Bowel Syndrome

What causes "leaky gut" or increased intestinal permeability?

- Chronic inflammation (can be from undereating and over-exercising all the way to low or high cortisol)

- Infection or dysbiosis
- Medications (such as NSAIDs, hormonal birth control, steroids, and antibiotics)
- Food poisoning
- Impaired digestion (i.e., low stomach acid, pancreatic enzymes, bile acids)
- Nutrient deficiencies
- Infections or viruses
- Stress and trauma
- Alcohol
- Environmental toxins
- Poor diet with low fiber and prebiotic intake
- Food sensitivities such as gluten (which can weaken tight junctions in susceptible people)

Sadly testing has it flaws, however assessing secretory IGA levels, LPS levels, and zonulin levels may be helpful.

How do you heal a "leaky gut"? Just like SIBO, you have to address the root cause of why it developed in the first place. Focus on the 4R approach (with professional help) to address it with a large focus on stress reduction and diet quality. Prebiotic rich foods and polyphenols will help support a healthy gut lining and assist in combatting inflammation. Prebiotics will specifically help to create short-chain fatty acids that fuel the maintenance and repair of your intestinal lining. My favorite supplements for reducing intestinal permeability include bovine immunoglobulins, glutamine, butyrate, partially hydrolyzed guar gum, zinc carnosine, saccharomyces boulardii, aloe vera, and collagen.

Bloating

Let's be real, it sucks to be bloated. Beating your bloat is all about identifying why you are bloated in the first place! Sometimes it's a quick fix, such as ensuring to chew your food thoroughly and eating more slowly. Other times, your bloating may be a sign that your thyroid needs some love, you have low stomach acid, or even that you have SIBO (small intestinal bacterial overgrowth).

The Common Causes of Bloating:

- Sugar alcohols or artificial sweeteners
- Food additives and preservatives (especially thickeners like xanthan gum)
- Too much fiber or raw vegetables
- Eating too quickly
- Not chewing food properly
- Drinking too much liquid with meals
- Dehydration
- Low stomach acid
- Low pancreatic enzymes
- Food Intolerances
- Constipation
- Hormonal or thyroid disorder
- Gut infection or overgrowth
- Stress
- PMS
- Dysbiosis

Remember this- it's normal to have mild bloat from food and water after eating, especially if you had a higher volume meal. Big salads are going to be harder to digest as the plant cell walls are harder for your body to break down. Higher fat meals take a longer time to digest in your GI tract. If you consume a lot of gas-producing foods such as cruciferous vegetables and beans, or eat too much fiber, you are also welcoming a bloat. However, if you struggle with consistent, constant bloating that creates pain or takes away from your day-to-day life- it's time to address it. That isn't normal.

To get rid of bloating- try asking yourself these questions and follow my recommendations:

1. Do you eat quickly? Do you drink too much water or carbonation with meals? Do you chew thoroughly or gulp down food? Focus on mindful eating!

2. How are your sleep and stress levels? Stress and lack of sleep can reduce the output of digestive enzymes, leading to gas and bloating as well as increasing water retention in the body. If stress may be a factor- hone in on self care and stress reduction techniques! Don't like who you're eating with? Fun fact.. that may stress you out and cause troubles digesting!

3. What does your diet look like? Do you eat lots of raw veggies and salads? Too much or too little fiber (which both can cause issues!), possibly have reflux or heartburn indicating low stomach acid, chew a lot of gum (and then swallowing air), or maybe have a food sensitivity? (Could be gluten, wheat, dairy, soy, eggs, or simply a food additive like xanthan gum, artificial sweeteners, or sugar alcohols). Make a food journal and start writing down when your bloating is better or worse. If you notice a pattern or trend, it may be a specific food causing you issues. If you notice a trend in types of foods (such as a higher fat meal or higher protein meal), that's an indicator that a specific digestive enzyme may be low.

4. How's your menstrual cycle? Do you have any heavy PMS or irregular cycles? It may be a hormonal imbalance! Head to Chapters 4 and 5.

5. Do you also have joint pain, muscle aches, brain fog, constipation, trouble with weight loss? Could be your thyroid! Head to Chapter 8.

Constipation

If your poop life isn't happy and consistent- neither are your hormones or metabolism. Pooping is one of the most important steps of natural detoxification. Can't poop? You can't get out any toxins or excess estrogen either. Weekly bowel movements may look different for everyone, but I say you should be pooping daily optimally! I don't know about you but if I don't crap daily... I feel like crap!

Chronic constipation is not only extremely uncomfortable, but it can lead to estrogen dominance, gut dysbiosis, SIBO, and the development of pelvic floor disorders. It also may worsen thyroid disorders, burden your liver, and cause nutrient deficiencies.

How can you fix it?

Always look to fix the root cause. This should be redundant to you by now. In many cases, constipation can be relieved by:

1. Increasing water intake - dehydration causes constipation! Drink 1 gallon a day, minimum. Low electrolyte intake can also cause constipation. Try using Nuun tablets, Ultima replenisher powder, or adding Himalayan salt to your foods.
2. Increase your activity - movement helps increase peristalsis of the large intestine, helping with gut motility. Walking after meals can help with digestion. Get outside after meals and go on a 5-10-minute walk. Note- over-exercising will not be helpful as it blunts digestion via the stress and cortisol connection! We want parasympathetic dominance- aka rest and digest mode.
3. Try to increase your fiber intake - 25-40 g is a good range, however everyone has a different "fiber sweet spot." Remember the different types of fiber here. Insoluble fiber helps move your digestion along and increases stool bulk, while soluble fiber slows things down and draws water into your intestines. Psyllium husk and citrus pectin are two fiber supplements that may be helpful, however try increasing your overall food fiber first. Great first addition could be 2 tbs chia or flax seeds!
4. Stress less - If you are constantly in fight-or-flight mode,

your body doesn't want to digest. You need to do more parasympathetic work and relaxing (or slothing, as I call it) to help get those digestive movements going.

5. Get sleep! Make sure to aim for 7-8 hours of sleep per night. Lack of sleep slows down intestinal motility and increases inflammation. I find that if I have disruptions in my sleep, I will always have disruptions in my poop life.

6. Make sure you aren't undereating. It can be common to get constipated if you aren't eating enough. It's also common to be mildly constipated when you are dieting, as your thyroid hormones naturally decline. Lower thyroid hormones can lead to slow gut motility. That doesn't make being constipated normal while dieting. It just means that if you are dieting, be aware that your poop motility may change.

7. Try adding a natural prokinetic such as ginger, triphala, or tryptophan or digestive bitters, which help to stimulate digestive juices, as well as can help relieve heartburn, support the liver, support blood sugar, and stimulate peristalsis. Digestive bitters include ginger, myrrh, orange peel, fennel, dandelion root, rhubarb, wormwood, and cinnamon. If the previous tips don't help, coffee or tea may help move things along. Caffeine can increase motility and so can the use of natural prokinetics like magnesium citrate. I would be cautious and avoid using supplements to enforce movements, as for some, they can become dependent and addicted to them. For example, senna (found in many "bowel movement regulator" supplements) is habit forming and the body becomes accustomed to it. Meaning that as you continue to take it, it will work less and less. The same may happen for magnesium citrate. Luckily, I have not seen dependency with caffeine, but that doesn't mean that it won't happen.

Just like any other condition, you want to find the root cause of the constipation. Look at lifestyle factors first to find what may be preventing you from happy daily bowel movements, then look at:

- Possible food intolerances
- Overgrowths (methane-dominant SIBO is a major cause)
- Lack of pancreatic enzymes or bile flow
- Cortisol dysregulation
- Hypothyroidism
- Intestinal adhesions
- Gut nerve damage
- Colonic muscle weakness

Low Stomach Acid-- Hypochlorhydria

Do these symptoms sound familiar?

- Bloating or belching immediately following a meal
- A sense of fullness after eating
- Itching around rectum
- Chronic candida infections
- Peeling or cracked fingernails
- Mineral deficiencies
- Acne
- Chronic parasite infection
- Weak, peeling, or cracked fingernails
- GERD (gastrointestinal reflux disease)
- Post-adolescent acne
- Undigested food in stool
- Morning diarrhea or diarrhea after big meals
- Iron, B12, or zinc deficiency
- Nausea
- Lack of desire to eat protein or meat
- Bloating
- Multiple food allergies or intolerances

If so- you might have low stomach acid. I suggest working with a health professional to confirm this, who can utilize both symptoms and lab work to confirm potential need for stomach acid support. A Betaine HCl challenge or baking soda challenge can also be done yourself, however these self-tests are not validated and cannot diagnose low stomach acid. Other tests to assess for HCl include the Heidelberg test, serum gastric (however not accurate with PPI or H2 blocker use), and autoantibodies to parietal cells (if autoimmune and pernicious anemia is expected).

How to perform a baking soda test:

- Drink a mix of 1/4 tsp in 4 oz water on empty stomach
- See if burping occurs within 5 minutes. If it does, it is likely you have adequate stomach acid. If your burp right away, you may have high stomach acid.
- How does it work? HCl + sodium bicarbonate $(NaHCO_3)$ = CO_2 gas = burping.

How to perform a betaine HCL test (do not use unless gastric ulcer and H pylori are ruled out):

- Start with consuming 1 betaine (300-400mg) at a protein containing meal. Add 1 pill per meal till a burning sensation occurs. If you reach over 3 betaines, you may have low stomach acid. (Burning can be neutralized with $\frac{1}{2}$ tsp baking soda in 4 oz water).

Low stomach acid can be caused by: hypothyroidism, infection or illness, autoimmune disease, stress, fasting, post-surgery, medications (such as proton pump inhibitors, antihistamines, antacids), gastroparesis, hiatal hernias, pyloric sphincter malfunction, and/or increased age.

Most often, I see hypochlorhydria stem from an H. pylori infection, however that is not always the case. Lack of stomach acid leads to the inadequate breakdown of proteins in your gut (which can increase your risk of overgrowths), reduction in antimicrobial activity (which reduces your gut immunity and increases risk of illness and infections), as well as nutrient deficiencies (which then feed into developing hormonal imbalances and chronic disease). Low stomach acid can lead to SIBO, chronic candida infections, H pylori, parasitic infection, mineral deficiencies, and iron and B12 deficiencies.

If you suffer from low stomach acid or GERD, there are some specific changes that may help with your symptoms!

Foods to avoid: high fatty/fried/greasy foods, chocolate, coffee, mints, high sugar, alcohol, onions, garlic, citrus fruits, tomato-based foods, spicy foods, and carbonation

Lifestyle changes to make: eat smaller meals, minimize liquids with meals, go on walks after meals, wear looser fitting clothing, don't lie down after meals, limit foot intake before sleeping, prioritize stress reduction, try chiropractic adjustments which may improve blood flow to the stomach to improve HCl production.

Supplementation: add in betaine HCL (if gastric ulcer and H pylori are ruled out), use digestive or Swedish bitters that help stimulate enzyme production (such as dandelion root, ginger, fennel, myrrh, rhubarb, wormwood, cinnamon, orange peel), or try apple cider vinegar. As bitters can also relieve heartburn, they can be helpful to use with GERB and H pylori infections without causing potential intestinal damage.

Low Pancreatic Enzymes

Common symptoms of low pancreatic enzymes include:

- Watery diarrhea
- Undigested food in stool
- Undesired weight loss or muscle wasting
- Chronic fatigue
- Chronic bloating

- Malnutrition or nutrition deficiencies
- Edema
- Indigestion/fullness 2-4 hours after meal
- Chronic bloating
- Slow digestive transit time

Pancreatic enzyme deficiencies can be caused by any alteration in the output or function of your pancreas, or by impaired or slow digestion due to bacterial overgrowths, infections, stress, alcohol abuse, environmental toxicity, inflammation, or hormonal imbalances. Additional enzyme deficiencies can also occur, including lack of lactose, fructose, and sucrose enzymes. These can be hereditary (as in the case for fructose) or developed over time (commonly occurring with lactose).

You can naturally support enzyme function by:

- Focusing on rest and digest: mindful and slow eating, ensuring proper mastification (aka chewing of your food), and prioritizing stress management
- Being cautious of your food choices: limit high fatty and processed foods, consume cooked vs raw vegetables, and avoid
- Add in herbal therapies and digestive bitters that help stimulate digestion such as ginger, fennel, mint, and natural proteolytic enzymes such as bromelain (from pineapple) or papain (from papaya)

Low Bile Acids

Bile acids help to emulsify fats from your food. Remember, bile is what helps to digest and absorb dietary fat and fat-soluble vitamins. It also plays a crucial role in helping to remove excess cholesterol, environmental toxins, and hormones from your body.

Think of bile like pac man- gobbling up toxins to remove and sweeping up to help vitamin absorption.

Primary bile acids are created in your liver, while secondary bile acids are created by your gut microbes in your large intestine. A problem with the creation of bile acids in your liver, release of bile acids from your gall bladder, or metabolism of bile acids within your microbiome can cause bile acid insufficiency.

If you say "yes" to the following symptoms- you may have issues with creating bile acids!

Symptoms:

- Fatty stools (bulky, pale/grey, oily stools)
- Floating stools
- Diarrhea
- Unintentional weight loss
- Constant feeling of fullness
- Nausea or pain after a high fat meal
- High cholesterol levels
- Malnutrition or nutrient deficiencies (especially of fat-soluble vitamins)

Inadequate bile can be caused by gallbladder removal (a cholecystectomy), bile sludge (in which the bile becomes too thick and alters bile release from the gallbladder), liver disease or blockage (which may inhibit bile creation), hypothyroidism, diabetes, and rapid weight loss. As bile is produced in the liver, a poor functioning liver can halt the creation of bile acids. On the other hand, without a gallbladder, production is not halted, but bile flow may be slowed.

Testing for bile insufficiency involves fecal steatocrit (elevated with fat malabsorption), endoscopies, or CT scans.

Treatment for low bile acids involves stimulating bile production and supplementing with bile salts if warranted. Bile stimulation can be triggered by digestive bitters such as dandelion or wormwood, or may the using of cholagogue foods like mustard greens, radishes, beets, turmeric, celery, turnip greens, and artichokes. If someone has liver disease, no gallbladder, or heavy malabsorption, bile salts or ox bile may be necessary.

Histamine Intolerance

Histamine is a natural compound produced by mast cells (immune cells) that is naturally found within foods and aids in regulating your immune and allergy responses. It triggers the beginning of an inflammatory response by helping to increase blood flow and marks as a red flag to your body that some "attacker" is present. It also helps to increase stomach acid and acts as a neutransmitter in your brain.

Symptoms of histamine intolerance include:

- Rashes or eczema
- Increased allergies
- Dry throat
- Sinus congestion
- Runny nose, water eyes
- Stomach aches and cramps
- Low blood pressure
- Flushing
- Headache
- Heartburn
- Diarrhea
- Rapid heart beat
- Insomnia

Histamine intolerance can be caused by lack of :

Treatment for histamine intolerance includes rebalancing the gut and restoring the immune system. Symptoms can be managed by removing high histamine foods such as fermented foods, alcohol, wine, aged cheeses, eggs, citrus fruits, seafood, spinach, processed meats, ripe bananas/avocadoes, tomato based products, vinegars, and even leftovers (in which histamine is produced with microbial fermentation and maturation). Histamine intolerance occurs when you have too much histamine in your body than it is able to break down. Histamine intolerance can be caused by: Lack of DAO or HNMT enzymes that help to degrade histamine, overgrowth of bacteria that produce histamine, and/or supplements and medications that black DAO production. An overburden of histamine containing foods can then lead to worsened histamine intolerance.

My favorite supplements for histamine intolerance include:

- Vitamin C: an antioxidant that helps to stabilize mast cells
- Quercetin & Stinging nettle: act as mast cell stabilizers
- Probiotics: Specific strains of probiotics may help to diminish your histamine responses and reactions including Bifidobacterium infantis, Bifidobacterium longum, Lactobacillus plantarum, Lactobacillus rhamnosus, and Bifidobacterium bifidum. Seeking Health has a great blend probiotic I love called ProBiota HistaminX that can be helpful for those with histamine or mast cell issues.
- Diamine Oxidase (DAO) supplements: help to degrade excess histamine in the body

Testing Bowel Transit Time

"Transit time" can be defined as the time it takes for you to eat, digest, and eliminate (aka poop) out the food that you eat. Testing your bowel transit time can tell you about a possible potential digesting your food. If you can't digest your food, you can't absorb

376 | THE WOMEN'S GUIDE TO HORMONAL HARMONY

your nutrients! An optimal transit time is between 12-24 hours. Less than 12 hours may indicate malabsorption or infection, while greater than 72 hours may indicate slow motility, which can predispose you to overgrowths due to increased colonic fermentation, as well as increase the reabsorption of toxins back into your bloodstream.

The Test:

Buy activated charcoal tablets and take about 1000mg. Write down when you took the charcoal. Monitor your poop for darkened stools (charcoal will turn your stool dark/black). Calculate the number of hours it took from taking the charcoal, to seeing the darkened stool. You may also do this test eating three to four beets, which will turn your poop a dark red color, or by consuming. This test can also be performed with your doctor with the use of an X-ray and marked gel capsules.

The best way to increase your bowel transit time? Increase your water intake, consume 30-40g fiber per day, exercise at least 30 minutes per day, and prioritize stress reduction.

Digestive Issue	What May Help
Low Stomach Acid	Products: -Betaine HCl -Apple Cider Vinegar -Digestive bitters (HCl not suggested if H. Pylori or stomach ulcers are present) Lifestyle Changes: -Stress reduction and vagal nerve/parasympathetic work Diet: -Consume easily digestible proteins -Choose smaller, more frequent meals
Low pancreatic enzymes	Products: -Over-the-counter pancreatic enzyme blends -Digestive bitters -PERTS (pancreatic enzyme replacement therapies) -Animal Derived pancreatins -Bromelain (from pineapple) -Papain (from papaya) Lifestyle changes: -Stress reduction and vagal nerve/parasympathetic work Diet: -Consume cooked vs raw vegetables -Incorporate probiotic foods -Choose soaked grains or seeds

GERD or Reflux	Products: -Baking soda -Apple Cider Vinegar -Digestive bitters Diet: -Focus on avoiding: high-fat meals, carbonation, citrus fruits, alcohol, chocolate, onions, garlic, peppermint Lifestyle changes: -Maintain a healthy weight -Walk 5-10 minutes after meals -Stop eating 2-3 hours before bed -Don't lie down after meals -Sleep on your left side (HCl not suggested if H. Pylori or stomach ulcers are present)

Slowed or Impaired Motility	Products: -Ginger root -Magnesium citrate or oxide -Digestive bitters -Triphala -Tryptophan -Senna (can be habit forming) -Psyllium husk -Citrus pectin Lifestyle changes: -Stress reduction and vagal nerve/parasympathetic work -Exercise -Acupuncture -Pelvic floor therapy -Visceral Manipulation therapy Diet: -Increase fiber -Probiotic rich foods -Green tea -Aloe Vera -Coffee (natural laxative) -Caffeine (natural laxative) -Flax or chia seeds -Omega-3s

Low Bile Acids	Products: -Bile acid sequestrants -Bile salts (Ox bile) -Dandelion root -Digestive bitters Lifestyle: -Avoid high-fat meals Diet: -Dandelion -Bitter greens -Artichoke -Coffee

Bloating	Products: -Antrantil or Iberogast (herbal tinctures) -Activated Charcoal -Ginger -Prokinetics (such as Motil Pro or Motility Activator) -Peppermint oil Lifestyle: -Walks after meals -Yoga -Meditation -Acupuncture -Abdominal massage Diet: -Mindful, slow eating -Limiting liquids with meals -Low FODMAP -Low volume meals/foods -Limiting carbonation -Smaller, frequent meals -Watch fiber intake -Ditch processed foods

Intestinal Lining Health / Intestinal Permeability	Products: -Partially Hydrolyzed Guar Gum (PHGG) -Bovine immunoglobulins -Colostrum -Zinc carnosine -Saccharomyces boulardii -Spore based probiotics (ex. Megaspore) -L-glutamine -Marshmallow root -Butyrate -Vitamin D3 -Full spectrum CBD oil -Prebiotics -Aloe vera -Deglycyrrhized licorice Lifestyle: -Prioritize stress reduction -Ensure adequate sleep -Limit exposure to environmental toxins Diet: -Remove food intolerances -Try going gluten-free -Limit artificial sweeteners, food preservatives, and gums such as xanthum gum -Eliminate alcohol and smoking -Power up the prebiotics in your diet -Focus on polyphenol rich foods (think color!)

A LETTER FROM THE AUTHOR

Thank you so much for taking your time to read my book. I hope it empowered, educated, and helped you to build the confidence that you need to become the true master of their own health and body. You deserve to not just survive, but thrive! I hope you can use every ounce of knowledge given to you and use it to be the best version of yourself.

To every woman that has every worked with me, thank you for being a part of this creation. Your stories, struggles, and trust in my guidance has helped me to be a better clinician and dietitian. To my family, you have been my rock throughout my entire life, and I couldn't be more thankful and blessed. And lastly, thank you to my amazing God that put every single passion in my heart and that gave me the strength and knowledge to be the person I am today.

FAQS & MYTHS DEBUNKED

1. Are organic foods healthier?

Being organic does not mean it is healthier. The term "organic" refers to how a product is made and processed through federal regulations. Organic farming uses lower amounts of pesticides (organic farming still allows pesticides!), no hormones, no antibiotics, follows specific agricultural practices, and has an increased focus on animal ethics.

Some facts:

- An organic product must be made without: genetic engineering (GMOs), ionizing radiation, sewage sludge, most synthetic pesticides and herbicides, antibiotics, and hormones.
- Organic products still allow the use of approved pesticides and vaccines. Many people choose organic products due to less pesticide use, no added hormones (note- hormones aren't allowed in poultry products anyway!), and sustainable agriculture practices. I myself choose organic meats and poultry, and avoid the dirty

dozen (listed by the EWG- Environmental Working Group) to help decrease my exposure to pesticides/herbicides (specifically Round Up), lower the bioaccumulation of those products in my meats, and maximize nutrient intake.

- Choosing organic can decrease your exposure to pesticides, but there is inconclusive evidence to fully answer whether the reduction of pesticides corresponds with a statistically significant health outcome (inconclusive doesn't mean there isn't a benefit- it just means the benefit and no benefit show mixed results). There is no arguing that consuming your fruits and veggies as non-organic outweighs skipping them altogether.

- The EPA regulates pesticide usage in conventional products. Most are below safety limits and washing your produce greatly further decreases pesticides exposure. Can't wash a product, such as in the case of oats, bread, or cereals? You may want to choose organic. These products, especially ones made with corn and wheat, may be sprayed with more levels of glyphosate, which you wouldn't be able to monitor or wash off.

- Do some organic foods have more nutrients than their conventional counterparts? Yes! But not all do, and some actually have lower amounts. For example- some organic meats have higher omega-3 fats than conventional meats, while some organic produce have higher nutrient content such as increased levels of vitamin C, magnesium, phosphorus, and iron. Keep in mind that this will depend on the specific produce, how it was grown, the soil quality, and how you cook it. As the more water you use in cooking, the more water-soluble nutrients can leach into the water.

Overall point- Choose organic based on your needs, budget, and priorities. Choosing organic meats, eggs, and dairy is my choice along with focusing on avoiding the Dirty Dozen.

2. Should I be avoiding dairy? Doesn't dairy have hormones in it?

If you are dairy or lactose intolerant, yes. If not, you don't need to unless it causes you specific inflammation such as acne or increased joint or muscle aches. Dairy is packed with beneficial micronutrients including Vitamin D, calcium, phosphorus, and protein!

3. What are the benefits and drawbacks to intermittent fasting?

Intermittent fasting, or "IF" for short, is a method and tool for dieting and a pattern of eating that involves time restricted feeding and fasting windows. There are many ways to implement it.

Common IF methods include:

- 16/8 (16 hours fasting, 8 hours eating)
- 12/12 (12 hour feeding with 12 hour fasting)
- Alternate day fasting (alternating "feast" days with "fast days")
- 5:2 (fasting 2 out of 5 days)

IF has potential benefits that include increasing insulin sensitivity and fat mobilization (aiding in metabolic flexibility), enhancing cognition, and decreasing blood lipid levels. It may also potentially help increase longevity (aka your life span), combat mitochondrial stress, aid in digestion, and decrease inflammation. However, these benefits are also seen with caloric restriction alone, and can be achieved through alternative diet and lifestyle changes. In addition, many studies that show these benefits result from studies that have been done on rodent species, not humans.

What about benefits for weight loss? In the literature, IF does not show a benefit for helping with fat or weight loss when compared to a normal eating schedule. What matters is energy balance. I have seen IF in my clients be helpful for those with insulin resistance, however, you can achieve insulin sensitivity through doing more than just IF, including adjusting your diet, lifestyle, and even supplementation.

Do keep in mind, IF may not be optimal for gaining muscle. A reduced feeding window means reductions in your protein feeding opportunities, and reductions in stimulating MPS. However, some studies show that doing IF with resistance training does not cause detrimental muscle loss or inhibit muscle growth. If you are a bodybuilder or want to gain muscle, you may want to focus on optimal eating for muscle growth, which would mean consuming at least 30 g protein with 3 meals a day spread out 3-4 hours.

Fasting can be detrimental to those with cortisol or adrenal dysfunction and can also make hormone imbalances worse, especially in women. Remember that stress is stress, and if you already have a half full stress bucket, doing IF could be the last drops of the bucket that you need for your bucket to overflow and cause hormonal chaos! Fasting can also spell a recipe for disaster if you struggle with overeating and binging. For some- it may help reduce snacking throughout the day. However, fasting during the day may set you up for failure by leading to overeating or binge eating late at night. Not good for your mental or physical health!

To review:

- Who it is good for: people who like larger meals, have a busy schedule, can plan their workouts around their fasting window (I always suggest breaking your fasting before a workout so you can have fuel for your workout and stimulate MPS!)

- Who should NOT do it: People with cortisol, adrenal, or some hormonal imbalances (IF could help some!), those with a history of disordered eating, or if you have digestion issues with larger meals

If intermittent fasting makes you feel good and fits your lifestyle, do it. It's not magical for weight loss. It won't help 'trick' your body into burning more fat. You do you, boo. Try it if you want to. I practice 16/8 hour fasting daily. That doesn't mean you should! Fun fact- technically everyone does IF in a way- cause when you sleep, you don't eat!

4. Do I need to worry about the "Anabolic Window"?

The "anabolic window" is typically defined as how long protein synthesis is elevated after weight training or resistance training. Many believe it's the time you have to build muscle, but this is not the sole truth. Your anabolic window can last up to 72 hours if untrained or a beginner trainee, or from 8 to 72 hours if advanced. Remember from my protein section, the longer you have trained, the lower response you have to MPS (muscle protein synthesis) with training. Therefore, post-workout nutrition may be more beneficial to advanced trainees than it is for beginners.

Facts- the amino acid levels in your muscle typically decline 3-4 hours after consuming a protein-rich meal. Essentially this means that for stimulating MPS, eating a pre-workout meal and post-workout meal within 3 hours of each other is redundant. Amino acids levels and MPS are already elevated. Why elevate what's already elevated?

As long as you had a protein-rich meal a few hours before working out, you don't have to worry about missing your "anabolic window" by eating right after your workout. Waiting 1-2 hours is fine! However- if you train fasted or you don't consume a protein rich meal within 1-2 hours prior to training, eating a quality protein post-workout is essential to maximize your MPS.

Keep this in mind- MPS elevation also changes based on the quality of the protein that you consume (remember- animal proteins are more easily digestible and more biologically available than most plant sources), and food sources, such as the presence of fat or fiber, will slow digestion and in turn, reduce MPS. If you didn't consume a high quality protein source a few hours before working out, you may want to strive for a low fat, low fiber, high biologically available protein source such as whey protein, Greek yogurt, egg whites, a brown rice/pea protein blend, or lean meat.

5. What about pre- and post-workout nutrition?

Multiple factors exist here- what are your goals? When was your last meal? (And what was it?) What type of training do you do? How insulin sensitive are you? What's your post-workout meal like and when do you have it? Refer to the anabolic window discussion.

Here are some scenarios for you:

- If you plan to eat within 1-2 hours before lifting, a mixed meal is adequate as long as it's not too high in fat or fiber to inhibit your digestion and performance (individual variances here). 10-15 g of fat and fiber should suffice. Keep in mind the more fat and fiber you eat, the slower your digestion. In this case, you may benefit from a small carbohydrate snack prior to lifting for additional energy. This is because if you ate 2 hours prior, your blood glucose levels may be lower, and without enough carbohydrate mid-workout, you are at an increased risk for going hypoglycemic. Not good in the middle of a training session! Consuming 15-30 g carbs prior to your workout or in the form of an intra-workout may be helpful.
- If you plan to eat an hour to 30 minutes prior to lifting, a meal with a quick digesting or a mix of slow and quick digesting carbohydrates, lean protein source, and low fat

and low fiber content may be optimal. This will help give you energy and not screw up your digestion during your lift. In this case, I suggested 25-50 g carbs and at least 25 g protein. Fiber and fat keep under 10 g.

- If you're insulin resistant- dividing up at least 50% of your daily carbs between pre- and post-workout would be beneficial, as you are most insulin sensitive during these times. If your daily carbohydrate goal is 150 g, this may mean dividing up your pre- and post-workout carbs to be at least 75 g total.
- If you're fasting- either lift fasted and have a low fat and fiber, moderate carbohydrate and protein meal post workout (with 25-35 g of each). Remember that fasted training is hard on the adrenals, and it also increases your risk of muscle loss. If you are worried about losing muscle, I suggest either drinking a protein shake at least before, or consuming a BCAA/EAA blend pre-workout.

Remember the goals of each macronutrient pre- and post-workout:

- Protein's goal- spike muscle protein synthesis, prevent muscle protein breakdown, aid in growth and recovery
- Carb's goal- provide immediate energy for training, fill glycogen stores, spike insulin, reduce cortisol, prevent muscle protein breakdown

Final note- eating carbs post workout doesn't enhance your protein synthesis. It enhances glycogen replenishment!

6. I had genetic testing done that shows that I have "XYZ" genes. What do I do with this information?

Your genes are not your destiny. Just because you have the "XYZ" gene does not mean that it is being expressed and influencing your health. Your risk of turning on or off a gene is influenced by your diet and lifestyle choices, as well as the presence of inflammation, infections, comorbidities, and your environment.

7. Are artificial sweeteners and sugar alcohols considered safe? Will they make me gain weight?

Let's go over quick facts:

- Fact 1: The high intensity sweeteners used in food products such as diet food, diet drinks, and sugar free syrups/products- are CALORIE FREE. Sucralose itself, Ace-K, aspartame, a stevia all have 0 calories. They can't directly contribute to energy and do not stimulate insulin levels. Therefore, they can't cause weight gain by contributing to a caloric surplus.
- Fact 2: The packets of sweetener such as Splenda, Equal, and Truvia/Purevia are not the same as Fact 1. They DO have calories (however very low calories). This is because they contain fillers such as maltodextrin (aka sugar) or additional sugar alcohols such as erythritol. 1 packet of equal = 4 calories. 1 packet of Splenda = 4 calories. Truvia contains mostly erythritol, not stevia, and is around 0.6 calories (aka nothing). You don't need to track these when consumed in small quantities (and they should be only consumed in small quantities!). Small amounts of these products will most likely not contribute to weight gain, as if you have 3 packets a day, that's a measly 12 calories.
- Fact 3: Safety of artificial sweeteners are based on the ADI (acceptable daily intake) which is established by the FDA (Food and Drug Administration). If you are below this amount, it's highly likely that they are safe to consume. However, even within the ADI, there is a potential for artificial sweeteners to contribute to alterations in your gut microbiome, leading to glucose intolerance and increased inflammation. These changes

MAY contribute to health concerns. The verdict is out on how much and how often you need to consume them to develop health issues. As I type this, I am off to grab me a Fresca now.

- Fact 4: Sugar alcohols have amazing low caloric values and many are deemed as safe for consumption under the ADI just like artificial sweeteners. However, many can produce really bad laxative effects and GI disturbance, even in small doses. For example- mannitol and sorbitol can cause major gas and bloating in small amounts, and diarrhea in larger amounts.

Each sugar alcohol has a different caloric value established based on their digestibility in your gut. For example, erythritol has 0.2 calories per gram, while sorbitol has 2.6, xylitol 2.4, and mannitol 1.6.

Sugar alcohols are a common reason why your food labels with processed foods (especially in protein bars or sugar free drinks), don't match your macros when inputting into an app like MyFitnessPal.

- Fact 5: Sugar alcohols can affect your blood glucose levels, however artificial sweeteners themselves do not. Diabetics should be aware of this.

8. **How should I handle dining out?**

Dining Out Distress? Take a breath, relax, it's just one meal- you got this. Meals are meant to be enjoyed and dining out is a social activity! Whether you track macros or not, my suggestion is to first ask yourself "What is my priority right now". If wellness is a priority, make sure your meal chosen matches that. If you want to enjoy some good grub, then pick what you want, enjoy it, and don't look back! The decision you make will cause a short term consequence- maybe that's curbing a craving, expanding your palette, or staying on top of your health and wellness goals. Choose your priority and go from there!

Some helpful tips to eat healthy dining out for you:

- Don't go into the meal starving. Make sure you had a good, normal meal a few hours before. If you take an untracked meal- I tell my clients to eat 1/2 of their daily macros at least outside of the untracked meal, then go enjoy your meal! Don't go in hangry or you're setting yourself up for overeating & making irrational choices.
- Look at the menu ahead of time if you can. Plan ahead! If you track macros, you can probably find a generic entry for your meal online. For example, with sushi you can use Pei Wei calories, or you can guesstimate by tracking the components & amounts in each meal. In the case of eating Mexican food and enchiladas- you could track corn tortillas, shredded chicken, 2-3oz shredded cheese, enchilada sauce, and any chips you may enjoy too.
- Don't be afraid to be picky and ask for what you want! I ask for no butter & steamed only vegetables, no dressing or dressing on the side, or order asking for no sauces (as some sauces can add lots of fat and calories easily!). Don't be afraid to ask for a side swap either. You can swap a potato or rice for extra vegetables or a side salad to lower carbs.
- Drink your water and eat slowly. Put your fork down between bites. Talk with your friends or family. Typically it takes a good 10 min for our bodies to realize we are full, so go slow.
- Play the portion game by using your palm as a 3 oz meat portion, or fist for 1 cup cooked whole grains or around 5-6 oz potato! Your thumb counts about 1 tbs of fats as well. (Pointer and middle finger together is about 1 oz avocado!). If there are large portions- eat half and save

half. Guess what? You can then save the other half for "meal prep".

- Stick with "baked, boiled, grilled, oven roasted" & limit "sauteed, marinated, smothered, fried"- those words typically mean added fats! Ask for steamed vegetables if available and don't be afraid to go simple. For salads, be cautious of added dried fruits, cheeses, or nuts that can add on calories quickly.
- What I personally like to do is track food based on eyeballed portion sizes. Most restaurant nutrition info is off anyways. I also take into account the fact that most restaurants cook in oils when grilling meats. Example if I get a chicken breast, I'll account for around 8gF. HOPE THIS HELPS!

ADDITIONAL RESOURCES & REFERENCES

"Lacey Approved Foods"

Oh wait… all are approved as long as you don't have specific food intolerances, allergies, or inflammation upon their consumption.

Foods to Include In Your Diet:

- Proteins: Chicken breast, ground turkey, ground beef, bison, steak, fish/seafood (salmon, tilapia, cod, halibut, mahi mahi, crab, shrimp), egg whites, eggs, tofu, tempeh, protein powder, low fat cheese, greek yogurt, cottage cheese
- Carbohydrates: Potatoes (red, purple, sweet, yellow, russet), all vegetables, rice (brown, wild, white, black, yellow, red), beans/legumes, low sugar cereal, oatmeal, quinoa, barley, cream of rice, cream of wheat, all fruits, 100% whole wheat breads and tortillas, 100% whole wheat pasta or lentil-based pasta, 100% whole wheat/oat/cassava flour
- Fats: Oils (olive, extra-virgin olive, avocado, coconut),

nuts (almonds, cashews, peanuts, walnuts), seeds (chia, flaxseed, sunflower, hemp, pumpkin), nut butters, coconut butter, coconut and almond flour, eggs, dark chocolate, full fat cheeses, flax seeds, chia seeds, avocado, olives, animal fat from meats

- Spices: cinnamon, clove, garlic, parsley, celery, ginger, turmeric
- Beverages: filtered water, unsweetened teas, herbal teas, black or unsweetened coffee, low calorie electrolyte drinks, seltzer, and diet sodas in moderation
- All fruits and vegetables

Foods to Limit In Your Diet: (limit does not mean 100% avoid!)

(obviously including any specific food intolerance or allergy you may have yourself)

- Highly processed vegetable oils (canola, soybean, sunflower, corn, safflower, margarine)
- Alcohol
- Hydrogenated oils and trans fat (avoid)
- Food additives and preservatives including: carrageenan, nitrates, nitrates, gums, sulfites,, artificial food dyes, BHA, BHT, polysorbates, sulfites, sodium benzoate, potassium bromate, EDTA
- Processed meats
- Canned fish unless low mercury (for example, Safe Catch)
- Sugary beverages or condiments
- Artificial sweeteners

References & Additional Reading:

Abraham GE. Nutritional factors in the etiology of the premenstrual tension syndromes. *J Reprod Med.* 1983;28(7):446-464.

Achufusi TGO, Sharma A, Zamora EA, Manocha D. Small Intestinal Bacterial Overgrowth: Comprehensive Review of Diagnosis, Prevention, and Treatment Methods. *Cureus*. 2020;12(6):e8860. Published 2020 Jun 27. doi:10.7759/cureus.8860

Adafer R, Messaadi W, Meddahi M, et al. Food Timing, Circadian Rhythm and Chrononutrition: A Systematic Review of Time-Restricted Eating's Effects on Human Health. Nutrients. 2020;12(12):3770. Published 2020 Dec 8. doi:10.3390/nu12123770

Alemyar A, van der Kooi ALF, Laven JSE. Anti-Müllerian Hormone and Ovarian Morphology in Women With Hypothalamic Hypogonadism. *J Clin Endocrinol Metab*. 2020;105(5):dgaa116. doi:10.1210/clinem/dgaa116

Alhamdan BA, Garcia-Alvarez A, Alzahrnai AH, et al. Alternate-day versus daily energy restriction diets: which is more effective for weight loss? A systematic review and meta-analysis. Obes Sci Pract. 2016;2(3):293-302. doi:10.1002/osp4.52

Allshouse A, Pavlovic J, Santoro N. Menstrual Cycle Hormone Changes Associated with Reproductive Aging and How They May Relate to Symptoms. *Obstet Gynecol Clin North Am*. 2018;45(4):613-628. doi:10.1016/j.ogc.2018.07.004

Ambrosini A, Di Lorenzo C, Coppola G, Pierelli F. Use of Vitex agnus-castus in migrainous women with premenstrual syndrome: an open-label clinical observation. *Acta Neurol Belg*. 2013;113(1):25-29. doi:10.1007/s13760-012-0111-4

Ardabilygazir A, Afshariyamchlou S, Mir D, Sachmechi I. Effect of High-dose Biotin on Thyroid Function Tests: Case Report and Literature Review. *Cureus*. 2018;10(6):e2845. Published 2018 Jun 20. doi:10.7759/cureus.2845

Arentz S, Smith CA, Abbott J, Bensoussan A. Nutritional supplements and herbal medicines for women with polycystic ovary syndrome; a systematic review and meta-analysis. *BMC Complement Altern Med.* 2017;17(1):500. Published 2017 Nov 25. doi:10.1186/s12906-017-2011-x

Arrieta MC, Bistritz L, Meddings JB. Alterations in intestinal permeability. *Gut.* 2006;55(10):1512-1520. doi:10.1136/gut.2005.085373

Asha MZ, Khalil SFH. Efficacy and Safety of Probiotics, Prebiotics and Synbiotics in the Treatment of Irritable Bowel Syndrome: A systematic review and meta-analysis. *Sultan Qaboos Univ Med J.* 2020;20(1):e13-e24. doi:10.18295/squmj.2020.20.01.003

Assiri AM, Elbanna K, Abulreesh HH, Ramadan MF. Bioactive Compounds of Cold-pressed Thyme (Thymus vulgaris) Oil with Antioxidant and Antimicrobial Properties. *J Oleo Sci.* 2016;65(8):629-640. doi:10.5650/jos.ess16042

Auborn KJ, Fan S, Rosen EM, et al. Indole-3-carbinol is a negative regulator of estrogen. *J Nutr.* 2003;133(7 Suppl):2470S-2475S. doi:10.1093/jn/133.7.2470s

Azziz R. Polycystic Ovary Syndrome. *Obstet Gynecol.* 2018;132(2):321-336. doi:10.1097/AOG.0000000000002698

Baker FC, Siboza F, Fuller A. Temperature regulation in women: Effects of the menstrual cycle. *Temperature (Austin).* 2020;7(3):226-262. Published 2020 Mar 22. doi:10.1080/23328940.2020.1735927

Bansal V, Costantini T, Kroll L, et al. Traumatic brain injury and intestinal dysfunction: uncovering the neuro-enteric axis. *J Neurotrauma.* 2009;26(8):1353-1359. doi:10.1089/neu.2008.0858

Barański M, Srednicka-Tober D, Volakakis N, et al. Higher antioxidant and lower cadmium concentrations and lower incidence of pesticide residues in organically grown crops: a systematic literature review and meta-analyses. Br J Nutr. 2014;112(5):794-811. doi:10.1017/S0007114514001366

Barański M, Srednicka-Tober D, Volakakis N, et al. Higher antioxidant and lower cadmium concentrations and lower incidence of pesticide residues in organically grown crops: a systematic literature review and meta-analyses. *Br J Nutr.* 2014;112(5):794-811. doi:10.1017/S0007114514001366

Baskin HJ, Cobin RH, Duick DS, et al. American Association of Clinical Endocrinologists medical guidelines for clinical practice for the evaluation and treatment of hyperthyroidism and hypothyroidism [published correction appears in Endocr Pract. 2008 Sep;14(6):802-3. Baskin, H Jack [added]; Cobin, Rhoda H [added]; Duick, Daniel S [added]; Gharib, Hossein [added]; Guttler, Richard B [added]; Kaplan, Michael M [added]; Segal, Robert L [added]]. *Endocr Pract.* 2002;8(6):457-469.

Bennett JW, Klich M. Mycotoxins. *Clin Microbiol Rev.* 2003;16(3):497-516. doi:10.1128/cmr.16.3.497-516.2003

Benvenga S, Bartolone L, Pappalardo MA, et al. Altered intestinal absorption of L-thyroxine caused by coffee. *Thyroid.* 2008;18(3):293-301. doi:10.1089/thy.2007.0222

Bertrand J, Ghouzali I, Guérin C, et al. Glutamine Restores Tight Junction Protein Claudin-1 Expression in Colonic Mucosa of Patients With Diarrhea-Predominant Irritable Bowel Syndrome. *JPEN J Parenter Enteral Nutr.* 2016;40(8):1170-1176. doi:10.1177/0148607115587330

Bi Z, Zheng Y, Yuan J, Bian Z. The Efficacy and Potential Mechanisms of Chinese Herbal Medicine on Irritable Bowel

Syndrome. *Curr Pharm Des*. 2017;23(34):5163-5172. doi:10.2174/1381612823666170822101606

Bischoff SC, Barbara G, Buurman W, et al. Intestinal permeability--a new target for disease prevention and therapy. *BMC Gastroenterol*. 2014;14:189. Published 2014 Nov 18. doi:10.1186/s12876-014-0189-7

Bitto A, Polito F, Atteritano M, et al. Genistein aglycone does not affect thyroid function: results from a three-year, randomized, double-blind, placebo-controlled trial. *J Clin Endocrinol Metab*. 2010;95(6):3067-3072. doi:10.1210/jc.2009-2779

Bonifácio BV, dos Santos Ramos MA, da Silva PB, Bauab TM. Antimicrobial activity of natural products against Helicobacter pylori: a review. *Ann Clin Microbiol Antimicrob*. 2014;13:54. Published 2014 Nov 19. doi:10.1186/s12941-014-0054-0

Brandt M, Brown C, Burkhart J, et al. Mold prevention strategies and possible health effects in the aftermath of hurricanes and major floods. *MMWR Recomm Rep*. 2006;55(RR-8):1-27.

Briden L. *Period Repair Manual: Natural Treatment for Better Hormones and Better Periods*.; 2018.

Brighten J. *Beyond the Pill*. HarperOne; 2020.

Brouns F. Overweight and diabetes prevention: is a low-carbohy-drate-high-fat diet recommendable? [published correction appears in Eur J Nutr. 2019 Apr 16;:]. *Eur J Nutr*. 2018;57(4):1301-1312. doi:10.1007/s00394-018-1636-y

Bueno NB, de Melo IS, de Oliveira SL, da Rocha Ataide T. Very-low-carbohydrate ketogenic diet v. low-fat diet for long-term weight loss: a meta-analysis of randomised controlled trials. *Br J Nutr*. 2013;110(7):1178-1187. doi:10.1017/S0007114513000548

Burrows LJ, Basha M, Goldstein AT. The effects of hormonal contraceptives on female sexuality: a review. *J Sex Med.* 2012;9(9):2213-2223. doi:10.1111/j.1743-6109.2012.02848.x

Byrne, N., Sainsbury, A., King, N. et al. Intermittent energy restriction improves weight loss efficiency in obese men: the MATADOR study. Int J Obes 42, 129–138 (2018). https://doi.org/10.1038/ijo.2017.206

Cadegiani FA, Kater CE. Adrenal fatigue does not exist: a systematic review [published correction appears in BMC Endocr Disord. 2016 Nov 16;16(1):63]. *BMC Endocr Disord.* 2016;16(1):48. Published 2016 Aug 24. doi:10.1186/s12902-016-0128-4

Campbell B, Kreider RB, Ziegenfuss T, et al. International Society of Sports Nutrition position stand: protein and exercise. *J Int Soc Sports Nutr.* 2007;4:8. Published 2007 Sep 26. doi:10.1186/1550-2783-4-8

Camps SG, Verhoef SP, Westerterp KR. Leptin and energy restriction induced adaptation in energy expenditure. *Metabolism.* 2015;64(10):1284-1290. doi:10.1016/j.metabol.2015.06.016

Chao AM, Quigley KM, Wadden TA. Dietary interventions for obesity: clinical and mechanistic findings. J Clin Invest. 2021;131(1):e140065. doi:10.1172/JCI140065

Chappell AJ, Simper T, Barker ME. Nutritional strategies of high level natural bodybuilders during competition preparation. J Int Soc Sports Nutr. 2018;15:4. Published 2018 Jan 15. doi:10.1186/s12970-018-0209-z

Charmandari E, Tsigos C, Chrousos G. Endocrinology of the stress response. *Annu Rev Physiol.* 2005;67:259-284. doi:10.1146/annurev.physiol.67.040403.120816

Chedid V, Dhalla S, Clarke JO, et al. Herbal therapy is equivalent to rifaximin for the treatment of small intestinal bacterial overgrowth. *Glob Adv Health Med.* 2014;3(3):16-24. doi:10.7453/gahmj.2014.019

Chen B, Kim JJ, Zhang Y, Du L, Dai N. Prevalence and predictors of small intestinal bacterial overgrowth in irritable bowel syndrome: a systematic review and meta-analysis. *J Gastroenterol.* 2018;53(7):807-818. doi:10.1007/s00535-018-1476-9

Chen C, Yu Z, Li Y, Fichna J, Storr M. Effects of berberine in the gastrointestinal tract - a review of actions and therapeutic implications. *Am J Chin Med.* 2014;42(5):1053-1070. doi:10.1142/S0192415X14500669

Chen K, Nakasone Y, Xie K, Sakao K, Hou DX. Modulation of Allicin-Free Garlic on Gut Microbiome. *Molecules.* 2020;25(3):682. Published 2020 Feb 5. doi:10.3390/molecules25030682

Chen XP, Li W, Xiao XF, Zhang LL, Liu CX. Phytochemical and pharmacological studies on Radix Angelica sinensis. *Chin J Nat Med.* 2013;11(6):577-587. doi:10.1016/S1875-5364(13)60067-9

Cheraghi E, Mehranjani MS, Shariatzadeh MA, Esfahani MH, Ebrahimi Z. N-Acetylcysteine improves oocyte and embryo quality in polycystic ovary syndrome patients undergoing intracytoplasmic sperm injection: an alternative to metformin. *Reprod Fertil Dev.* 2016;28(6):723-731. doi:10.1071/RD14182

Ciotta L, Pagano I, Stracquadanio M, Di Leo S, Andò A, Formuso C. Aspetti psichici del disturbo disforico della fase luteale: nuove prospettive terapeutiche, il vitex agnus castus. Nostra esperienza [Psychic aspects of the premenstrual dysphoric disorders. New therapeutic strategies: our experience with Vitex agnus castus]. *Minerva Ginecol.* 2011;63(3):237-245.

Clark A, Mach N. Exercise-induced stress behavior, gut-microbiota-brain axis and diet: a systematic review for athletes. *J Int Soc Sports Nutr*. 2016;13:43. Published 2016 Nov 24. doi:10.1186/s12970-016-0155-6

Cole JA, Norman H, Doherty M, Walker AM. Venous thromboembolism, myocardial infarction, and stroke among transdermal contraceptive system users [published correction appears in Obstet Gynecol. 2008 Jun;111(6):1449]. *Obstet Gynecol*. 2007;109(2 Pt 1):339-346. doi:10.1097/01.AOG.0000250968.82370.04

Cui Y, Cai T, Zhou Z, et al. Health Effects of Alternate-Day Fasting in Adults: A Systematic Review and Meta-Analysis. Front Nutr. 2020;7:586036. Published 2020 Nov 24. doi:10.3389/fnut.2020.586036

Dağlı Ü, Kalkan İH. The role of lifestyle changes in gastroesophageal reflux diseases treatment. *Turk J Gastroenterol*. 2017;28(Suppl 1):S33-S37. doi:10.5152/tjg.2017.10

Davison G, Marchbank T, March DS, Thatcher R, Playford RJ. Zinc carnosine works with bovine colostrum in truncating heavy exercise-induced increase in gut permeability in healthy volunteers. *Am J Clin Nutr*. 2016;104(2):526-536. doi:10.3945/ajcn.116.134403

de Andrade KQ, Moura FA, dos Santos JM, de Araújo OR, de Farias Santos JC, Goulart MO. Oxidative Stress and Inflammation in Hepatic Diseases: Therapeutic Possibilities of N-Acetylcysteine. *Int J Mol Sci*. 2015;16(12):30269-30308. Published 2015 Dec 18. doi:10.3390/ijms161226225

Dhabhar FS. Effects of stress on immune function: the good, the bad, and the beautiful. *Immunol Res*. 2014;58(2-3):193-210. doi:10.1007/s12026-014-8517-0

Dhabhar FS. The short-term stress response - Mother nature's mechanism for enhancing protection and performance under conditions of threat, challenge, and opportunity. *Front Neuroendocrinol.* 2018;49:175-192. doi:10.1016/j.yfrne.2018.03.004

Diamanti-Kandarakis E, Bourguignon JP, Giudice LC, et al. Endocrine-disrupting chemicals: an Endocrine Society scientific statement. *Endocr Rev.* 2009;30(4):293-342. doi:10.1210/er.2009-0002

Dirlewanger M, di Vetta V, Guenat E, et al. Effects of short-term carbohydrate or fat overfeeding on energy expenditure and plasma leptin concentrations in healthy female subjects. Int J Obes Relat Metab Disord. 2000;24(11):1413-1418. doi:10.1038/sj.ijo.0801395

Elbini Dhouib I, Jallouli M, Annabi A, Gharbi N, Elfazaa S, Lasram MM. A minireview on N-acetylcysteine: An old drug with new approaches. *Life Sci.* 2016;151:359-363. doi:10.1016/j.lfs.2016.03.003

Facchinetti F, Borella P, Sances G, Fioroni L, Nappi RE, Genazzani AR. Oral magnesium successfully relieves premenstrual mood changes. *Obstet Gynecol.* 1991;78(2):177-181.

Foster C, Farland CV, Guidotti F, et al. The Effects of High Intensity Interval Training vs Steady State Training on Aerobic and Anaerobic Capacity. *J Sports Sci Med.* 2015;14(4):747-755. Published 2015 Nov 24.

Frank-Herrmann P, Heil J, Gnoth C, et al. The effectiveness of a fertility awareness based method to avoid pregnancy in relation to a couple's sexual behaviour during the fertile time: a prospective longitudinal study. *Hum Reprod.* 2007;22(5):1310-1319. doi:10.1093/humrep/dem003

Fruzzetti F, Fidecicchi T. Hormonal Contraception and Depression: Updated Evidence and Implications in Clinical Practice. *Clin Drug Investig.* 2020;40(12):1097-1106. doi:10.1007/s40261-020-00966-8

Fulghesu AM, Ciampelli M, Muzj G, et al. N-acetyl-cysteine treatment improves insulin sensitivity in women with polycystic ovary syndrome. *Fertil Steril.* 2002;77(6):1128-1135. doi:10.1016/s0015-0282(02)03133-3

Geller SE, Studee L. Botanical and dietary supplements for menopausal symptoms: what works, what does not. *J Womens Health (Larchmt).* 2005;14(7):634-649. doi:10.1089/jwh.2005.14.634

Gibson S, Gunn P, Wittekind A, Cottrell R. The effects of sucrose on metabolic health: a systematic review of human intervention studies in healthy adults. Crit Rev Food Sci Nutr. 2013;53(6):591-614. doi:10.1080/10408398.2012.691574

Gullo D, Latina A, Frasca F, Le Moli R, Pellegriti G, Vigneri R. Levothyroxine monotherapy cannot guarantee euthyroidism in all athyreotic patients. *PLoS One.* 2011;6(8):e22552. doi:10.1371/journal.pone.0022552

Günalan E, Yaba A, Yılmaz B. The effect of nutrient supplementation in the management of polycystic ovary syndrome-associated metabolic dysfunctions: A critical review. *J Turk Ger Gynecol Assoc.* 2018;19(4):220-232. doi:10.4274/jtgga.2018.0077

Gunnar MR, Vazquez DM. Low cortisol and a flattening of expected daytime rhythm: potential indices of risk in human development. *Dev Psychopathol.* 2001;13(3):515-538. doi:10.1017/s0954579401003066

Guo S, Al-Sadi R, Said HM, Ma TY. Lipopolysaccharide causes an increase in intestinal tight junction permeability in vitro and in vivo by inducing enterocyte membrane expression and localization of TLR-4 and CD14. *Am J Pathol*. 2013;182(2):375-387. doi:10.1016/j.ajpath.2012.10.014

Hall KD, Bemis T, Brychta R, et al. Calorie for Calorie, Dietary Fat Restriction Results in More Body Fat Loss than Carbohydrate Restriction in People with Obesity. *Cell Metab*. 2015;22(3):427-436. doi:10.1016/j.cmet.2015.07.021

Hall KD, Guo J. Obesity Energetics: Body Weight Regulation and the Effects of Diet Composition. Gastroenterology. 2017;152(7):1718-1727.e3. doi:10.1053/j.gastro.2017.01.052

Harrison JJ, Rabiei M, Turner RJ, Badry EA, Sproule KM, Ceri H. Metal resistance in Candida biofilms. FEMS Microbiol Ecol. 2006;55(3):479-491. doi:10.1111/j.1574-6941.2005.00045.x

Harvie MN, Pegington M, Mattson MP, et al. The effects of intermittent or continuous energy restriction on weight loss and metabolic disease risk markers: a randomized trial in young overweight women. Int J Obes (Lond). 2011;35(5):714-727. doi:10.1038/ijo.2010.171

Haugen BR. Drugs that suppress TSH or cause central hypothyroidism. *Best Pract Res Clin Endocrinol Metab*. 2009;23(6):793-800. doi:10.1016/j.beem.2009.08.003

Hawrelak JA, Myers SP. The causes of intestinal dysbiosis: a review. *Altern Med Rev*. 2004;9(2):180-197.

Helms E, Morgan A, Valdez A. *The Muscle & Strength Pyramid: Nutrition*. San Bernardino, CA: Muscle and Strength Pyramids; 2019.

Hendrickson-Jack L, Briden L. *The Fifth Vital Sign: Master Your Cycles and Optimize Your Fertility*. Fertility Friday Publishing Inc.; 2019.

Hodges RE, Minich DM. Modulation of Metabolic Detoxification Pathways Using Foods and Food-Derived Components: A Scientific Review with Clinical Application. *J Nutr Metab*. 2015;2015:760689. doi:10.1155/2015/760689

Hodges RE, Minich DM. Modulation of Metabolic Detoxification Pathways Using Foods and Food-Derived Components: A Scientific Review with Clinical Application. J Nutr Metab. 2015;2015:760689. doi:10.1155/2015/76068

Hsu H, Sheth CC, Veses V. Herbal Extracts with Antifungal Activity Against Candida albicans: A Systematic Review [published online ahead of print, 2020 Jun 27]. *Mini Rev Med Chem*. 2020;10.2174/1389557520666200628032116. doi:10.2174/1389557520666200628032116

Hu T, Mills KT, Yao L, et al. Effects of low-carbohydrate diets versus low-fat diets on metabolic risk factors: a meta-analysis of randomized controlled clinical trials. *Am J Epidemiol*. 2012;176 Suppl 7(Suppl 7):S44-S54. doi:10.1093/aje/kws264

Iraki J, Fitschen P, Espinar S, Helms E. Nutrition Recommendations for Bodybuilders in the Off-Season: A Narrative Review. Sports (Basel). 2019;7(7):154. Published 2019 Jun 26. doi:10.3390/sports7070154

Irving SA, Vadiveloo T, Leese GP. Drugs that interact with levothyroxine: an observational study from the Thyroid Epidemiology, Audit and Research Study (TEARS). *Clin Endocrinol (Oxf)*. 2015;82(1):136-141. doi:10.1111/cen.12559

Jacquet P, Schutz Y, Montani JP, Dulloo A. How dieting might make some fatter: modeling weight cycling toward obesity from a perspective of body composition autoregulation. *Int J Obes (Lond).* 2020;44(6):1243-1253. doi:10.1038/s41366-020-0547-1

Jaishankar M, Tseten T, Anbalagan N, Mathew BB, Beeregowda KN. Toxicity, mechanism and health effects of some heavy metals. *Interdiscip Toxicol.* 2014;7(2):60-72. doi:10.2478/intox-2014-0009

Janegova A, Janega P, Rychly B, Kuracinova K, Babal P. The role of Epstein-Barr virus infection in the development of autoimmune thyroid diseases. *Endokrynol Pol.* 2015;66(2):132-136. doi:10.5603/EP.2015.0020

Janegova A, Janega P, Rychly B, Kuracinova K, Babal P. The role of Epstein-Barr virus infection in the development of autoimmune thyroid diseases. Endokrynol Pol. 2015;66(2):132-6. PubMed PMID: 25931043

Janegova A, Janega P, Rychly B, Kuracinova K, Babal P. The role of Epstein-Barr virus infection in the development of autoimmune thyroid diseases. *Endokrynol Pol.* 2015;66(2):132-136. doi:10.5603/EP.2015.0020

Järvinen KM, Konstantinou GN, Pilapil M, et al. Intestinal permeability in children with food allergy on specific elimination diets. *Pediatr Allergy Immunol.* 2013;24(6):589-595. doi:10.1111/pai.12106

Johnston CS, Tjonn SL, Swan PD, White A, Hutchins H, Sears B. Ketogenic low-carbohydrate diets have no metabolic advantage over nonketogenic low-carbohydrate diets. *Am J Clin Nutr.* 2006;83(5):1055-1061. doi:10.1093/ajcn/83.5.1055

Johnstone A. Fasting for weight loss: an effective strategy or latest dieting trend?. Int J Obes (Lond). 2015;39(5):727-733. doi:10.1038/ijo.2014.214

Jonklaas J, Bianco AC, Bauer AJ, et al. Guidelines for the treatment of hypothyroidism: prepared by the american thyroid association task force on thyroid hormone replacement. *Thyroid*. 2014;24(12):1670-1751. doi:10.1089/thy.2014.0028

Juruena MF. Early-life stress and HPA axis trigger recurrent adulthood depression. *Epilepsy Behav*. 2014;38:148-159. doi:10.1016/j.yebeh.2013.10.020

Kaewrudee S, Kietpeerakool C, Pattanittum P, Lumbiganon P. Vitamin or mineral supplements for premenstrual syndrome. *Cochrane Database Syst Rev*. 2018;2018(1):CD012933. Published 2018 Jan 18. doi:10.1002/14651858.CD012933

Kamenov Z, Gateva A. Inositols in PCOS. *Molecules*. 2020;25(23):5566. Published 2020 Nov 27. doi:10.3390/molecules25235566

Katagiri R, Yuan X, Kobayashi S, Sasaki S. Effect of excess iodine intake on thyroid diseases in different populations: A systematic review and meta-analyses including observational studies. *PLoS One*. 2017;12(3):e0173722. Published 2017 Mar 10. doi:10.1371/journal.pone.0173722

Kawai N, Sakai N, Okuro M, et al. The sleep-promoting and hypothermic effects of glycine are mediated by NMDA receptors in the suprachiasmatic nucleus. *Neuropsychopharmacology*. 2015;40(6):1405-1416. doi:10.1038/npp.2014.326

Keating SE, Johnson NA, Mielke GI, Coombes JS. A systematic review and meta-analysis of interval training versus moderate-intensity continuous training on body adiposity. *Obes Rev*. 2017;18(8):943-964. doi:10.1111/obr.12536

Keenan S, Cooke MB, Belski R. The Effects of Intermittent Fasting Combined with Resistance Training on Lean Body Mass:

A Systematic Review of Human Studies. *Nutrients.* 2020;12(8):2349. Published 2020 Aug 6. doi:10.3390/nu12082349

Kelesidis T, Pothoulakis C. Efficacy and safety of the probiotic Saccharomyces boulardii for the prevention and therapy of gastrointestinal disorders. *Therap Adv Gastroenterol.* 2012;5(2):111-125. doi:10.1177/1756283X11428502

Kerdivel G, Habauzit D, Pakdel F. Assessment and molecular actions of endocrine-disrupting chemicals that interfere with estrogen receptor pathways. *Int J Endocrinol.* 2013;2013:501851. doi:10.1155/2013/501851

Kerksick CM, Arent S, Schoenfeld BJ, et al. International society of sports nutrition position stand: nutrient timing. *J Int Soc Sports Nutr.* 2017;14:33. Published 2017 Aug 29. doi:10.1186/s12970-017-0189-4

Kerksick CM, Wilborn CD, Roberts MD, et al. ISSN exercise & sports nutrition review update: research & recommendations. *J Int Soc Sports Nutr.* 2018;15(1):38. Published 2018 Aug 1. doi:10.1186/s12970-018-0242-y

Kim S, Jo K, Hong KB, Han SH, Suh HJ. GABA and l-theanine mixture decreases sleep latency and improves NREM sleep. *Pharm Biol.* 2019;57(1):65-73. doi:10.1080/13880209.2018.1557698

Kimura K, Ozeki M, Juneja LR, Ohira H. L-Theanine reduces psychological and physiological stress responses. *Biol Psychol.* 2007;74(1):39-45. doi:10.1016/j.biopsycho.2006.06.006

Konturek PC, Brzozowski T, Konturek SJ. Stress and the gut: pathophysiology, clinical consequences, diagnostic approach and treatment options. *J Physiol Pharmacol.* 2011;62(6):591-599.

Koutras DA. Disturbances of menstruation in thyroid disease. *Ann N Y Acad Sci.* 1997;816:280-284. doi:10.1111/j.1749-6632.1997.tb52152.x

Langeveld M, de Vries JH. Het magere resultaat van diëten [The mediocre results of dieting]. *Ned Tijdschr Geneeskd.* 2013;157(29):A6017.

Layman DK. Protein quantity and quality at levels above the RDA improves adult weight loss. *J Am Coll Nutr.* 2004;23(6 Suppl):631S-636S. doi:10.1080/07315724.2004.10719435

Leung AM, Braverman LE. Consequences of excess iodine. *Nat Rev Endocrinol.* 2014;10(3):136-142. doi:10.1038/nrendo.2013.251

Li Z, You Y, Griffin N, Feng J, Shan F. Low-dose naltrexone (LDN): A promising treatment in immune-related diseases and cancer therapy. *Int Immunopharmacol.* 2018;61:178-184. doi:10.1016/j.intimp.2018.05.020

Liew WP, Mohd-Redzwan S. Mycotoxin: Its Impact on Gut Health and Microbiota. *Front Cell Infect Microbiol.* 2018;8:60. Published 2018 Feb 26. doi:10.3389/fcimb.2018.00060

Liu Y, McKeever LC, Malik NS. Assessment of the Antimicrobial Activity of Olive Leaf Extract Against Foodborne Bacterial Pathogens. *Front Microbiol.* 2017;8:113. Published 2017 Feb 2. doi:10.3389/fmicb.2017.00113

Lopetuso LR, Scaldaferri F, Bruno G, Petito V, Franceschi F, Gasbarrini A. The therapeutic management of gut barrier leaking: the emerging role for mucosal barrier protectors. *Eur Rev Med Pharmacol Sci.* 2015;19(6):1068-1076.

Lucidi RS, Thyer AC, Easton CA, Holden AE, Schenken RS, Brzyski RG. Effect of chromium supplementation on insulin resistance and ovarian and menstrual cyclicity in women with poly-cystic ovary syndrome. *Fertil Steril.* 2005;84(6):1755-1757. doi:10.1016/j.fertnstert.2005.06.028

MacLean PS, Higgins JA, Giles ED, Sherk VD, Jackman MR. The role for adipose tissue in weight regain after weight loss. Obes Rev. 2015;16 Suppl 1(Suppl 1):45-54. doi:10.1111/obr.12255

Martin VT. Ovarian hormones and pain response: a review of clinical and basic science studies. *Gend Med.* 2009;6 Suppl 2:168-192. doi:10.1016/j.genm.2009.03.006

Martin WF, Armstrong LE, Rodriguez NR. Dietary protein intake and renal function. Nutr Metab (Lond). 2005;2:25. Published 2005 Sep 20. doi:10.1186/1743-7075-2-25

McArthur JO, Tang H, Petocz P, Samman S. Biological variability and impact of oral contraceptives on vitamins B(6), B(12) and folate status in women of reproductive age. *Nutrients.* 2013;5(9):3634-3645. Published 2013 Sep 16. doi:10.3390/nu5093634

McFarland LV. Systematic review and meta-analysis of Saccharomyces boulardii in adult patients. *World J Gastroenterol.* 2010;16(18):2202-2222. doi:10.3748/wjg.v16.i18.2202

McLachlan JA, Simpson E, Martin M. Endocrine disrupters and female reproductive health. *Best Pract Res Clin Endocrinol Metab.* 2006;20(1):63-75. doi:10.1016/j.beem.2005.09.009

McNulty KL, Elliott-Sale KJ, Dolan E, et al. The Effects of Menstrual Cycle Phase on Exercise Performance in Eumenorrheic Women: A Systematic Review and Meta-Analysis. *Sports Med.* 2020;50(10):1813-1827. doi:10.1007/s40279-020-01319-3

Melby CL, Paris HL, Foright RM, Peth J. Attenuating the Biologic Drive for Weight Regain Following Weight Loss: Must What Goes

Down Always Go Back Up?. *Nutrients.* 2017;9(5):468. Published 2017 May 6. doi:10.3390/nu9050468

Mesen TB, Young SL. Progesterone and the luteal phase: a requisite to reproduction. *Obstet Gynecol Clin North Am.* 2015;42(1):135-151. doi:10.1016/j.ogc.2014.10.003

Messina M, Redmond G. Effects of soy protein and soybean isoflavones on thyroid function in healthy adults and hypothyroid patients: a review of the relevant literature. *Thyroid.* 2006;16(3):249-258. doi:10.1089/thy.2006.16.249

Michielan A, D'Incà R. Intestinal Permeability in Inflammatory Bowel Disease: Pathogenesis, Clinical Evaluation, and Therapy of Leaky Gut. *Mediators Inflamm.* 2015;2015:628157. doi:10.1155/2015/628157

Mohn ES, Kern HJ, Saltzman E, Mitmesser SH, McKay DL. Evidence of Drug-Nutrient Interactions with Chronic Use of Commonly Prescribed Medications: An Update. *Pharmaceutics.* 2018;10(1):36. Published 2018 Mar 20. doi:10.3390/pharmaceutics10010036

Monastra G, Unfer V, Harrath AH, Bizzarri M. Combining treatment with myo-inositol and D-chiro-inositol (40:1) is effective in restoring ovary function and metabolic balance in PCOS patients. *Gynecol Endocrinol.* 2017;33(1):1-9. doi:10.1080/09513590.2016.1247797

Morris G, Berk M, Walder K, Maes M. The Putative Role of Viruses, Bacteria, and Chronic Fungal Biotoxin Exposure in the Genesis of Intractable Fatigue Accompanied by Cognitive and Physical Disability. *Mol Neurobiol.* 2016;53(4):2550-2571. doi:10.1007/s12035-015-9262-7

Mullin GE, Clarke JO. Role of complementary and alternative medicine in managing gastrointestinal motility disorders. *Nutr Clin Pract*. 2010;25(1):85-87. doi:10.1177/0884533609358903

Naude CE, Schoonees A, Senekal M, Young T, Garner P, Volmink J. Low carbohydrate versus isoenergetic balanced diets for reducing weight and cardiovascular risk: a systematic review and meta-analysis [published correction appears in PLoS One. 2018 Jul 2;13(7):e0200284]. PLoS One. 2014;9(7):e100652. Published 2014 Jul 9. doi:10.1371/journal.pone.0100652

Nicolopoulou-Stamati P, Pitsos MA. The impact of endocrine disrupters on the female reproductive system. *Hum Reprod Update*. 2001;7(3):323-330. doi:10.1093/humupd/7.3.323

Obi N, Vrieling A, Heinz J, Chang-Claude J. Estrogen metabolite ratio: Is the 2-hydroxyestrone to 16α-hydroxyestrone ratio predictive for breast cancer?. *Int J Womens Health*. 2011;3:37-51. Published 2011 Feb 8. doi:10.2147/IJWH.S7595

Ottillinger B, Storr M, Malfertheiner P, Allescher HD. STW 5 (Iberogast®)--a safe and effective standard in the treatment of functional gastrointestinal disorders. *Wien Med Wochenschr*. 2013;163(3-4):65-72. doi:10.1007/s10354-012-0169-x

Palmery M, Saraceno A, Vaiarelli A, Carlomagno G. Oral contraceptives and changes in nutritional requirements. *Eur Rev Med Pharmacol Sci*. 2013;17(13):1804-1813.

Pandey KR, Naik SR, Vakil BV. Probiotics, prebiotics and synbiotics- a review. *J Food Sci Technol*. 2015;52(12):7577-7587. doi:10.1007/s13197-015-1921-1

Panzer C, Wise S, Fantini G, et al. Impact of oral contraceptives on sex hormone-binding globulin and androgen levels: a retrospective study in women with sexual dysfunction. *J Sex Med.* 2006;3(1):104-113. doi:10.1111/j.1743-6109.2005.00198.x

Pascoe MC, Thompson DR, Ski CF. Yoga, mindfulness-based stress reduction and stress-related physiological measures: A meta-analysis. *Psychoneuroendocrinology.* 2017;86:152-168. doi:10.1016/j.psyneuen.2017.08.008

Patrick L. Thyroid disruption: mechanism and clinical implications in human health [published correction appears in Altern Med Rev. 2010 Apr;15(1):58]. *Altern Med Rev.* 2009;14(4):326-346.

Pereira HM, Larson RD, Bemben DA. Menstrual Cycle Effects on Exercise-Induced Fatigability. *Front Physiol.* 2020;11:517. Published 2020 Jun 26. doi:10.3389/fphys.2020.00517

Quartarone G. Role of PHGG as a dietary fiber: a review article. *Minerva Gastroenterol Dietol.* 2013;59(4):329-340.

Rafieian-Kopaei M, Movahedi M. Systematic Review of Premenstrual, Postmenstrual and Infertility Disorders of Vitex Agnus Castus. *Electron Physician.* 2017;9(1):3685-3689. Published 2017 Jan 25. doi:10.19082/3685

Rani A, Sharma A. The genus Vitex: A review. *Pharmacogn Rev.* 2013;7(14):188-198. doi:10.4103/0973-7847.120522

Rao R, Samak G. Role of Glutamine in Protection of Intestinal Epithelial Tight Junctions. *J Epithel Biol Pharmacol.* 2012;5(Suppl 1-M7):47-54. doi:10.2174/1875044301205010047

Rees WD, Rhodes J, Wright JE, Stamford LF, Bennett A. Effect of deglycyrrhizinated liquorice on gastric mucosal damage by aspirin. *Scand J Gastroenterol.* 1979;14(5):605-607. doi:10.3109/00365527909181397

Rees-Jones RW, Larsen PR. Triiodothyronine and thyroxine content of desiccated thyroid tablets. *Metabolism.* 1977;26(11):1213-1218. doi:10.1016/0026-0495(77)90113-5

Rezaie A, Pimentel M, Rao SS. How to Test and Treat Small Intestinal Bacterial Overgrowth: an Evidence-Based Approach. *Curr Gastroenterol Rep.* 2016;18(2):8. doi:10.1007/s11894-015-0482-9

Roberts BM, Helms ER, Trexler ET, Fitschen PJ. Nutritional Recommendations for Physique Athletes. J Hum Kinet. 2020;71:79-108. Published 2020 Jan 31. doi:10.2478/hukin-2019-0096

Rondanelli M, Infantino V, Riva A, et al. Polycystic ovary syndrome management: a review of the possible amazing role of berberine. *Arch Gynecol Obstet.* 2020;301(1):53-60. doi:10.1007/s00404-020-05450-4

Rothman, M. S., & Wierman, M. E. (2008). *Female hypogonadism: evaluation of the hypothalamic–pituitary–ovarian axis. Pituitary, 11(2), 163–169.* doi:10.1007/s11102-008-0109-3

Rushworth GF, Megson IL. Existing and potential therapeutic uses for N-acetylcysteine: the need for conversion to intracellular glutathione for antioxidant benefits. *Pharmacol Ther.* 2014;141(2):150-159. doi:10.1016/j.pharmthera.2013.09.006

Russell G, Lightman S. The human stress response. *Nat Rev Endocrinol.* 2019;15(9):525-534. doi:10.1038/s41574-019-0228-0

Rusu AV, Penedo BA, Schwarze A-K, Trif M. The Influence of *Candida* spp. in Intestinal Microbiota; Diet Therapy, the Emerging Conditions Related to *Candida* in Athletes and Elderly People. https://www.intechopen.com/online-first/the-influence-of-candida-spp-in-intestinal-microbiota-diet-therapy-the-emerging-conditions-related-t. Published June 11, 2020. Accessed January 26, 2021.

Saad RJ, Chey WD. Breath testing for small intestinal bacterial overgrowth: maximizing test accuracy. *Clin Gastroenterol Hepatol.* 2014;12(12):1964-e120. doi:10.1016/j.cgh.2013.09.055

Schomburg L. Treating Hashimoto's thyroiditis with selenium: no risks, just benefits?. *Thyroid.* 2011;21(5):563-565. doi:10.1089/thy.2010.0416

Schug TT, Johnson AF, Birnbaum LS, et al. Minireview: Endocrine Disruptors: Past Lessons and Future Directions. *Mol Endocrinol.* 2016;30(8):833-847. doi:10.1210/me.2016-1096

Sears ME, Kerr KJ, Bray RI. Arsenic, cadmium, lead, and mercury in sweat: a systematic review. *J Environ Public Health.* 2012;2012:184745. doi:10.1155/2012/184745

Seelig MS. Consequences of magnesium deficiency on the enhancement of stress reactions; preventive and therapeutic implications (a review). *J Am Coll Nutr.* 1994;13(5):429-446. doi:10.1080/07315724.1994.10718432

Sharma AK, Basu I, Singh S. Efficacy and Safety of Ashwagandha Root Extract in Subclinical Hypothyroid Patients: A Double-Blind, Randomized Placebo-Controlled Trial. *J Altern Complement Med.* 2018;24(3):243-248. doi:10.1089/acm.2017.0183

Shi L, Zhang J, Lai Z, et al. Long-Term Moderate Oxidative Stress Decreased Ovarian Reproductive Function by Reducing Follicle Quality and Progesterone Production. *PLoS One.* 2016;11(9):e0162194. Published 2016 Sep 27. doi:10.1371/journal.pone.0162194

Simmons RG, Jennings V. Fertility awareness-based methods of family planning. *Best Pract Res Clin Obstet Gynaecol.* 2020;66:68-82. doi:10.1016/j.bpobgyn.2019.12.003

Singh N, Bhalla M, de Jager P, Gilca M. An overview on ashwagandha: a Rasayana (rejuvenator) of Ayurveda. *Afr J Tradit Complement Altern Med*. 2011;8(5 Suppl):208-213. doi:10.4314/ajt-cam.v8i5S.9

Skovlund CW, Mørch LS, Kessing LV, Lidegaard Ø. Association of Hormonal Contraception With Depression [published correction appears in JAMA Psychiatry. 2017 Jul 1;74(7):764]. *JAMA Psychiatry*. 2016;73(11):1154-1162. doi:10.1001/jamapsychiatry.2016.2387

Smith SM, Vale WW. The role of the hypothalamic-pituitary-adrenal axis in neuroendocrine responses to stress. *Dialogues Clin Neurosci*. 2006;8(4):383-395. doi:10.31887/DCNS.2006.8.4/ssmith

Stavropoulou E, Bezirtzoglou E. Probiotics in Medicine: A Long Debate. *Front Immunol*. 2020;11:2192. Published 2020 Sep 25. doi:10.3389/fimmu.2020.02192

Srivastava JK, Shankar E, Gupta S. Chamomile: A herbal medicine of the past with bright future. *Mol Med Rep*. 2010;3(6):895-901. doi:10.3892/mmr.2010.377

Stipanuk MH, Caudill MA. *Biochemical, Physiological, & Molecular Aspects of Human Nutrition*. St. Louis: Elsevier; 2019.

Studer-Rohr I, Dietrich DR, Schlatter J, Schlatter C. The occurrence of ochratoxin A in coffee. *Food Chem Toxicol*. 1995;33(5):341-355. doi:10.1016/0278-6915(94)00150-m

Sturniolo G, Mesa J. Selenium supplementation and autoimmune thyroid diseases. *Endocrinol Nutr*. 2013;60(8):423-426. doi:10.1016/j.endonu.2013.07.001

Su T, Lai S, Lee A, He X, Chen S. Meta-analysis: proton pump inhibitors moderately increase the risk of small intestinal bacterial overgrowth. *J Gastroenterol*. 2018;53(1):27-36. doi:10.1007/s00535-017-1371-9

Sun J, Shen X, Liu H, Lu S, Peng J, Kuang H. Caloric restriction in female reproduction: is it beneficial or detrimental?. *Reprod Biol Endocrinol.* 2021;19(1):1. Published 2021 Jan 4. doi:10.1186/s12958-020-00681-1

Sun X, Shan Z, Teng W. Effects of increased iodine intake on thyroid disorders. *Endocrinol Metab (Seoul).* 2014;29(3):240-247. doi:10.3803/EnM.2014.29.3.240

Sworczak K, Wiśniewski P. The role of vitamins in the prevention and treatment of thyroid disorders. *Endokrynol Pol.* 2011;62(4):340-344.

Ta N, Walle T. Aromatase inhibition by bioavailable methylated flavones. *J Steroid Biochem Mol Biol.* 2007;107(1-2):127-129. doi:10.1016/j.jsbmb.2007.01.006

Tähkämö L, Partonen T, Pesonen AK. Systematic review of light exposure impact on human circadian rhythm. *Chronobiol Int.* 2019;36(2):151-170. doi:10.1080/07420528.2018.1527773

Takeuchi H, Trang VT, Morimoto N, Nishida Y, Matsumura Y, Sugiura T. Natural products and food components with anti-Helicobacter pylori activities. *World J Gastroenterol.* 2014;20(27):8971-8978. doi:10.3748/wjg.v20.i27.8971

Talbott SM, Talbott JA, Pugh M. Effect of Magnolia officinalis and Phellodendron amurense (Relora®) on cortisol and psychological mood state in moderately stressed subjects. *J Int Soc Sports Nutr.* 2013;10(1):37. Published 2013 Aug 7. doi:10.1186/1550-2783-10-37

Tchounwou PB, Yedjou CG, Patlolla AK, Sutton DJ. Heavy metal toxicity and the environment. *Exp Suppl.* 2012;101:133-164. doi:10.1007/978-3-7643-8340-4_6

Thakker D, Raval A, Patel I, Walia R. N-acetylcysteine for polycystic ovary syndrome: a systematic review and meta-analysis of randomized controlled clinical trials. *Obstet Gynecol Int.* 2015;2015:817849. doi:10.1155/2015/817849

Thompson LA, Darwish WS. Environmental Chemical Contaminants in Food: Review of a Global Problem. *J Toxicol.* 2019;2019:2345283. Published 2019 Jan 1. doi:10.1155/2019/2345283

Tosini G, Ferguson I, Tsubota K. Effects of blue light on the circadian system and eye physiology. *Mol Vis.* 2016;22:61-72. Published 2016 Jan 24.

Trepanowski JF, Kroeger CM, Barnosky A, et al. Effect of Alternate-Day Fasting on Weight Loss, Weight Maintenance, and Cardioprotection Among Metabolically Healthy Obese Adults: A Randomized Clinical Trial. JAMA Intern Med. 2017;177(7):930-938. doi:10.1001/jamainternmed.2017.0936

Trexler ET, Smith-Ryan AE, Norton LE. Metabolic adaptation to weight loss: implications for the athlete. J Int Soc Sports Nutr. 2014;11(1):7. Published 2014 Feb 27. doi:10.1186/1550-2783-11-7

Triantafyllidi A, Xanthos T, Papalois A, Triantafillidis JK. Herbal and plant therapy in patients with inflammatory bowel disease. *Ann Gastroenterol.* 2015;28(2):210-220.

Turakitwanakan W, Mekseepralard C, Busarakumtragul P. Effects of mindfulness meditation on serum cortisol of medical students. *J Med Assoc Thai.* 2013;96 Suppl 1:S90-S95.

Vanuytsel T, van Wanrooy S, Vanheel H, et al. Psychological stress and corticotropin-releasing hormone increase intestinal permeability in humans by a mast cell-dependent mechanism. *Gut.* 2014;63(8):1293-1299. doi:10.1136/gutjnl-2013-305690

Varady KA. Intermittent versus daily calorie restriction: which diet regimen is more effective for weight loss?. Obes Rev. 2011;12(7):e593-e601. doi:10.1111/j.1467-789X.2011.00873.x

Ventura M, Melo M, Carrilho F. Selenium and Thyroid Disease: From Pathophysiology to Treatment. *Int J Endocrinol.* 2017;2017:1297658. doi:10.1155/2017/1297658

Walker AF, De Souza MC, Vickers MF, Abeyasekera S, Collins ML, Trinca LA. Magnesium supplementation alleviates premenstrual symptoms of fluid retention. *J Womens Health.* 1998;7(9):1157-1165. doi:10.1089/jwh.1998.7.1157

Wan MLY, Ling KH, El-Nezami H, Wang MF. Influence of functional food components on gut health. *Crit Rev Food Sci Nutr.* 2019;59(12):1927-1936. doi:10.1080/10408398.2018.1433629

Wang X, Ran S, Yu Q. Optimizing quality of life in perimenopause: lessons from the East. *Climacteric.* 2019;22(1):34-37. doi:10.1080/13697137.2018.1506435

Williams NT. Probiotics. *Am J Health Syst Pharm.* 2010;67(6):449-458. doi:10.2146/ajhp090168

Yarnell, E, Abascal, K. Botanical Medicine for Thyroid Regulation. Alternative and Complementary Therapies. 2006; 12: 107-112. dos: 10.1089/act.2006.12.107.

Yavuz S, Salgado Nunez Del Prado S, Celi FS. Thyroid Hormone Action and Energy Expenditure. *J Endocr Soc.* 2019;3(7):1345-1356. Published 2019 May 16. doi:10.1210/js.2018-00423

Yonkers KA, Simoni MK. Premenstrual disorders. *Am J Obstet Gynecol.* 2018;218(1):68-74. doi:10.1016/j.ajog.2017.05.045

Zhang H, Tong TK, Qiu W, et al. Comparable Effects of High-Intensity Interval Training and Prolonged Continuous Exercise Training on Abdominal Visceral Fat Reduction in Obese Young Women. *J Diabetes Res.* 2017;2017:5071740. doi:10.1155/2017/5071740

Zhao X, Jiang Y, Xi H, Chen L, Feng X. Exploration of the Relationship Between Gut Microbiota and Polycystic Ovary Syndrome (PCOS): a Review. *Geburtshilfe Frauenheilkd.* 2020;80(2):161-171. doi:10.1055/a-1081-2036

Zhu JL, Chen Z, Feng WJ, Long SL, Mo ZC. Sex hormone-binding globulin and polycystic ovary syndrome. *Clin Chim Acta.* 2019;499:142-148. doi:10.1016/j.cca.2019.09.010

Zimmermann MB, Köhrle J. The impact of iron and selenium deficiencies on iodine and thyroid metabolism: biochemistry and relevance to public health. *Thyroid.* 2002;12(10):867-878. doi:10.1089/105072502761016494

ABOUT THE AUTHOR

Lacey Dunn, MS, RD is a functional medicine dietitian who helps women to reclaim their health and become the boss of their own bodies. She specializes in hormonal disorders, thyroid struggles, and metabolic resistance. In her virtual practice, UpliftFit Nutrition, she uses a personalized, holistic approach to help her clients to feel their best, transform their lives, and go from surviving to thriving.

You can find Lacey online at:

Website: https://www.upliftfitnutrition.com

Instagram: @faithandfit

Twitter: @laceyadunn